SPACE EXPLORATION AND ASTRONAUT SAFETY

7/05

Amazon 06/07

SPACE EXPLORATION AND ASTRONAUT SAFETY

by
Joseph N. Pelton
George Washington University

with

Peter Marshall
Dorset, United Kingdom

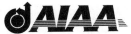

American Institute of Aeronautics and Astronautics, Inc.
1801 Alexander Bell Drive
Reston, Virginia 20191
Publishers since 1930

American Institute of Aeronautics and Astronautics, Inc., Reston, Virginia

1 2 3 4 5

Library of Congress Cataloging-in-Publication Data

Pelton, Joseph N.
   Space exploration and astronaut safety / by Joseph N. Pelton with Peter Marshall.--1st ed.
      p. cm.
   Includes index.
   ISBN 1-56347-844-7 (hardcover)
   1. Astronautics--United States--Planning. 2. Manned space flight--United States--Safety measures.
 3. Outer space--Exploration. I. Title.

   TL789.8.U5.P385 2006
   363.12'472--dc22

FOREWORD

B ack when I flew in space on Apollo 9 the tenor of the times was quite different from what it is now. NASA was a young shiny agency involved in a sprint to the finish in a race called by John F. Kennedy, our glamorous President. The country was alarmed in the early 60s by the Soviet Union not only beating us into space, but also walking off time and again with a seemingly unending list of "firsts".

The United States had been shocked out of its complacency. We were being challenged directly, and in a field which exemplified America's satisfied image of itself... technology, engineering, manufacturing, and yes, even pioneering. NASA was the agency coming to the rescue, and the astronauts were the embodiment of the American can-do spirit that invited every citizen to directly identify with the effort personally.

"We choose to go to the moon in this decade and do the other things, not because they are easy, but because they are hard,..." Ringing words from the President's speech at Rice University on September 12, 1962 that, to this day, cause shivers to run up my spine. These were heady days in the space program, days when the President, the Congress, and the American people were ready to take substantial risks to regain our self-image and our leadership position in the world.

The President set a goal; clear, easy to understand, and with a very specific and challenging time table. We were to send a man to land on the moon and bring him safely back to Earth by the end of the decade. It was bold; it was terribly costly; and it was exciting!

How different are the times now! The Cold War and the race with the Soviets are over. We won. We successfully met President Kennedy's goal, and by the deadline set. The attitude of the country turned around to one of great pride. Not only was there pride here at home, but the whole world was excited and happy for us. One couldn't travel anywhere abroad, even in the Soviet Union, without people expressing their excitement and feeling as if just meeting an American put them closer to being a part of it.

So why are things so different now? And is there anything that we can or ought to do to reestablish that sense of excitement and involvement on the part of the American people? President George W. Bush's Vision for Space Exploration did not exactly galvanize the citizenry of the country to throw their hearts and pocketbooks into the collection plate as it passed. Not only was the "vision" a good bit less specific than landing on the moon and returning safely to Earth by the end of the decade, but there in the foreground, like an elephant in the middle of the room, were the unfinished International Space Station (ISS) and the crippled and tainted Space Shuttle, its necessary partner. This pesky, largely unwanted-in-the-first-place megaproject, and its associated international contractual agreements, would have to be disposed of first, before going back to the moon, let alone on to Mars or Beyond could really get underway. And, of course, to get past this elephant blocking the far door into deeper space would require a toll payment of something like $80 billion!

This, and a hundred other niggling considerations have blocked the enthusiasm and support for our national space program. The nation no sooner looks up from its enthusiasm for our cute little Sojourner rover on Mars and we've got a series of disasters crashing into that planet. We get past that hiccup and into a series of very capable Mars orbiters and the Eveready Bunny rovers Spirit and Opportunity and look up again to see space science cut to and beyond the bone in order to feed the insatiable appetite of the ISS and Shuttle.

Nor did the public appreciate the incredibly risk-averse decision, now thankfully abandoned, to forego a manned repair mission to the Hubble Telescope! Thank heaven the new NASA Administrator, Mike Griffin, revisited and corrected that gutless faux pas. But the original decision stuck in the public mind and justifiably caused many otherwise enthusiastic supporters of space exploration to question just how was it that this same NASA got us to the moon in less than a decade?

And then, from an unexpected direction, comes a breath of fresh air. With fits and starts, backfires and belching smoke, but breath-taking leaps into the unknown as well comes the private sector space "program". Peter Diamandes and the X-Prize, the Ansari family and their space dreams, Elon Musk and his doggedly determined and visionary SpaceX launch vehicles, Paul Allen with his courage and checkbook in hand supporting the irreverent, irascible and brilliant Burt Rutan and Space Ship 1, and not least that irrepressible future-sniffing Richard Branson and his Virgin Galactic. These and many more like them, most of them deeply influenced and inspired by the Apollo experience, are boldly, even brazenly stepping into the vacuum, filling the public imagination with hope that the dream isn't really dead. In fact, not only is it alive, but it's now in *our* hands... or at least hands like ours. And all without a penny of tax money being spent.

So along come Joe Pelton and his editor, Peter Marshall, two experienced and involved space advocates and contributors to wrestle with the big questions... what's going on here? What are proper roles and responsibilities in this new and different era? What has to be done for NASA to regain support for itself? And what should the future investment in space development be, and by whom?

There are a million questions and several times as many options to consider. In these comments I've not even scratched the surface. But between the covers of this book, Joe Pelton delves into most of it and teases out the multiplicity of possibilities to hold them before the light to be examined. For anyone interested in the future of humankind as we slowly but surely emerge from the Earth into the awaiting cosmos, this investigation into the current state of space exploration affairs and where we ought to be going from here is must reading. Whether one agrees or disagrees with the authors, the issues raised cannot be avoided. Private initiatives are slowly pushing up into near space, despite the fact that it's a monster step from four minutes of euphoria to continuous weightless-ness. To what extent and how should the government retreat in the face of this upslaught? How does NASA avoid future black holes in space that suck the vital juices out of public enthusiasm for exploration? These and many other critical issues deserve your attention if you, like me, see the human future emerging from the womb of Earth into the cosmos.

Russell L. (Rusty) Schweickart
Apollo Astronaut
Chairman, B612 Foundation
Chairman, Association of Space Explorers
Committee on NEOs

TABLE OF CONTENTS

ACKNOWLEDGMENTS

This book was made possible by the research and assistance of many people who contributed to an earlier study conducted at George Washington University entitled Space Safety 2005. In particular I would like to thank John Logsdon of the Space Policy Institute, especially for his contributions to Chapter 2, as well as David Smith and Neil Helm my colleagues at the Space and Advanced Communications Research Institute at George Washington University for their many contributions. There was other key input as well—by Philip Caughran (assistance with interviews) and Peter MacDoran (key research and input on GPS systems) in the original study. In addition there were many who helped with specific research and graphics, and these included Justin Borodinsky, Mark Evan Green, C. Vyas, Alexander Pelton, and Mamta Sodikumar. Finally the editor of the original study and my colleague who did extensive editing of this book, i.e. Peter Marshall, made this a much better, more readable and certainly a crisper product.

I would also like to thank all of those just mentioned as well as others who provided advice and counsel such as Dick Kline, Lewis Peach, Tommaso Sgoba, Delbert D. Smith, and D. K. Sachdev among others helped with factual corrections. A special thanks goes to Astronaut Rusty Schwieckart who I have known and admired for many years. His profound thoughts and endorsement are truly treasured. Finally I would like to thank the Arthur C. Clarke Foundation and the Space Shuttle Children's Trust Fund for their past support.

As always, any errors are those of the author. I could not have written this book without the assistance of all of those that I acknowledge here and more.

CHAPTER 1
A New Beginning
for U.S. Space Exploration?

"One small step for a man, one giant leap for mankind."

—Astronaut Neil Armstrong,
the first man to walk on the moon, 1969

"We have had a failure of national leadership."

—Admiral Gehman, Chairman of the Columbia
Accident Investigation Board, 2003

Towards a New Space Agenda

Exploration is one of the hallmark characteristics of a dynamic civilization. From Lewis and Clark's travels to the first moon landing, this willingness by courageous explorers to define and explore new frontiers is a basic American trait. The probing of space by humans, like any frontier exploration, is not risk free. Nor will major risks soon be eliminated from ventures into space.

Yet, we believe that if the findings and recommendations in this book about the U.S. space program, the space shuttle, the International Space Station, and Project Constellation are considered and acted on, it could help strengthen NASA and make space exploration less risky. It could also help NASA build public support, make its program more relevant to Americans in all walks of life, and help to make future U.S. space activities more effective and astronaut travel safer. The chapters that follow thus explore safety concerns related to the space shuttle program, the International Space Station, and Project Constellation from a technical, operational, and management perspective and relate these findings to a possible new space agenda that is more international, more compelling, more cost effective, and more risk free.

This ultimately leads in the final chapter to a five-point program to "re-envision" NASA, in which a basic goal is to help sustain human existence on this planet and beyond. This five-point plan suggests that agency can help to identify and make better use of scarce resources and use space science and technology to make life on Earth safer and more sustainable—including the reduction of global warming. This would in turn create greater public support for a "NASA that is working for you."

From High to Low

NASA has had a wild ride—from the high exhilaration of the first moon landing in July 1969 to the low ebbs of the *Challenger* and *Columbia* disasters in 1986 and 2003. NASA's path into space has been bumpy indeed. Since 1969, NASA has seemingly gone from national icon to national question mark. The troublesome reflight of the *Discovery* shuttle orbiter in August 2005 has raised more questions than it answered. The deadly "missile of foam" that broke off the external tank at liftoff just cleared the critical thermal protection tiles that shield the Shuttle on reentry. Because estimated direct and indirect expenditures, in the neighborhood of $2 billion, have been spent on shuttle recovery since February 2003 to prevent "foam shedding," American's confidence in the shuttle program has lagged. The recurring problem after billions have been spent has raised questions in the court of public opinion. The NASA reflight program was supposed to "find it, fix it and fly safely again." Thus the *Discovery*'s reflight in August 2005 flight raised a host of new concerns about whether the shuttle could ever be made a reasonably safe vehicle. Indeed former Astronaut Michael Mullane in a new book has spoken out to say just how "dangerous" the shuttle is. Mullane suggests that without a "full envelope" escape capability that the shuttle carries a higher risk than a more prudent design would provide. He further claims that the *Challenger* and the *Columbia* accidents were the same in that both shuttle missions were launched with known defects that were not corrected [1,2].

> Since 1969, NASA has seemingly gone from national icon to national question mark.

Indeed the question of the day is whether, under the leadership of new Administrator Michael Griffin, NASA—or indeed the shuttle—can truly soar again? At this point only one thing is clear: it will not be easy.

NASA is an agency being torn by conflicting agendas complicated by a host of near-term, medium-term, and long-term objectives. The Presidential vision of going back to the moon and on to Mars is currently not backed by needed resources to get to either destination for a goodly time to come. Indeed, the demands on the U.S. tax base represented by overseas military operations, the huge cost of recovery of the Katrina- and Rita-ravaged Gulf Coast, Medicare, and Social Security at a time when baby boomers are retiring is enormous—as in HUGE.

With an ongoing large federal deficit, new appropriations for space seem very unlikely. The space science community continues to feel that manned space programs take away vital resources for key research into the basic mechanics of the sun, planetary evolution, and the still unknown secrets of astrophysics. A recent survey undertaken by the Planetary Society showed that many space enthusiasts agree with the early and permanent grounding of the aging shuttle fleet. Many also feel that most of the missions slated for astronauts could be accomplished better and at much lower cost by robotic space probes.

The newly announced crew exploration vehicle (CEV) launch system, based on a design that stays within NASA's current ongoing budget of $15–16 billion/year will nevertheless cost an estimated $104 billion over the next 12 years, has already drawn a bevy of detractors. Even Jay Leno of the Tonight Show has asked whether we should spend over a $100 billion to go to the moon when we cannot even cope with the rain and wind of Gulf Coast hurricanes? Leno and the average American on the street are now asking: "Are these the right priorities?"

Today we know there are limited options. Little can be done to make the remaining three shuttles, as designed in the 1970s, fundamentally safer. Former Houston Space Center Director George Abbey and former Presidential Science Advisor Dr. Neal Lane have recently spelled out very cogently the key issues that NASA Administrator Griffin must face. Their report goes well beyond space safety and manned space programs and provides very useful advice about where the U.S. space agency should go. After exploring the issues of U.S. space safety in some depth here and in following chapters, we too set forth recommendations about where the U.S. space program could go and how to get there. These include findings that NASA must explore innovative solutions that accomplish several objectives in parallel:

1) Develop an overall space agenda that has more relevance to practical space applications related to saving the Earth's biosphere, improving communications and information systems, better education and healthcare, and protecting our planet from hazards such as meteorites, comets, and global warming. [Recent new information about large numbers of near-Earth objects (NEOs) suggests that saving our species from extinction through the avoidance of celestial bodies might be one of the most important part of our space program. The dinosaurs did not have a space program, and look what happened to them.]

2) Find ways to conduct space sciences and space exploration more cheaply and with greater "safety" through the use of robotics and new space vehicle technology.

3) Adapt to the evolution of new private space initiatives so that certain space functions, transport systems, and activities can transition to corporate or industrial activities. (New private space vehicles can provide one of the most significant ways forward in human space activities over the next two decades after 20 years of sluggish progress.)

4) Streamline and give sharper definition to the role and mission of the various NASA centers, and thus make the U.S. space agency leaner and more focused.

5) Explore how to make international cooperation more meaningful. (Perhaps if NASA developed new and more effective models of cooperation and clearer goals and objectives, there could be cost savings and better use of human resources by leveraging international resources.)

6) Accomplish targeted and specific objectives in a competent manner that could restore faith in the NASA organizational abilities to accomplish major new goals without cost overruns, major schedule delays, and unfortunate loss of life.

NASA was once the place where young people in the United States, and indeed from all over the world, most wanted to work. To be an astronaut was a higher aspiration than to be President of the United States. One might assume that the *Columbia* disaster in 2003 and the *Challenger* disaster in 1986 were perhaps just bad luck or isolated failures. But no! There is solid evidence that these accidents were symptomatic of larger issues and problems. Ultimately this was not the failure of NASA but of national leadership.

> To be an astronaut was a higher aspiration than to be President of the United States.

The Gehman Commission that followed the *Columbia* accident tells us so in exactly those words. U.S. national leadership and the people that led NASA for at least the last 20 years, through both Republican and Democratic administrations, as well as the U.S. Congress must bear a great deal of the responsibility for the decline of the U.S. space agency. We have had not only a failure of management and national policy, but a failure of imagination. Just as we have seen the rise and decline of U.S. Steel, of RCA, of IBM, and most recently of AT&T, NASA has seemingly succumbed to the fate of overly large institutions that lose their agility, their innovative spark, and their ability to shift to new circumstances and new needs. Better management and streamlining of staff might accomplish a great deal.

The detailed review of space safety that follows not only examines both the space shuttle and the International Space Station (ISS), but also puts the findings of these reviews into a larger context. Space safety cannot improve unless the basic operations of NASA improve. NASA needs to revitalize its culture and refind the innovative mindset that found enormous success in the Apollo age. Its new leaders must find a way of setting a new course within the many demands on its limited resources. The creation of a new program evaluation office at NASA, under the leadership of Dr. Scott Pace, is certainly a step in the right direction. A new initiative to see how to improve and expand international space cooperation as recommended by Abbey and Lane, also seems imperative. Support for the new initiatives of the International Association for the Advancement of Space Safety (IAASS) would be an important further step that NASA should certainly take in tandem with it sister space agencies around the world. The biggest questions of all still remain. When to ground the space shuttle? What to do with the ISS and to make it more productive for the United States and its international partners? To what extent must we rely on the Russian Soyuz vehicle, the European ATV and the Japanese HTV? Are the new designs for Project Constellation that include the CEV, the crew launch, return and escape vehicles, and the new heavy lift solid rocket booster system the best way forward?

Thus clearly NASA's problems are manifold. Yet what to do with the International Space Station remains perhaps the biggest immediate issue.

The ISS (see Figure 1.1) has in many ways become the albatross that has pulled NASA down. It is the all-consuming desire to finish the huge, complex, increasingly expensive megaproject that has fueled the need to keep the

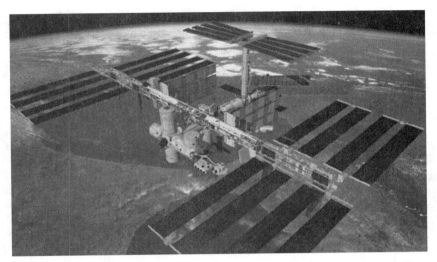

Figure 1-1 NASA cannot truly advance until it focuses on the issues presented by the International Space Station and how much of the system can be completed. (Graphic courtesy of NASA)

obsolete space shuttle flying years beyond its reasonable lifetime. This *idée fixe* to complete the ISS, which was at one time to have been completed by 1994, has clearly delayed the creation of safer, more cost efficient, and more flexible manned space vehicles, and it has created new hazards for astronauts and cosmonauts in orbit without having clear-cut scientific or exploratory goals. Ironically, carrying on with the ISS is key to international cooperation in space, yet it also represents a huge financial burden to all of its partners. All of the space agencies around the world that signed on to this megaproject find the programmatic costs and continuing delays, at least to some degree, a huge drain on resources, a difficult series of ongoing demands on research scientists, and in some cases virtually a national embarrassment. For both the United States and its international space partners alike, it is difficult to abandon such a huge commitment of time, money, and human resources, but it also embarrassing to explain why this project has taken so long, cost so much, and returned so few significant results.

Fortunately Congress has restored some funding to at least allow some scientific benefits to flow from ISS operations, but the truth is that the onboard two-person skeleton crew over the past three years has little time for scientific experiments because they must spend all of their time maintaining the ISS in orbit.

The Rogers Commission and the Paine Commission that followed on the heels of the *Challenger* failure in 1986 told a story of failed leadership and faulty NASA management. These high-level commissions urged NASA to replace the space shuttle with newer and better technology—and to do so before the time of its projected obsolescence—namely, 2001.

The Paine Commission noted the need for rapid completion of the International Space Station before costs spiraled out of control and set forth the case to establish new goals and aspirations. Most of all, the Rogers Commission of 1986 noted that NASA management was out of step with its engineers and scientists. The distinguished scientists and engineers of the Rogers Commission emphasized the dangers of NASA managers being indifferent to the safety risks that came from waivers they had routinely granted to defects in their space systems [3,4].

Is this to say that NASA is obsolete? Is there is no hope for a resurgence of space research, exploration, and applications in the United States and around the world? No! There is still time for NASA to chart new courses. There is still time to define Project Constellation in such a way that the new crew vehicles can be safer and more cost efficient. There is still time to use robotic systems more exten-sively to reduce costs and advance program objectives. And there is still time to achieve a better balance among and between NASA's goals for scientific discovery, exploration, and the development of new applications for the betterment of humankind. NASA's recently announced designs for Project Constellation represent a move in this direction, but Congress and the U.S. public still experienced considerable "sticker shock" when the $104-billion price tag for the moon mission was announced. Critics like Dr. Robert L. Park of the American Physical Society and Warren Leary of the *New York Times* [5] have sharply criticized the program and the lack of focus on robotic probes to do more for less. Indeed the charts found at the end of the three chap-ters that follow outline safety concerns related to both the space shuttle and the International Space Station as well as possible remedial actions that might be undertaken to increase safety and system performance.

The future of space, space exploration, and space safety, of course, goes beyond NASA programs, not only to other space agencies, but also increasingly to the emerging space-related private enterprises in the United States and other parts of the world.

The U.S. Congress passed new legislation that was signed into law in January 2005 to authorize the Federal Aviation Administration (FAA) to oversee the commercial development of new space technology and "manned commerce" from the entrepreneurial and aerospace sectors of the U.S. economy. The FAA has sent proposed detailed regulations governing those private organizations that plan to send people into space out for public comment and to Congress for hearing. Final action is antici-pated by midyear 2006, and a new space tourism business is expected to burgeon in the next few years with most planning to begin in 2008.

New entities such as Space X, Bigelow Aerospace, SpaceDev, SpaceOne, Scaled Composites, Rocketplane Ltd., Space Adventures, and now Virgin Galactic are promising new and innovative approaches to space. Reservations are can even be made on Virgin Galactic, Space

Adventures, and Rocketplane today by those who want to be among the first 1000 or so humans in space.

Scaled-composite guru Burt Rutan's explanation of how he let safety concerns drive the development of his innovative SpaceOne enterprise in the June 2005 issue of *Ad Astra* is but one case in point as to how entrepreneurial talent can complement the thinking of space agency engineers [6]. The Aldridge Commission rendered its report in late 2004. This commission had a mandate from President George W. Bush to define the specifics of the new U.S. space vision. Former Astronaut Pete Aldridge's Commission went beyond this charge to set forth ideas not only about how to go to the moon but also about how NASA might be reorganized and how the NASA research centers might be redeployed as federally financed research and development centers (FFRDCs). In this new form the NASA centers hopefully might receive clearer goals, more specific performance measures, yet with the flexibility to develop new technology in more innovative ways and for additional parts of the federal government. In short, the time might well have come to reshape NASA to 21st-century needs, and one can hope that NASA's leadership has the vision and the political skills to make this happen.

This would mean redefining the mission of NASA and its centers and to release the intellectual energy of entrepreneurial enterprises that can most likely find innovative new applications, open the road to space tourism, and provide cost-effective new transportation systems. This redefined NASA would still be left with plenty to do—something we will address in the later stages of this book.

In this new environment there would be a redefined and symbiotic relationship between the new NASA and the new entrepreneurial companies that will build a new pathway to space. For 20 years space applications, research, and exploration have stagnated; in the *next* two decades we can at least hope to build a new pathway to the stars. This means recognizing past failures—not only in space safety but also in the broader aspects of the NASA space program.

In short, it is imperative to undertake broad-based and creative planning for a new pathway to space. This new pathway could include private spacehabs in Earth orbit and even lunar colonies. It also might involve highly innovative international ventures involving new technology such as nanotube-based space elevators and or solar sails. It could also take a new and creative role in seeking a resurgence in space applications that could help with space-based health and educational systems, environmental monitoring, and enhanced space navigational systems to allow us to more safely fly and land aircraft, decongest our highways, and aid in diminishing the effects of global warming. The greatest pathway forward in the U.S. space program might well not be in technology, but in innovative management and entrepreneurial talent. On this new pathway NASA must be both a leader and a partner with other space agencies and private enterprise.

The key to the future of space might well have more to do with entrepreneurs such as Burt Rutan, Paul Allen, Bob Bigelow, Peter Diamandis, and Sir Richard Branson than it does with the so-called "Old NASA." The "New NASA" could, however, be a source of innovation and inspiration if it truly sought to reinvent itself and its mission as outlined in the five-point program outlined in Chapter 10.

NASA: at Its Zenith

In late July 1969 Neil Armstrong and Buzz Aldrin climbed out of their spaceship and walked into history. Humans would, for the first time, explore not a new frontier but a totally alien world. Billions of years of history laid beneath their footsteps on an ancient moonscape. These now famous spacefarers alighted from their lunar exploration module, took a few steps down a ladder, and began to explore the surface of the moon. Exciting! Electrifying! Almost unimaginable! Five hundred million people all around the world—some of them staying up all night—watched in amazement as this incredible event unfolded "live via satellite" [7].

It was so amazing, in fact, that some people still claim the Apollo moon landings were all faked in a studio in England under the direction of Sir Arthur Clarke—to the great amusement of both NASA and Arthur C. Clarke!

Everyone seeing that satellite telecast knew the future of the human species had altered—and in a significant and irreversible way. What it meant for humans to be true spacefarers no one yet truly knew. Yet we sensed that this was a new stage upon which *homo sapiens* would act—foolishly, wisely, or, as it turns out over time, rather ineptly. This was a new opportunity to think not only about the exploration and settlement of space but also to think globally in ways that our forefathers could never have imagined.

Humans for the first time had actually escaped their gravity well and flown beyond the ties of Mother Earth. Astronauts had escaped Gaia's womb. Amazingly this happened less than a dozen years after the Sputnik launch in 4 October 1957. We the descendants of apes had become space explorers, and humans began to dream of Mars and beyond.

> We the descendants of apes had become space explorers, and humans began to dream of Mars and beyond.

Humanity had now reached a new stage of evolution. It was one thing for Galileo, Tycho Brahe, Kopernicus, William Herschell, Percival Lowell, and many other astronomers over the centuries to look to the planets and the stars through telescopes and imagine amazing foreign worlds. Certainly astronomers could survey the constellations, chart imagined "canals," on Mars and envision journeying into space. Edward Everett Hale, H. G. Wells, Jules Verne, Robert Heinlein, Isaac Asimov, Arthur C. Clarke, and other speculative writers fueled our imagination of what might be. But now this was real. This was no longer scientific musing, but real living and breathing people were walking on another world. Human technology had made distant dreams a reality—and the world watched as if we were indeed all one on Spaceship Earth.

Thus in late July 1969, almost 40 years ago, we humans gave thought to conquering new worlds. It was no longer science fiction but science fact. Humanity saw new possibilities. For the first time we witnessed the Earth as it rose above the lunar plain. It signaled the oneness of all the people that inhabit our small planet we call Earth. Or at least it signaled new possibilities for space exploration.

Phrases like "the sky is the limit" suddenly seemed frightfully quaint. People began talking about what we should do next. Could there be permanent colonies on the moon? Space tourism? Might we not transform the surface and atmosphere of Mars to become a place for humans to live? Surely lunar colonies might become possible, could they not? Journeying to the outer planets or even to the stars suddenly did not seem preposterous.

People like Dr. Francis Clauser, chairman of the College of Engineering at Cal Tech, said outrageous things at the time. He proclaimed: "I believe that we can place men on Mars before 1980." He also predicted in late 1969 that "...in the coming decade we will see the cost of space transportation reduced to the point that the average citizen can afford a trip to the Moon." In the mid-1970s, Max Hunter of Lockheed foresaw, with stupendous inaccuracy, a shuttle program that would support "95 flights a year at a per launch cost of $350,000 and $7 per pound of payload to low earth orbit" [8]. At the start of the 1970s, enthusiasm soared, and incredible conquests in outer space seemed possible. NASA was the place where young people dreamed to work and becoming an astronaut was the most awe-inspiring ambition.

NASA Today

But now, nearly four decades later, the dream has faded. Our aspirations that soared at the start of the 1970s have sunk as we have staggered into a new millennium of anemic space exploration and a series of setbacks. Indeed, not only space programs have changed, but the entire world has changed too. Our globe is now a scarier place. Computer viruses, AIDS, terrorism, Al Qaida, genocide and starvation in Africa, and new forms of bacteria and epidemics with new names like SARS and ebola threaten global society. Natural disasters, such as the great tsunami in the Indian Ocean and Hurricanes Katrina and Rita that devastated the U.S. Gulf Coast, have signaled the need to use technology to save lives at home before trying to trek into space.

Aspirations to go where "no man has gone before" have shrunk almost to obscurity. The wonderful dreams of what NASA could deliver in our lifetime have gradually faded. Yet humans are ultimately seekers, explorers, and problem solvers, and space represents not only the next frontier, but, in many ways, it can also be a pathway to a better future. Space can allow us to protect against natural disasters, cope with global warming and ozone depletion, and alert us to asteroids or comets that could spell catastrophic destruction.

Yet, dramatic new goals in space now seem further away than in 1969. NASA, by essentially abandoning the field of space applications, has led many to conclude that the space agency is irrelevant to the everyday human condition. The Cold War "dissolved" in the 1980s, and the "missile gap" has become an obscure factoid of the presidential race of 1960. The space race to outdo the Soviet Union no longer motivates us toward the ultimate frontier. China and Japan are now seriously planning to send their own astronauts to the moon, perhaps before the United States can return there. The slow but now steady retrograde motion of the U.S. space program is greeted with overwhelming indifference among the American populace and indeed around the world. The space programs that receive the greatest attention today in the U.S. budget relate to the strategic uses of space for defensive and potentially offensive purposes. How did things go so wrong? Why has NASA apparently become lost in space and its once brilliant accomplishments faded away?

New Space Entrepreneurs

Today space entrepreneurs have stolen the headlines. Players like Peter Diamandis (the X-Prize founder), Burt Rutan (the designer of SpaceOne), Sir Richard Branson (now planning Virgin Galactic), and Paul Allen (of Microsoft fame and backer of SpaceOne) are the new space pioneers who are offering us hope and excitement and the promise of space commercialization. Dr. Peter Diamandis is not only father of the X-Prize and cofounder of the International Space University, but he is now offering rides via his new company at $2700 a ride to those space enthusiasts seeking 40 s of weightlessness aboard the so-called "vomit comet." Burt Rutan, of Voyager and SpaceOne rocket fame, is currently offering more excitement about space than NASA. He and his coinventors are designing the commercial craft for space tourism of the future. When we think of exciting space firsts, we now seem to look to people like Bob Bigelow of Bigelow Aerospace who wants to create a private space station. Certainly, we think of Sir Richard Branson of Virgin Atlantic who wants to create private space vehicles for tourists who wish to fly into protospace and see the big blue marble and know once and for all that the Earth is not flat. Branson is already doing commercials and taking reservations to fly into space via Virgin Galactic with the projected cost of such a space flight being pegged at $25,000!!! Space Adventures and Rocketplane claim on be on their own exciting parallel tracks.

Jim Benson, chief executive officer (CEO) of SpaceDev, whose company developed the engines for SpaceOne has become an ongoing critic of what he calls the old NASA. SpaceDev figured out that a particular neoprene rubber and laughing gas (nitrous oxide) was a cheap and safe fuel for the world's first private space plane. The engine that SpaceDev developed for SpaceOne was not only cheap but safe in that it could be "throttled" to a stop in the event of a problem. Benson has claimed that he has been unable to bid on NASA contracts, not because his proposals are too high but too low and thus under the minimum levels that NASA has set for safety.

Likewise, Peter Diamandis has labeled conventional space agencies and conventional giant aerospace companies as "dinosaurs" and proclaimed the new breed of space entrepreneurs "the furry mammals" of the future. The truth is probably more complicated. There is reason to believe that NASA can chart a new course to the future, and its new administrator seems ready to let innovative thought, space applications, partnership with entrepreneurs, and global partnerships be a part of the future—but under new types of models based on stimulus packages and competition prizes. However, there is concern that shortcuts to safety should not be a part of the future that ends in a devastating blow to NASA's very existence.

Ongoing Problems

Certainly NASA's space programs and the great enthusiasm they once generated have withered away. The accidents with the *Challenger* (in 1986) and the *Columbia* (in 2003) were the mega-events that captured worldwide media attention. These two spectacular shuttle failures and the loss of life of over a dozen astronauts have shaken U.S. and even world public opinion of the once "heroic" NASA. The Rogers Commission report after *Challenger* and the Gehman Commission after *Columbia* both confirmed a NASA that had made mistakes, overridden the advice of engineers and scientists to maintain schedule and budget, and authorized "waivers" to proceed when there were known problems—problems that led to deadly results. There were some 5800 waivers granted during just the last flight of the *Columbia* prior to its destruction.*

But there is more to the story than two failures of the space shuttle. There are a number of parallel failures such as the ongoing termination of a number of experimental development programs—all geared to develop the so-called "space plane" or a space escape or return vehicle. And yes, one after the other, all were cancelled without success.

All of the so-called X-programs have gotten X-ed out of the NASA budget one by one as the space shuttle and the ISS have consumed funds (almost literally breathed all the oxygen out of the American space program) that might have been spent on new initiatives. Indeed, the ISS looms large in much of NASA's problems over the last 20 years. To many, it is the grinch that ate NASA.

The mission and rationale for the International Space Station, some two decades after it was launched in the Reagan years, is now extremely murky. This is not surprising in that this program (once planned for completion in 1991 and then readjusted to 1994 when it became the ISS) is now over a decade behind schedule and still counting for at least another five

---

*Data available online at http://www.nasa.caib.gov.

years. The ISS is more than late. It has also swollen to a total cost of some $100 billion. This is a huge price tag even for NASA and its international partners. It is now vying for the honor of being the U.S.'s most expensive public project—perhaps ultimately more expensive than the Boulder Dam, the Tennessee Valley Authority (TVA) initiative, or the Arkansas River navigation projects. Yet oddly enough as the cost of building the ISS has zoomed and construction schedule expanded, the experimental program budget (presumably the reason the ISS was built in the first place) has been cut in size. Apparently, we need to spend many more resources and risk many astronaut lives to build something for which we have a shrinking need. The costs of the ISS are so high that NASA has called into question its ability to service and resupply the Hubble Telescope—the one megaspace project that has provided enormous knowledge of our universe and is of proven value. Go figure.

These types of failures go on. There is the incident where NASA crashed a satellite into Mars because the orbital parameters somehow got confused in the calculations as between miles vs kilometers. These events and accidents have all taken their toll. Today NASA expects over 25% of its workforce to retire in the next five years, and it has many fewer workers under 30 than over 55. In many people's minds it is an "old guy" government bureaucracy that has run out of steam.

NASA's 240 Astronauts—But Will They Fly in Space?

Young people still think being an astronaut would be neat, but here too questions arise. The NASA astronaut corps has now swollen to 240 astronauts in training. One does not truly become an astronaut until one has flown into space. Currently NASA says it will not have a new "human-rated" vehicle ready for some time. The new NASA Administrator, Michael Griffin, has promised to advance the date for the CEV to be able to fly with crew aboard to the ISS from the first announced date of 2014 to as soon as 2012. This accelerated schedule comes, in part, from eliminating the "fly-off" competition between the two teams of Lockheed Martin vs Boeing/Northrop Grumman. This new schedule came partially in response to new congressional strictures to have a replacement vehicle fly before the shuttle is permanently grounded or very nearly so. However, recent shuttle program deficits can possibly return the schedule for the CEV back to 2014 [9]. We do know that the previously published flight manifests for 28 flights of the space shuttle in order to complete the ISS no longer hold. The latest number is probably some 18 further flights. Only after the next flight of the shuttle, sometime in 2006, will it become clearer as to what will be final design and scope of the ISS and the number of additional shuttle flights that will fly.

Whatever the number of remaining flights, the most salient point is that only a small fraction of NASA's astronaut corps will fly into outer space. Instead NASA astronauts and astronauts in training have become highly paid and visible public relations people who speak in public forums to promote space programs. Only a few of these young, willing, and able astronauts will actually be able to go into space. A booking on Virgin Galactic, Rocketplane, or Space Adventures might get you into space more surely than being one of today's astronauts in Houston, Texas.

A Billion Here and a Billion There—After a While It Adds up to Real Money

Remarkably, when NASA was in "can do" mode it took only 12 years to go from the jolt of the Sputnik launch in October 1957 to landing humans on the moon in July 1969. Since then, we have not made any "great leaps for mankind" but only small steps into near Earth orbit. In audits in 2004, NASA seemingly mislaid $2 billion in funds. At least this is the amount of loose cash that they seem to be having a tough time locating. Many speculate that the resignation of Sean O'Keefe's as NASA administrator was related to this financial fiasco as much as NASA's other problems. Certainly, it was thought by the George W. Bush White House that made the appointment that O'Keefe, who was formerly the deputy director of the Office of Management and Budget, would at least know how to manage money and finally get all of the NASA centers and Headquarters operating on the same computerized budgeting system.

> Since then, we have not made any "great leaps for mankind" but only small steps into near Earth orbit.

The New York Times in an editorial summed up the frustration of many. They expressed the view that NASA, under O'Keefe's leadership, had apparently set a course to complete the International Space Station without serious review or new assessment. This, they stated, was little more than "stubborn determination to finish a project once started" [10]. They went on to say that this result was really not an acceptable answer to U.S. taxpayers. In fact, they suggested that the U.S. space program had faded in a fog of financial crisis that includes some $2 billion in misallocated funds that NASA accountants seem unable to find [10]. In another month as 2004 grinded to a halt, Administrator Sean O'Keefe's resignation was on "W's" desk.

Certainly in today's uncertain world, no one would put the space program at the top of our priority list. Indeed we are now plagued with problems of huge imbalances in trade with China and other trading partners, soaring petroleum costs, environmental concerns with melting ice caps and ever more polluted air and oceans, global epidemics from AIDS and SARS to the Asian bird flu, and now a never-ending War on Terrorism that has spread to wars in Iraq and Afghanistan. Americans swim in seas of red ink with record annual deficits seemingly stuck at well over $400 billion. Young people born in the United States today arrive with a "birth tax" of $36,000 of national debt per person. National debt seems to be spiraling out of control, and space programs are only one of the victims.

Clearly NASA's woes must be seen in perspective. Resolving problems in Iraq, Iran, North Korea, and elsewhere around the world is clearly more important to U.S. national political leaders. Environment, global warming, energy, health care, and education are higher priority issues—yet a dynamic and responsive NASA could be front and center in addressing all of these issues. NASA could be helping with new space-based solutions to environmental, energy, education, and health care issues. The key to the future thus remains finding balance between applications, scientific discovery, and "safe" and effective exploration of space (using a combination of astronauts and more capable and cost-effective robotic devices).

Does the American Public Still Find NASA's Space Programs Relevant?

In short, could and should we ask NASA, and Administrator Griffin in particular, to make the U.S. space agency more relevant, more accountable, and more effective? In the last 20 years, NASA has managed to redesign its programs to be irrelevant to social and economic needs and remote from public interests. Today, NASA's base of support is found largely among the lobbyists of aerospace conglomerates and legislator's representing districts with NASA centers or high-tech installations. Many government bureaucracies, in response to efforts during the Clinton and Bush administrations to reinvent government, are finding ways to make themselves more cost efficient, less bureaucratic, and more productive. But NASA has seemingly become increasingly hidden behind a high-tech cloud of abstruse research objectives and organizational inefficiency. NASA has not only major accounting problems, and soaring costs for an International Space Station that is now many, many years behind schedule and with a price tag of $100 billion, but an aging and expensive fleet of shuttle orbiters now reduced to only three in number [11]. How did this happen? How could we have moved to a position so far away from the thrill

"Has the Shuttle Become NASA's 1976 Dodge Dart?"

of the Apollo program that we find a newspaper headline asking the embarrassing question: "Has the Shuttle Become NASA's 1976 Dodge Dart?"

How could we have come to a point reminiscent of a Naders' Raiders investigation of what went wrong at NASA. But instead of "unsafe at any speed" with General Motors and its Corvair being the prime suspect, we have now gone to "unsafe at hyperspeed" with NASA and the space shuttle as the focus of attention [12].

What Way Forward?

We know the shuttle is aging technology conceived in the 1970s and first flown in the early 1980s. To continue these systems after the failure of the *Challenger* (1986) and *Columbia* (2003) through until 2010 to even 2012 is a daring risk. After the crash of the Concorde SST in Paris, enormous expense was undertaken to bring this vehicle back to flight only to find the system was not financially or operationally viable to fly. The remaining aircraft were sent off to the museums. The likelihood that the shuttle might be following the same historical pattern should be a major worry for the new NASA administrator, the White House, and Congress. As Astronaut Mike Mullane, who logged some 156 hours of flight time on three different shuttle flights, has said, the space transportation system (STS) has never lived up to its billing as a safe vehicle. Without an effective escape system Astronaut Mullane maintains that the shuttle is the most dangerous of vehicles flying because it offers no escape capability during critical periods of each mission [2].

Most 1970s technology (whether from the field of telecommunications, computers, robotics, aviation, or astronautics) is more suited for museums rather than operational use. Certainly systems designed in the 1970s are highly questionable for flying astronauts into Earth orbit. What then is the next step beyond the shuttle? Are today's programs to go to the moon and Mars, based on a new crew exploration vehicle and a new crew launch vehicle, going to repeat some of the very same mistakes we made with the shuttle? The early previews by some critics say "yes," even as NASA officials are saying "no."

Should NASA be allowing private enterprise to take a greater role in developing new 21st-century space technology? Does the NASA organization, which has grown like topsy since its birth in 1958, need to be revamped to become more relevant to today's needs and opportunities? Thomas Jefferson once suggested a revolution is needed every 20 years. Perhaps NASA, as it nears 50, is long overdue at least for reinvention.

To understand how the past links to the future, we must understand the history of the shuttle and NASA's increasing difficulties over the last few decades. The initial design problems and budgetary issues that called for economies in the design of the so-called STS have already been a subject of controversy. Then, outrageous claims were made about the reliability, the performance, the refurbishment, and turnaround period for relaunch of the shuttle. This was all done to sell a new program to Congress and a reluctant space communications industry. These claims included outrageous statements about how safe the shuttle would be and how little it would cost to launch either crew or cargo into space. Some of those estimates as to costs were off by over two orders of magnitude. Journalists, however, in the early days believed that the space shuttle would be something like a commercial airline flight in terms of safety and operational performance. After the *Challenger* accident, engineers and managers were asked about shuttle safety. The managers tended to describe the space shuttle as many times safer than the engineers. This result alone should indicate that NASA's management and structure needed fundamental change.

The greatest problem of all, however, has been the decision to greatly extend the operation of the space shuttle well past its reasonable lifetime. Even the Paine Commission's report, presented after the *Challenger* disaster in 1986, tells us the straight story. This distinguished panel, headed by former NASA Administrator Thomas O. Paine and which included Neil Armstrong, Ambassador Jeanne Kirkpatrick, military generals, and aerospace experts clearly stated that the top priority was to develop new space vehicles and that the shuttle would be "obsolete" certainly by 2001 [13]. The shuttle and the gummy bear we call the "International Space Station" has managed to claim more and more of NASA resources, and the safety risks—for both the space shuttle and the ISS—have risen as we rely on technology that is more and more out of date. The overriding budgetary demands of the space station certainly have contributed greatly to the many hapless and now failed attempts to develop a working spaceplane that could carry a small crew to orbit with greater reliability and certainly greater economy than the space shuttle.

NASA's various development programs (the X-program projects) started and then stopped one after another without success. First it was the X-33, and then the X-34, followed by the X-37, and most recently the X-47A & X-47C programs. One after the other they were going to give astronauts tremendously safer access to orbit and much greater cost efficiency of operation, or in the case of the HL-20 or the X-38 that were also cancelled, they were going to provide an escape capability from the space station. One after another NASA cancelled these programs. The reasons varied. Cost overruns! Schedule delays! Not enough progress! More promising approaches! But there are many who believe that the real bugaboo for the various X-programs that were cancelled was the $100-billion financial vacuum cleaner in the sky that we call the ISS. And here the culprit might be not so much NASA leadership but the overseers in Congress that failed to provide leadership and program priorities as it reviewed and revised NASA's program year after year. The design and building of the ISS has sucked all of NASA's financial resources dry for over a decade and Congress as much as NASA must share the blame.

These misadventures with the shuttle, the ISS, and the space plane are all part of a story about why today's NASA seems lost in space. It is certainly too early to tell if the cautious approach to design the crew exploration vehicle as an "Apollo Program on steroids" is the best route forward. Nevertheless, there is very little new technology being developed under Project Constellation. Yet, there is a huge budget that exceeds $100 billion, and a 12-year timetable is involved. Further some would question if there is a clearly defined mission for returning to the moon and what the exploratory objectives are once we get there. In basic terms the capsule that will ride aboard the new crew launch vehicle is about a meter and a half greater in diameter than the Apollo Command Capsule and will house four astronauts rather than three, but the engineering and the design is not greatly different from the system the United States deployed in the 1969 Moon mission. See Fig. 1.2 for an artist's impression of the crew launch vehicle carrying the crew exploration vehicle (CEV) into space.

These types of questions are red flags that suggest Project Constellation needs clearer strategic direction. We need serious answers to the preceding issues and more. Specific lunar exploration goals must be addressed before we design very expensive hardware at a cost that exceeds $100 billion. The most fundamental questions are: are we trying to go to the moon or Mars? Why do we want to go to either location? What

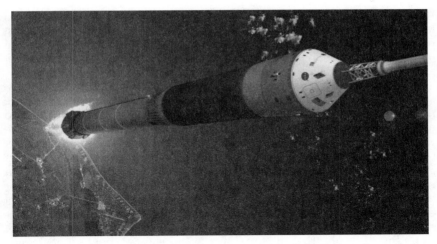

Figure 1-2 New space vehicle being designed and built for Project Constellation. (Graphic courtesy of NASA)

are our specific goals in terms of exploration, establishing permanent bases, setting up observatories, establishing material processing factories, or other objectives perhaps of national prestige, employment, or just exploring the unknown? What can best be done by crew and what by robotic probes and machines.

All of the preceding suggests that the NASA story and its answers to the questions badly needs to be told to the U.S. public and the rest of the world as we move forward with both American and international space programs. Clearly Administrator Griffin must define some new priorities and use the new project evaluation office to achieve focus on what NASA's objectives should be going forward. It is not too late to redirect human and financial resources to different space goals, to restructure NASA to be better able to achieve 21st-century goals, and to align technical programs with the primary needs of the American public.

This might mean that NASA needs a new structure for itself and all of its centers, creative leadership from within the executive and legislative branches, and most certainly revamped goals and objectives. Nearly 50 years have now gone by since President Eisenhower hastily formed the new National Aeronautical and Space Administration out of the precursor NACA organization based in Ohio. Times and goals have changed! NASA needs an overhaul! The bright young people that undertook the Mercury, Gemini, Skylab, and Apollo programs did not have a job. They were zealots on a mission. They were willing to give their all to succeed in a campaign to bring America into the space age.

The NASA of the 1960s, 1970s, and even 1980s was America's poster child for success—pretty much up to the *Challenger* disaster of 1986, things seemed to be going right. But since that time NASA, despite a few shiny moments such as with the Mars rovers, has become a humdrum story of failure. It is now a full-fledged government bureaucracy plagued by budgetary overruns, a couple of billions of dollars unaccounted for in recent audits, and sudden and questionable program terminations. Most of all, NASA's human space exploration program is of questionable safety and is more space construction than it is discovery.

It is an agency driven by unrealistic expectations and a sense of disappointment both within and without. There needs to be a fresh start. We need a new sense of direction in Congress, by agency employees and management, and certainly the public at large. The new Vision for Space Exploration presented by George W. Bush was an attempt to infuse direction into NASA, and the Aldridge commission had been seen by many as an opportunity for innovation. Indeed many of the highly competent and well-trained NASA personnel involved with either the shuttle program or the ISS are scrambling to get into the new and more exciting Project Constellation initiative. This is at a time when these now geriatric programs need all of the help they can get. But fundamental change cannot be imposed simply from the top down or by placing a new set of slogans on the NASA web site.

The space shuttle and the ISS represent familiar stories often heard in Washington, D.C. Archaic concepts and outdated technology can only be pushed so far. Budgetary resources cannot be strained too thin—by NASA, by the White House, or by Congress. Most of all, neither large bureaucracies, nor huge aerospace corporations, succeed well in introducing new ideas, fresh concepts, and breakthrough technologies.

A Failure of National Leadership?

Indeed if there is a villain to be found in this story of NASA's fading glory, it is not in the dedicated scientists and engineers of NASA but a fault of leadership and bureaucratic process. Certainly we must see current issues in the context of national leadership, not just that of NASA. The *Columbia* Accident Investigation Board (CAIB), in reporting its findings, pointed an accusing finger at the entire national leadership, at congressional oversight and budgeting, at Office of Management and Budget (OMB) and General Accounting Office (GAO), the White House, and everyone who kept asking NASA to do everything—stretch the budget, keep on schedule and, oh yes, keep everything very safe too.

There has been a lack of reasonable guidance, expectation, and goal setting within the leadership of NASA, of Congress, the OMB, the Office of Science and Technology Policy at the White House, and even at the presidential level itself. One can examine the zigzags in NASA's so-called Comprehensive Space Transportation Policy to see that it should not be called "a comprehensive policy" at all but rather an "ad hoc," "cursory," and even "slap dash" set of plans always responding to the last budgetary cycle or political directive. The problems are not partisan, and one cannot fault the Bush or Clinton or Bush-again years in particular.

Certainly NASA has suffered from political intervention, compounded by the lobbying on behalf of aerospace giants who have garnered large contracts and sizable profits. These were profits that came when NASA succeeded, which is as it should be. But there were profits and sizable awards that did not falter even when NASA failed. NASA has maintained and funded centers and programs not central to its core mission, maintained programs that distributed geographic largesse (some might call it "pork"), and stretched out and maintained an aging shuttle program well past its prime in order to achieve impossible goals. Thus the space shuttle will apparently live decades beyond its reasonable lifetime. In the process NASA will thus likely continue to shift priorities at the beck and call of congressional mandates. President George W. Bush has announced a two-decades-long vision for space exploration. Many cynics believe it might not even last through until the end of 2008—the end of his term of office.

Who now remembers that when the space station was first announced by President Reagan it was to be finished by 1991? This is a date now past due by almost 15 years. Who now remembers that when the space station became the International Space Station and Russia, Europe, Canada, and Japan joined the effort that the completion date moved to a more realistic date of 1994? But, under current planning, and blissfully assuming a "perfect launch schedule" for the space shuttle, it would still take many years to finish the ISS as it was planned at the time of the *Columbia* failure. With the problems exposed by the most recent launch in August 2005, a scaling back of the ISS program seems very likely, and the shuttle launch manifest was scaled back to 18. New congressional authorization that will allow the United States to purchase additional Soyuz vehicles certainly provides new options beyond the shuttle, but the cost issues for the ISS still remain even if the shuttle is permanently grounded.

At last count, NASA had poured an estimated $1.75 billion over a 2.5-year period (i.e., Feb. 2003–August 2005) of direct and indirect costs into the reflight program in order to make the space shuttle safe. Now, in the wake of the problems with the latest *Discovery* launch (STS-114), many more hundreds of millions are being spent to solve the foam-shedding problem all over again. We have, in effect, poured good money after bad to make a number of fixes to get the shuttle back into space. The mantra instilled by Admiral Readdy who headed this mammoth effort was "find it, fix it, and fly safely." This was an excellent mission statement—brief, short, and easily understood. But as explained in the chapters that follow, all that was found was not or could not be fixed. Further the cost of fixing what was found has gone from an initial estimate of some three quarters of a billion dollars in 2003 to nearly $2 billion in 2006—and perhaps more. Meanwhile the crew that is responsible for servicing and preparing the shuttle for flight after a space mission has gotten older. Many have indeed now retired, and the workforce has shrunk in size and capability. Meanwhile the parts for retrofitting the space shuttle become harder and harder to obtain because suppliers have gone out of business or stopped making the parts. Some of the test equipment for the shuttle even contains radio tubes—a testament to the age not only of the shuttle but its retrofit

20

Table 1-1 Cumulative Risk of a Category One Failure of a Shuttle Flight Assuming Different Possible Failure Rates

Calculated "Cumulative Risk" of a Category One Failure Based on Number of Additional Shuttle Launches			
Number of Further Shuttle Flights	If there is a 1 in 50 Risk of Failure	If there is a 1 in 55 Risk of Failure	If there is a 1 in 60 Risk of Failure
20	35%	33.5%	32.0%

and maintenance program. The strategic planning elements of how to get through another five to seven years of space shuttle operations are woefully missing.

You only have to read the report of the CAIB to learn that the basic risk factors of a category one failure for the space shuttle is high and certainly worse than the 1 in 200 category one accident rating recently cited for the shuttle's reliability. This conclusion is simply reached based on experience to date (i.e., two failures in just over 110 launches). Or one can undertake calculations based on the rated reliability of a hugely complex system with over two million parts that must be integrated together and work in tandem with near perfection in a hostile and demanding environment. Just based on the law of statistics, as seen in the Table 1.1, the chances of another catastrophe with some 20 more launches might be estimated to be in the 30 to 35% probability range. The reduction of shuttle flights from 28 to 18 flights, in a statistical sense, would likely reduce the chance of another category one failure from around 50/50 to 1/3.

There are a host of questions that remain unanswered about the shuttle and the ISS, and these go beyond questions of safety. These questions involve costs, astronaut safety, competent management, and reasonable goals and objectives. Some of the more important questions are as follows:

Why should we spend billions of dollars on a thoroughly antiquated launch system, that is, the space shuttle, that has already gone into triple overtime?

Why does it make sense to spend billions more to complete an increasingly obsolete space station (with an estimated total price tag of $100 billion) when Congress and NASA are also cutting back on funding for ISS experimental programs and when there are not enough astronauts onboard to conduct experimental research?

Advancing and retreating at the same time seems the strangest policy of all. Further, there are key questions about whether planning for new astronaut-rated launch systems are well conceived or not. There is indeed some danger that we can and will replicate problems and pitfalls already encountered in the shuttle program.

As noted earlier, *The New York Times* has likened NASA's current program as being akin to Daimler-Chrysler bringing out in 2006 a 30-year-old

1976 Dodge Dart and trying to sell it to the public as a safe new, state-of-the-art product with modern fuel efficiency. Who in their right mind would buy it? Yet the American taxpayer is at this time still paying their hard-earned taxes to support an "obsolete" space vehicle that was designed in the mid-1970s. Furthermore, they could potentially spend billions more to complete a space station that will be almost two decades overdue when finished [12].

Certainly the United States has international obligations to other countries, and these obligations should not be lightly ignored. But other countries also have their own concerns and misgivings. A truly international effort to explore new options and solutions might well produce better answers than ignoring the elephant in the living room that no one seems willing or able to talk about.

In early 2006, new concerns about NASA have emerged in the form of an FBI investigation into the NASA Inspector General's 200-person office that monitors wrongdoing, financial mismanagement, and safety violations. This investigation is focused on NASA's Inspector General, Robert W. Cobb, who is alleged to have hindered inquiries into major safety violations related to shuttle launches in 2002 and 2003, including the *Columbia* launch. This investigation, reported on later in this book, again raises questions about the so-called broken safety culture within NASA [14,15].

So how do we untangle the massive tangle of problems that seem to ensnare current U.S. space policy? Where to begin? Certainly a new NASA administrator has been put in place—one with a great deal of experience and relevant training. Further, a new project evaluation office that has been needed for some time is up and running. But still to come is the need for a new and pragmatic focus on priorities. There needs to be a clearer explanation and integration of NASA efforts in the areas of space science, space application, and space exploration as well as a clearer definition of its role with regard to strategic space objectives *vis-à-vis* the U.S. Department of Defense. We believe that within this process there needs to be a new emphasis on astronaut space safety, a restructuring of NASA to focus on top priorities, a spin-off of functions best left to others in the private sector or other government agencies, a restructuring of the NASA centers, and a fresh look at international cooperation. We believe all of these actions are key to NASA's future success.

References

1 Schwartz, J., "A Wide-Eyed Astronaut Becomes a NASA Critic," *New York Times*, 24 Jan. 2006, pp. D1, D4.
2 Mullane, M., "Riding Rockets—The Outrageous Tales of a Space Shuttle Astronaut," *New York Times*, 19 Jan. 2006, D-1.
3 *Pioneering the Space Frontier*, Report of the National Commission on Space, Bantam Books, New York, May 1986.
4 The Presidential Commission on the Space Shuttle Challenger Accident Report, Government Printing Office, Washington, DC, 1986.

5 "NASA Planning Return to the Moon Within the Next 13 Years," *New York Times*, 20 Sept. 2005, A1, A12.

6 Rutan, B., "Minimizing Risk," *Ad Astra*, June 2005, p. 12.

7 Pelton, J. N., and Alper, J., *The Intelsat Satellite System*, AIAA, New York, 1984, p. 79.

8 Heppenheimer, T. A., *The Space Shuttle Program*, Vol. 1, NASA, Washington, DC, 1999, p. 245.

9 Gugliotta, G., "Bush's Space Plan in Danger," *Washington Post*, 24 Nov. 2005, pp. A1, A11.

10 "NASA's Budgetary Gift Horse," *New York Times*, 29 Nov. 2004, p. A24.

11 Osbourne, D., and Gaebler, T., *Re-Inventing Government*, Plume Books, New York, 1993.

12 Glanz, J., with Broad, W. J., "Has the Space Shuttle Turned into NASA's '76 Dodge Dart," *New York Times*, 27 Jan. 2004, pp. D1, D2.

13 Paine Commission Report, NASA, Washington, DC, 1986, pp. 1–15.

14 Gugliotta, G., "NASA's Inspector General Probed," *Washington Post*, 3 Feb. 2004, pp. A1, A8.

15 Leary, W., "Investigator at NASA Faces Inquiry over Safety," *New York Times*, 4 Feb. 2006, p. A9.

Additional Reading

"FAA Guidelines for Private Space Travel," 2006, http://www.faa.gov.

Pelton, J. N., Oslund, R. J., and Marshall, P. (eds.), *Communications Satellites: Global Change Agents*, LEA Publications, Mahwah, NJ, 2004.

"Rules Proposed for Space Travelers," *Washington Post*, 30 Dec. 2005, p. A-5. [Note, this is a book!]

"Space Safety Report: Vulnerabilities and Risk Reduction in US Human Space Flight Programs," George Washington Univ., Washington, DC, March 2005.

CHAPTER 2
U.S. Astronaut Programs: Past, Present, and Future—from Mercury to Project Constellation*

> "Objections to the pilot range from the engineer who semi-seriously notes that all the problems of Mercury would be tremendously simplified if we did not have to worry about the bloody astronaut, to the military man who wonders if a college trained chimpanzee or a village idiot might not do as well in space as an experienced test pilot."
>
> —*Astronaut Deke Slayton*

Then There Were Three ...

As of early 2006, the once powerful space shuttle fleet was down to three in number ... and grounded. The once proud and vaunted U.S. astronaut program was in a state of considerable disarray. The total estimated direct and indirect cost of restoring the three aging vehicles to flight-worthiness following the *Columbia* disaster ballooned to about $1.75 billion from February 2003 up until the relaunch of the *Discovery* in August 2005. Despite these huge expenditures, we now know that serious safety concerns still remain. Some members of the *Columbia* Accident Investigation Board (CAIB), the editorial staff of the *New York Times*, and the former head of the Massachusetts Institute of Technology (MIT) Lincoln Laboratories (among others) were calling for the grounding of the space shuttle and a curtailment of the International Space Station (ISS) in early to mid-2005. This was even before the reflight of the *Discovery* (STS 114) exhibited continuing problems eerily parallel to those that led to the *Columbia* disaster.

---

*This chapter derives in large part from the *Space Safety 2005 Report* and the research originally carried out for that study. In particular, text related to the Mercury through the Apollo Program was originally researched and written by Dr. John Logsdon, director of the Space Policy Institute, George Washington University. We thus give special thanks to Professor Logsdon for his contributions to this chapter. All substantive and editorial errors, however, are those of the author.

When the heat-insulating foam material broke off (i.e., so-called foam shedding), nearly missing the fragile tiles of the *Discovery* Orbiter's thermal protection system (TPS), shuttle operations were again halted. And then in December 2005 cracks were found in the PAL ramp that was designed after the *Columbia* accident to ensure that no blown-off foam could damage the vulnerable TPS that coats the underbelly of each orbiter. The "fix" of adding the ramp thus surfaced as an additional problem.

Indeed, the flight of the *Discovery* in August 2005 served to renew fears that the shuttle TPS might not ever be made as thoroughly safe for future missions as NASA had sought to achieve during the past two and half years of downtime. This downtime will now apparently stretch a number of months into the future before another shuttle flies.

The new video cameras installed on the *Discovery* in the aftermath of the *Columbia* accident showed live yet another near-fatal accident in the making with the insulation foam rocketing at supersonic speeds perilously close to the *Discovery*'s TPS at liftoff. This potentially lethal projectile could have punctured the thermal protection system and thus created another deadly situation, remarkably close to the *Columbia* mission. This is particularly shocking given the multibillion dollars that NASA had spent from 2003 to 2005 to correct this very problem—apparently to no avail.

The 2005 George Washington (GW) University study of the performance and the safety of the space shuttle and ISS itemized a number of concerns that went well beyond the thermal protection system. It addressed many other subsystems as well. This led to the recommendations in the GW University study, as of March 2005, to proceed to phase out the space shuttle just as soon as possible. This study recommended limiting the full scope of the ISS where possible and supporting the construction and operation of the ISS via other launch systems, a robotically operated shuttle. It particularly reduced the number of launches from the then planned number of 28 launches.

Today some of these shifts in NASA schedule and program planning are indeed taking place. This is not to say that NASA action was in response to the GW or any particular study because many others, both within and outside the U.S. space agency, have made similar recommendations. Some former NASA astronauts—and particularly Mike Mullane—have now gone public and expressed concerns about the space shuttle safety. Mullane in a book about his astronaut experience explains that the lack of an escape capability for critical parts of the mission, that is, at launch and during reentry, makes the shuttle a dangerous vehicle [1].

In the wake of the *Columbia* disaster and the near miss with the *Discovery*, there remain questions that the U.S. public and the world space community want to know:

1) How safe is the shuttle program?
2) Should the shuttle fly again and at what cost?
3) Is it still a reasonable objective to try to complete the entirety of the ISS?
4) What should NASA Administrator Michael Griffin, who is faced with a number of increasingly difficult choices, do to recover from the current

problems that surround NASA's space exploration program—the space shuttle program, the ISS, and major space agency budgetary shortfalls?

To answer these questions, a recap of the history of NASA's spaceflight program is highly pertinent. Indeed a review of astronaut history suggests that a number of critical "lessons" were never learned—or at least not thoroughly applied to the space shuttle design in terms of enhancing safety.

But before reviewing this history, some basic observations about NASA's safety record and the next steps forward seem even more pertinent.

> Indeed a review of astronaut history suggests that a number of critical "lessons" were never learned—or at least not thoroughly applied to the space shuttle design in terms of enhancing safety.

U.S. astronauts have died since the early 1960s in three separate incidents—the Apollo fire and the *Challenger* and the *Columbia* accidents. It is not clear exactly how many Russian cosmonauts have perished, but it seems that about 5% of the 434 astronauts and cosmonauts that have flown have given their lives to space exploration. Flying in space is not equivalent to boarding an aircraft or bungee jumping in terms of risk. Space exploration has been and will likely continue to be a relatively high-risk enterprise for some years to come, although current efforts aimed a space tourism have geared their engineering to reduce this risk to much lower levels.

When the space shuttle flies again, sometime in 2006, our own assessment is that with each launch there will be something like a one in 60 chance of another catastrophic failure—not the one in 200 chance that some in NASA announced even after the 2005 flight of *Discovery*. The GWU team's prolonged and in-depth review of the space shuttle program, and the many performance and safety issues that it represents, concluded that the STS is indeed now essentially obsolete.

This is hardly a startling conclusion since the Payne and Rogers Commissions in 1986 unanimously concluded that the shuttle would be obsolete within 15 years, that is, by 2001. What is abundantly clear is that much of the STS technology is three decades old and based on outmoded designs, materials, and parts. Also, the design is overly complex, and a full-envelope escape capability is lacking. The thermal protection system is particularly complex, potentially hazardous, and very costly to maintain. (A passive part of a rocket launcher, i.e., something with no moving parts, should never require some 30 to 40% of the time, energy, and cost of operating a launch system. It is the rocket motors and the "active" part of a reusable launcher system that should require the major part of the refurbishment time and energies and not the "passive" thermal protection system. A simple breakdown of time and cost to refurbish the shuttle orbiters alone is a clear indication of a critical path problem that has not been solved in the reflight efforts for the space transportation system.)

In short, these safety studies conducted in 2003 through early 2005 concluded that, for many reasons, the shuttle program should be brought to an end as soon as possible, together with the design and deployment of replacement launch systems. This is a conclusion that rather uncannily resembles the findings of the Payne and Rogers Commissions 20 years ago.

This finding leads rather ineluctably to the conclusion that the ISS deployment and ongoing operation also needs to be curtailed, at least to some reasonable degree.

Today, plans continue for the buildout of the ISS to accommodate international commitments to deploy the Canadarm2 and Japanese and European scientific modules, but there are options. One approach would be to use expendable launch vehicles. Another would be to operate the shuttle by remote control without astronauts aboard. Either option might make more sense than continuing to operate the remaining three orbiters as fully crewed freighters to low Earth orbit. It is certainly clear that if the estimated nearly $2 billion spent on shuttle retrofits and safety measures, through Spring of 2006, had been used instead on expendable rockets and/or on converting the shuttles to automated operation, the U.S. space program might be well ahead. Even expenditures to increase the capacity and capability of the Soyuz/Progress vehicles or even upgrading the European ATV so that it could carry crew to and from the ISS might have made more sense—and certainly less "dollars and cents."

Shuttle's Checkered History

NASA, despite $15 to $16 billion a year of public expenditures in recent years, has achieved much less than critics or enthusiasts would have hoped since the failure of the *Challenger* in 1986 brought NASA to its current era of uncertainty and difficulty. Creditable critics in the press, the Governmental Accounting Office, and the Members of the Gehman Commission, that is, the Columbia Accident Investigation Board, have all seen the space agency as falling short in terms of a less than stringent safety culture, management problems, and also noted a lack of coherent public policy and leadership at the national level. Despite the work of the CAIB and NASA's estimated nearly $2-billion return-to-flight program, the critical review by the GW University study, and others, have found major safety risks with the shuttle, risks with the ISS and envisioned the very real possibility of parallel mistakes being made in future programs related to going to the moon and Mars.

The crew exploration vehicle and the Project Constellation undertaking have benefited by reviewing past history. The designers of this new system have learned from past experience and mistakes and have come up with some innovative ideas. Yet at the end of this chapter we note some lessons yet to be learned that apply to the next generation of launch systems.

Lessons from Past Space Programs

After the successes of the Apollo missions to the moon from 1969 to 1972, the space shuttle was quickly designed by NASA in consultation with the

White House in a period when Richard Nixon was in power and about to win a landslide victory over George McGovern. White House officials Peter Flannigan and Clay "Tom" Whitehead were charged with negotiating with NASA to develop a new reusable vehicle that provided access to low Earth orbit and not break the budget in the process. During these discussions, the lift capability of the shuttle was reduced, and a solid fuel booster was added to keep costs under control [2].

Then the Watergate scandal hit the headlines, and this ultimately led to Nixon's resignation from office in 1974. But the space shuttle program was launched, and Congress committed to fund this next step forward in space.

Five operational shuttles were built and successfully flown—the *Atlantis*, the *Columbia*, the *Challenger*, the *Discovery*, and the *Endeavor*. The *Enterprise* was used for atmospheric tests and was never an operational vehicle. In the early days, from 1981 up until the first failure with *Challenger* in 1986, NASA managed to claim success despite critics who said the economic performance of the space shuttle was not even close to that which had been initially advertised. The claim that the shuttle could be refurbished to refly in a matter of weeks proved dramatically wrong. Claims that a mission might be accomplished at costs below $1000 per kilogram also were also off by a huge margin as well.

> The claim that the shuttle could be refurbished to refly in a matter of weeks proved dramatically wrong. Claims that a mission might be accomplished at costs below $1000 per kilogram also were also off by a huge margin as well.

In those first five years from 1981 to 1986, however, the shuttle was still seen by the general public as a triumph of American enterprise and ingenuity. The fact that the costs were high and the refurbishment process took a long time was not something the general public found to be of concern because the shuttles appeared to work flawlessly.

After the *Challenger* tragedy in 1986 with the explosive loss of seven astronauts "live via satellite television," this all changed in an instance. The investigating Rogers Commission found fault with NASA management and indicted space officials for cavalier judgments and leniency in granting waivers on key mission-related decisions. Most of all, the Paine and the Rogers Commissions noted the increasingly urgent need to find a replacement vehicle to continue effective 21st-century space exploration in light of the perceived approaching obsolescence of the space shuttle.

The remaining shuttle orbiters, after two-and-a-half years of investigation and reengineering, resumed their flight program. Also, the *Endeavor* Orbiter was ordered to be constructed by President Reagan, using available spare parts, to replace the *Challenger*.

But in time problems reemerged, key management issues arose, and again too many waivers were granted as concerns of safety engineers were overridden.

The *Columbia* accident in February 2003, with the loss of seven more lives, led to the grounding of the remaining three shuttles while the accident was investigated, the cause of the failure of the thermal protection system identified, and retrofits undertaken.

NASA then spent an estimated $1.75 billion on direct and indirect costs on a return-to-flight program at a time the agency was preparing for a further 25–30 shuttle flights. The CAIB report outlined the detailed steps recommended to be taken to make the shuttle program safe again. These efforts to "engineer in" additional safety for the remaining shuttles inspired new public confidence that if the CAIB recommendations were followed the shuttle would perform with a high level of safety when restored to flight. These steps, however, were essentially to revamp the thermal protection system and to install new video monitoring and management systems within NASA. The CAIB recommendations did nothing to reengineer the basic design of the shuttle, and the many other safety concerns that are discussed in Chapter 3 were not addressed.

The narrow focus of the Gehman Commission (i.e., the CAIB) is not surprising in that the charge to this group of experts was to discover the specific reason for the *Columbia* accident and recommend corrective action, rather than to review the safety of the shuttle program from top to bottom. NASA did indeed revamp the structure and nature of its safety program, sought to alter its institutional culture regarding safety, and undertook ambitious plans for the future. Thus the agency's mission ultimately turned out to be not only steps to improve shuttle safety and deploy the ISS but also, since early 2004, to launch a new "Moon, Mars and Beyond" exploration program, now known as Project Constellation.

This new Presidential Space Vision, announced in January 2004, included not only plans to go to the moon and Mars but also envisioned the full-scale build out of the ISS. Thus NASA, in the 2004 time frame, was still planning a full flight manifest of 28 shuttle flights to test the performance of the revamped orbiters, finish the International Space Station, and possibly resupply the Hubble Telescope. At this time, the shuttle reflight program was expected to be fully successful, with no more failures. This meant that NASA would be able to support perhaps as many as five shuttle launches each year until at least the end of 2010 when the shuttle fleet would be finally grounded. Only the mission to repair and resupply the Hubble Telescope was called into question until Congress restored funding to accomplish this mission as well.

This planning in early 2004, therefore, was based on the assumption that the remaining shuttle flights would be near faultless with no more category one accidents. There was no evidence on the public record of a fall-back option if any one of the remaining three orbiters should fail. The *Discovery* flight in the summer of 2005 signaled that the "total success" formula was not necessarily viable.

The main purpose of the return-to-flight program for the shuttle was the continuing construction of the International Space Station. Yet the ISS, currently manned by a skeleton crew of one U.S. and one Russian astronaut, has virtually no time scheduled in its daily calendar of events to conduct experiments. In short, NASA for the last three years has been able to do little more than maintaining the ISS as an outpost in space and occasionally boosting its orbit so that it does not reenter the Earth's atmosphere.

Amazingly, this project, when first conceived under the Ronald Reagan administration, was originally intended for completion in 1991/1992. Then, when it was redesigned to become the International Space Station, the date was repegged for full construction by the end of 1994. But now, after six more years of delay associated with the space shuttle reflight campaign and other budget and management difficulties, the ISS completion target date is the end of 2010, even after the scope is scaled down. At the same time, inflation and maintaining a standing army of support staff for the shuttle on the ground have led to skyrocketing costs.

Without the shuttle, or a new replacement, the Russian Soyuz spacecraft provides the only link to Earth for astronauts, equipment, and supplies. Although six new manned personal spacecraft projects (i.e., the various developments in the X series) were commissioned and then abandoned by NASA over the past two decades at a cost of billions of dollars (see Chapter 6), no new replacement for the shuttle will be available until the crew exploration vehicle and its new launch system for the Constellation Program are tested and flying perhaps as early as 2012. The exception to this statement is that NASA has, as of December 2005, asked the aerospace industry to propose ways that "private vehicles," as opposed to NASA vehicles, might provide launch services under contract to support ferrying astronauts and materials to the ISS as a stop-gap measure.

The NASA 2006 fiscal year budget was approved at the increased level of $16.5 billion, but new disclosures indicate that even this budget will not be enough. This is because program problems for the shuttle and the ISS are even more severe than first disclosed. The manifest of space shuttle launches has now been pared to 18 launches. This manifest schedule presumably can allow for one mission to resupply the Hubble telescope and also allow enough flights to "finish" the ISS. This bare-bones schedule will not cut back too much in the design and will be sufficient to meet most of the U.S. international obligations to Europe and Japan. The problem is that there is an estimated $4–6 billion additional needed to complete these flights over the next five years based on the current calculations. (At this point NASA is saying $4 billion for 18 flights and White House and OMB experts are saying $6 billion.) To stay within foreseen budgets, NASA would presumably have to cut shuttle flights to two a year and support only 10 flights or defer the development of new launch systems for Project Constellation by two to four years. Such a cutback to 10 launches would endanger U.S. commitments to launch the European Space Agency's Columbus space lab (a $1.4-billion investment on the part of the Europeans) and also possibly endanger the Japan Engineering Module (JEM) and even more so the Centrifuge Accommodation Module (CAM). The JEM and the CAM collectively represent an even larger net development cost on the part of the Japanese than the European Space Agency.

The options currently being discussed thus include the downsizing of the ISS and possible renegotiation of international commitments to reduce the remaining launches of the shuttle, the delay of the new launch system and CEV for Project Constellation, or other serious cuts to other parts of NASA programs. None of these options is appealing, and, because of the huge standing army that supports the space shuttle program, reducing the number of launches at this time saves proportionately little money [3].

A former astronaut as well as a top official from the Nixon White House, who contributed to the GW University study, both agreed that the initial shuttle decisions in the 1970s were made on the basis that this was to be an "experimental or prototypal first generation reusable launch vehicle system." They also believed as of the late 1980s that the STS would be replaced with more modern technology and that the shuttle was in no way designed for an operational lifetime of more than 30 years. Just as General Motors, U.S. Steel, and other large U.S. corporations did not adapt to changing markets and rapid technological change, it would seem that NASA also is in need of restructuring and major innovation in order to cope with today's challenges.

After the *Challenger* and *Columbia* disasters, the safety and reliability of the shuttle both remain a subject of debate. The nature—and the size— of the safety risks for both the shuttle and the ISS is still not widely understood. The *Challenger* failure study showed that administrators in the space program rated the safety of the shuttle much higher than did the engineers and scientists associated with it.

Today, in the context of Project Constellation, aerospace scientists and engineers in industry and at NASA now maintain that much greater safety can be achieved using new 21st-century technology and systems. Certainly, if one were to design today a new human-rated launch vehicle using the latest technology (such as advanced thermal protection systems, complete launch-to-land mission escape capability, improved propulsion systems capable of instant shutdown, etc.) this system would be much higher rated than the shuttle in terms of safety. At one time, NASA officials estimated safety factors for such a new vehicle as high as one critical accident in 10,000 flights, as opposed to the shuttle system that is, at best, one in 100. The new launchers for Project Constellation announced in late September 2005 were projected to have a safety objective of a one in 1000 accident rate. Indeed the Project Constellation launch and exploration vehicle is notable in that its design has taken a very cautious approach and returned to the roots of safety developed in the early days of the manned space program through Project Apollo. Unlike the shuttle, Project Constellation has chosen simplicity over complexity in many of its design concepts, but at enormous expense. The budget that NASA has estimated to develop the new vehicles and the moon landings has soared to $104 billion [4]. It is ironic that the Russian Space Agency has, as of February 2006, announced that it will build, at significantly less cost than NASA's program, a new "shuttle-like" reusable vehicle that can fly to the ISS as of 2012. They have indicated that this new vehicle can sustain the ISS as an international space port for the longer term future and that the ISS can by that time be frequented by not only Russian vehicles but the European ATV and the Japanese HTV.

The sheer complexity of the shuttle, with millions of parts and tens of thousands of them in the thermal protection system alone, does not allow for significantly higher safety ratings, especially when many of these parts and wiring systems are used over and over again [5]. Space safety has a great deal to learn from basic principals derived ever since the Mercury project—principals that were partially overridden or neglected in the shuttle program.

How Safe Is Space?

From the 1950s, the U.S. and Russian space programs have worked on the development of manned spacecraft with the capability to lift humans into outer space. Then in 2004, China became the third nation to successfully launch a man into space—a feat that was repeated again in October 2005 with the Chinese providing live television coverage of this latest launch. Also in the fall of 2004, Burt Rutan, head of Scaled Composites, with private backing, designed the SpaceOne vehicle that flew into low Earth orbit twice within an eight-day schedule to collect the Ansari X-Prize. When Rutan's craft landed, it was greeted by an impromptu sign that read simply: "SpaceOne, NASA Zero!!"

Since the triumph of Yuri Gagarin's first flight in the late 1950s, only 434 individuals have flown in orbit—271 of them from the United States. The American manned spaceflight program began with Project Mercury over 40 years ago and has continued with Gemini, Apollo, the Skylab space station, the space shuttle, and the International Space Station. Now with the CEV, NASA's astronaut programs are again thinking of moving beyond earth's low Earth orbit, but questions as to the reason, purpose, and cost efficiency of these plans remain. The NASA exploration program features the words "the Moon, Mars and Beyond," but the next 12 years of U.S. space exploration seemingly anticipate only going to the moon.

> The NASA exploration program features the words "the Moon, Mars and Beyond," but the next 12 years of U.S. space exploration seemingly anticipate only going to the moon.

To put U.S. astronaut programs and astronaut safety into perspective and learn key lessons from the past, one should examine how manned spaceflight has evolved since it began with the Mercury program and continued through the Gemini, Apollo, and Skylab programs.

Mercury Program

The ability of humans to withstand the stresses associated with spaceflight was extensively tested during 1959 and 1960. These tests included the now well-known seven Mercury astronauts themselves. However, in January 1961, President Kennedy's science adviser, Jerome Weisner, who headed a transition task force on space, was asked to recommend to President Kennedy whether Project Mercury should be manned or not. (At the time the concept of an astronaut who would "pilot" space systems had not even emerged.) Rather than giving a specific answer, Weisner requested NASA undertake a complete range of further tests to prove the feasibility and safety of putting a human onboard Mercury. Weisner specifically recommended the following:

> A thorough and impartial appraisal of the MERCURY program should be urgently made. The objectives of the various phases of this program (including the proposed physiological tests) should be critically examined. The margins of safety should be realistically estimated. If our present man-in-space program appears unsound, we must be prepared to modify it drastically or even cancel it [6].

Christopher Kraft, NASA's first director of flight operations, played a key role in this assessment. He established an approach to managing human spaceflight. The guidelines he oversaw for the Mercury project set the precedents that have been followed by NASA ever since. Those precedents "took on the elements of a philosophy," and a key principle was that "the crew must be protected from dying" [7]. These key principles, however, were in part abandoned with the space shuttle program. The most important change was the elimination of the launch-to-land full-envelope escape possibility. There was also some loss of redundancy of critical subsystems. Finally there was a loss of attitude that applied to constant vigilance, which was to be applied at all times to safety concerns in the early astronaut program. (It is these vigilance issues that translate into finding and correcting problems rather than just granting of waivers.)

However, a differentiation existed between the riskiest portion of the mission, the launch phase, and in-orbit operations. In the launch phase, everything possible was done to ensure crew survival. But a failure in orbit leading to a mission abort might mean that another crew had to undergo the risks of launch in order that the mission's objectives could be achieved. Thus there was a need for balancing risks against gains in a decision to abort a mission.

Nevertheless, the investigations into the loss of the 18 astronauts who have died during Apollo/Saturn and space shuttle missions have indicated that the cause of their death essentially relates to the approval of waivers to program safety guidelines.

An early view from the astronaut corps came in October 1959 when Donald "Deke" Slayton told the Society of Experimental Test Pilots that there were many who thought that the pilot's role should be minimized. He stated a much different viewpoint that emphasized the role of the trained pilot as follows: "Objections to the pilot range from the engineer who semiseriously notes that all the problems of Mercury would be tremendously simplified if we did not have to worry about the bloody astronaut, to the military man who wonders if a college trained chimpanzee or a village idiot might not do as well in space as an experienced test pilot" [8].

Slayton went on to explain his case as to why "a highly trained test pilot is desirable" because such an individual is best able to "collect maximum valid data in a minimum time under adverse circumstances." However, he prudently added that he supported the idea that Mercury was also being designed to support an "automated abort capability." In short, Mercury was designed to operate without astronaut input if need be. Thus he acknowledged that "the astronaut is essentially a backup to the automatic systems and would normally not override automatic systems unless necessary."

The extent to which most space missions are indeed automated and can operate without astronauts aboard is a fact not well understood by the public. Space scientists from the Planetary Society and other sources have argued for years that automated space probes could obtain much more information at much lower cost and obviously reduce risk to astronauts. The politics and public dynamics of space exploration have consistently shown that putting people into space is essential to support among the general populace, but rebalancing the ratio of robotic missions to manned missions and giving astronauts more robotic assistants seems to make a great deal of sense going forward.

Project Mercury Problems

The Project Mercury program consisted of two suborbital missions first, followed by four orbital flights. These missions were completed in the 1961–1963 time period. This program began with the rather simple suborbital flights and ended with a 34-h mission that took astronaut Gordon Cooper on 22 orbits around the Earth. However, on three of these flights dangerous situations were encountered.

On the occasion of the second suborbital flight in July 1961, with astronaut Gus Grissom aboard, a life-threatening problem occurred after splashdown. On Grissom's return to an ocean landing, explosive bolts detonated unexpectedly and thus blew off the hatch cover. Water began to enter the spacecraft, and Grissom decided to evacuate. Water then began to seep into his space suit. At virtually the last minute, the rescue helicopter dropped a lifeline to Grissom, and he was hauled aboard and thus avoided drowning.

Next came two problems on the first orbital mission by John Glenn in February 1962. The automatic stabilization and control system malfunctioned at the end of the first orbit, and Glenn had to take over manual control of the spacecraft for the rest of the three-orbit mission, confirming the logic of Deke Slayton's arguments in support of allowing the astronaut to actually pilot the spacecraft as an emergency backup. The second problem related to data that indicated that the all-important heat shield and landing bag had become detached from the spacecraft. If correct, this created a very real danger of the heat shield coming loose during reentry and the capsule and its occupant being burned up. Ground managers decided to continue, and the indication proved to be false. The heat shield had not become detached during orbital flight, but the incident reinforced the need for detailed mission rules for all possible scenarios. These rules were progressively developed over the years, and by the time of Apollo they filled several volumes that formed the basis for the ground-based training and simulations that were an essential element of mission success [7].

The final Mercury flight, in May 1963, experienced a loss of power to the automatic stabilization and control system during the 21st orbit. The astronaut, Gordon Cooper, took over manual control and guided the spacecraft successfully through the retro-fire and reentry process.

The success of Project Mercury provided many precedents for NASA to follow to maximize astronaut safety. These included the need for good initial and not overly complex designs, extensive testing of designs, redundancy in critical systems, scrupulous quality control at every step, extensive training for all contingencies, means of escape from all possible situations, and an effective human–machine partnership. This program was the evolution of the astronaut's role from little more than a passenger in a fully automatic system to a fully integrated part of the mission.

Lessons from Gemini

There were 10 Gemini missions between March 1965 and November 1966, and these missions achieved the great majority of their objectives. But again, crew members were at considerable risk on several occasions during these flights.

The first extravehicular activity (EVA) by a U.S. astronaut was added at a late stage in the planning for Gemini IV, partially in reaction to the first-ever EVA by Soviet cosmonaut Alexy Leonov on 18 March 1965 and partially because the needed equipment was ready and preparations accomplished in time to make this possible. The mission was launched on 3 June 1965, and astronaut Ed White carried out this historic space walk without any major problem.

During the launch attempt of Gemini VI in December 1965, the Titan II engines shutdown 1.2 s after ignition and before the launch vehicle had lifted off. Judging that the vehicle had not actually left the launchpad and that he and his colleague Tom Stafford were not in immediate danger, astronaut Wally Schirra did not pull the D-ring that would have triggered the ejection seats. All astronauts were hesitant to actually use the ejection seats after tests showed that they would experience up to 20 g of acceleration in the process and thus risk considerable injury from the escape process. (Of course, if the alternative were death as a result of launch-vehicle explosion, they *were* willing to eject, but only as a last resort.) The mission was successfully launched three days later, but this was only possible because of Schirra's cool decision not to eject—although strict adherence to mission rules said that he should have done so.

In March 1966, Gemini VIII was making a rendezvous with its Agena target when one of the thrusters on the spacecraft's orbital maneuvering system stuck in the open position. The crew immediately undocked from the Agena, but the spacecraft revolutions increased to almost one per second, and the crew (Neil Armstrong and David Scott) was in danger of losing their ability to function. They decided to use their reentry control system, a redundant means of spacecraft attitude control, to stop the revolutions. They were successful in doing so, but had to abort their mission and return to Earth as soon as possible. Again this problem confirmed the wisdom of active discretionary astronaut system control.

The Gemini IX mission in June 1966 included a planned 167-min EVA. But astronaut Gene Cernan discovered that working in space was much more difficult than anticipated and just over 60 min into the space walk his helmet faceplate began to fog. He continued with the EVA, but after two hours he was exhausted and almost unable to see through his fogged faceplate. He and spacecraft commander Tom Stafford decided to cancel the rest of the space walk, and Cernan safely returned to the spacecraft.

Apollo Program and Much Higher Risk Factor

Projects Mercury and Gemini demonstrated that humans could enter space and return safely to Earth. These initial programs provided an essential bridge to the much more demanding astronaut activities needed to carry out Project Apollo and the sending of people to the moon. Parallel programs conducted by the Soviet Union at the time had demonstrated even more complex operations and longer-duration missions. These lent confidence to the idea that a moon mission was possible in terms of astronaut-related requirements of endurance, radiation exposure, and interaction with mission control.

Gemini and Mercury astronauts had been exposed to life-threatening risks, but all of these had fortunately been overcome. Everyone acknowledged that these risk factors were going to be almost minor in comparison to those associated with landing on the moon and returning to Earth.

A representative of the Martin Company, who calculated that the risks were much higher with Apollo than with previous programs, approached the White House in May 1965 with a proposal for a National Orbital Rescue Service. Presidential Assistant Bill Moyers asked Secretary of Defense Robert McNamara and NASA Administrator James Webb to comment on the need for space rescue, and Deputy Secretary of Defense Cyrus Vance answered for the Pentagon. He noted that the U.S. Department of Defense (DOD) was familiar with such proposals by industry but added that "any genuine rescue service separate from the basic flight hardware would be useful only if it could be sustained for quick launch by the manned program; could be capable of rendezvous and docking under uncertain conditions; and could be assured of higher reliability than the orbital vehicle requiring help." Vance went on: "It is very likely that astronauts will be killed, though stranding them is one of the less likely ways.

"The nation must expect such a loss of life in the space program .... We would be untruthful if we were to present anything different to our citizens."

The nation must expect such a loss of life in the space program .... We would be untruthful if we were to present anything different to our citizens."
    NASA Administrator James Webb told the president:

> Our concern for the safety of United States astronauts means that we take steps to reduce risks by every conceivable means. We maintain intense efforts in the fields of reliability, crew training, equipment check-out, design redundancy, safety margins, and the use of abort systems. We have also given careful consideration to the practicability of space rescue within the current or immediately predictable state-of-the-art.

Webb went on to suggest: "It is our judgment that the knowledge needed to begin the design of such a space rescue system is not yet available, but will come from our present developmental and flight program."
    A formal independent rescue capability has never been pursued by the United States; however, during the Skylab program there was an effort to have an Apollo capsule ready for a rescue effort if needed. Despite the decision not to undertake a formal rescue operation, one of the guiding principles for all of the low Earth operations was to provide to the maximum extent possible a complete "launch-to-land" or full-envelope escape capability.
    During the investigation of the *Columbia* accident in 2003, NASA studies suggested that a shuttle rescue mission to the stranded orbiter might have been feasible if it had been known that the vehicle was unlikely to survive reentry. The problem is that the rescue vehicle would have been subject to the same type of failure mode as experienced by *Columbia*, much as predicted by the Cyrus Vance memorandum many years before.

Apollo Fire

The first fatal accident of the space program was on 27 January 1967 when a launchpad fire killed Apollo 1 astronauts Gus Grissom, Ed White, and Roger Chafee.
    During the preceding months, George Mueller, NASA's assistant administrator for manned spaceflight, had reported to North American Aviation (NAA) President Leland Atwood that "positive and substantial actions" were needed "immediately ... to meet the national objectives of the Apollo program." Mueller told Atwood that it was his conclusion that "a good job has not been done" and that he had "absolutely no confidence that future commitments will be met."
    In spite of these stern warnings, the local Apollo program manager had to complain about the amount of unfinished engineering work in the command module for the first crew-carrying Apollo flight when it was delivered to the Kennedy Space Center in August 1966. However, even though there were problems with the module's environmental control system, reaction control system, and crew couches, top Apollo management declared the spacecraft "flightworthy" in October, provided these and other problems were corrected. Preparations for the Apollo 1

mission went forward in parallel with completing the work on the mission's spacecraft.

The crew also had substantial problems related to both the availability and performance of the command module simulator, with those problems eventually leading Gus Grissom to hang a lemon on the simulator door!

In early December, NASA gave up on its hopes of launching the mission in 1966 and set a February 1967 launch date. In a paper he planned to present at an Apollo Executives Conference scheduled for 28 January, Apollo Program Manager Sam Phillips listed quality assurance as one of the top problems being faced by the Apollo program.

One of the final prelaunch tests was set for 27 January 1967, with the fully suited crew sealed in the command module. At 1831 hours one of the crew members exclaimed, "There is a fire in here!" Efforts to rescue Grissom, White, and Chaffee were to no avail, and they became the first U.S. astronauts to perish during a space-related activity. NASA immediately organized an intense internal investigation of the causes of the accident. Administrator Webb was able to prevent an external review by telling President Lyndon Johnson that NASA was in the best position to understand those causes. Floyd Thompson, director of NASA's Langley Research Center, led the investigation. In its summary report, issued on April 5, the Board said:

> Although the Board was not able to determine conclusively the specific initiator of the Apollo 204 fire, it has identified the conditions which led to the disaster - 1. A sealed cabin, pressurized with an oxygen atmosphere. 2. An extensive distribution of combustible materials in the cabin. 3. Vulnerable wiring carrying spacecraft power. 4. Vulnerable plumbing carrying a combustible and corrosive coolant. 5. Inadequate provisions for the crew to escape. 6. Inadequate provisions for rescue or medical assistance. [9]

Having identified the conditions that led to the disaster, the Board also addressed the question of how these conditions came to exist. This led the Board to the conclusion that in its devotion to the many difficult problems of space travel the Apollo team failed to give adequate attention to certain mundane but equally vital questions of crew safety. The investigation revealed many deficiencies in design and engineering, manufacture, and quality control. Essentially, the problem can be traced to such seemingly common-sense issues as an incredibly unwise decision to grant a waiver to allow paper into the capsule in the pure-oxygen highly combustible environment. If the combustible material had not been allowed into the astronauts' cabin, for instance, the fatal accident might have never occurred. As noted by former astronaut Senator John Glenn during a speech at the National Air and Space exhibit facility near Dulles Airport, the connecting link between the Apollo command module fire, the *Challenger* launch catastrophe, and the *Columbia* burn-up during reentry can all be directly traced to the granting of waivers. Senator Glenn noted that if waivers had not been granted to allow highly combustible paper on the Apollo capsule, if the *Challenger* had not been authorized for launch under adverse and extremely cold weather conditions and if the *Columbia* had not been granted many thousands of waivers—many of them related to the thermal protection system—then it is possible that none of these U.S. space fatalities would have occurred [10].

One of the accounts of the Apollo program [7] suggests that "... the history of Apollo is divided into two time periods, Before the Fire and After the Fire." It suggests that the fire was "a demarcation of the loss of innocence. Never again would individuals be allowed to take so much responsibility unto themselves, to place so much faith in their own experience and judgment ...." Instead, "the people who had written the rules would themselves be governed by them." When asked how the experience of the fire changed the way that NASA managed Apollo, one senior person replied tersely: "We tightened up."

Director of Flight Operations Chris Kraft added that "it changed the way we did business ... we were running our fannies off trying to do Apollo. And it was difficult for us to take the lessons learned from Mercury and Gemini and apply them back into Apollo as we designed it and as we built it." He added that after the fire Apollo managers asked "what are these lessons ... What lessons have we learned from this horrible tragedy? ... Let's pump that back and be doubly sure we are going to do it right."

George Mueller added: "It wasn't just that we fixed [what caused] the fire, we fixed everything else we could find that had any possibility of being fixed."

Astronaut Walter Cunningham wrote as follows about the investigation into the cause:

> The investigation's conclusions became a virtual indictment of everyone connected with Apollo, including those of us who were to fly it. We contributed to the disaster by our willingness to tolerate questionable designs, equipment, and testing procedures; by ignoring our own good sense and accepting borderline safety margins; in short, by our eagerness to blow our bolts and get off the ground. All of us who participated in the design and testing at North American Rockwell felt that there were deficiencies in some of the systems and that crew safety had been given a lower priority than in the past .... The birthing pains of Mercury and the just-completed Gemini program seemed like perfection alongside Apollo. A great number of things had needed improving but changes meant delays. The Program Manager weighed the crew's demands for performance, safety, and other operational improvements against the payload of the spacecraft, schedules, and, not least, cost.

This comment suggests that maximizing astronaut safety during the Apollo program was more a case of following the precedents established during the Mercury and Gemini programs than it was introducing new safety-related design features into the Apollo hardware. Unfortunately, it took the deaths of three astronauts to remind NASA of that reality.

Between the January 1967 Apollo 1 fire and the Apollo 7 mission, which carried Walter Schirra, Walter Cunningham, and Don Eisle into Earth orbit in October 1968, NASA did indeed do everything possible to ensure that there would be no more accidents. Even so, sending humans to the moon was an extremely risky undertaking. Despite all of the renewed attention after the fire to make sure that the Apollo equipment met quality and safety standards, despite the development of a flight operations approach that built on, but went well beyond, the lessons of Mercury and Gemini, and despite the intense training that preceded each of the Apollo missions, there were still "close calls" during several of the eight flights from the Earth to the moon.

The first lunar landing, on the Apollo 11 mission, was not without problems. As the lunar module made its final approach to the moon's surface, there were several computer alarms. The flight guidance mission controller recognized the alarms from a preflight simulation and, supported by the guidance "back room," decided not to abort the landing. It took almost to the time of liftoff from the moon to understand what had caused the computer alarm and how to fix it. An overactive radar system on the lunar module was identified, and the liftoff and rendezvous with the command module went off smoothly once this issue was resolved.

On the Apollo 12 mission, the command module was hit by two lightning strikes just at liftoff, temporarily disabling the module's electrical systems and causing its guidance platform to lose alignment. Again, a flight controller recognized the situation from an earlier test and suggested a remedial action. This solution indeed worked and both restored electrical power and allowed the mission to proceed. Further analysis showed that the temporary loss of power had not negatively affected critical systems, and after 90 min in Earth orbit the crew was cleared to start their journey to the moon.

Fateful Apollo 13

Apollo 13 was more than 200,000 miles from Earth on the third evening of the mission when an oxygen fuel tank in the service module exploded, damaging adjacent equipment and effectively ending the generation of electrical power for the command module. This was thus a single point of failure and meant that the moon landing had to be aborted. The issue quickly became the survival of the crew. The lunar excursion module (LEM) was designed with the capability to act as a "lifeboat" for the crew if they had to abandon the command module. It also had enough power in its descent engine to maneuver both it and the command module, once they neared the moon, into a trajectory that would put them on a return path to Earth.

However, because the accident took place virtually at the time the spacecraft was approaching the moon, it would take four days to return to Earth, and it was not clear that the LEM had enough electricity and water to sustain the crew for that period of time. To conserve these precious supplies, all possible equipment was turned off or operated at minimum power. Also, the LEM did not have the capability by itself to remove the carbon dioxide generated by the crew's breathing from the cabin air. Thus another critical concern was that the crew could be asphyxiated before they got home. Over the next day, an improvised solution was developed on the ground, using storage bags, tape, plastic covers, and a hose. The astronauts assembled the ad hoc equipment, and it worked, thereby eliminating excess carbon dioxide as a problem.

After firing the LEM engine, Apollo 13 was successful in achieving a trajectory that would take them to a recovery area in the Pacific Ocean. The ground had to develop a reentry procedure for the unprecedented situation, and the command module and its parachute system worked properly and ended with a safe landing. During the 87 h between the explosion and splashdown, those involved in improvising and approving the procedures to get the Apollo 13 crew back to Earth had their doubts about the chances of success. Only the flight controllers seemed confident throughout the crisis period, and all agreed that the safe return of the crew had been a close call.

After Apollo 13, there were four more missions to the moon without mishap, and two additional missions were cut by the Nixon administration in a budget reduction move. Ironically these would have been accomplished at much less expense than the currently projected costs of a moon landing under the Project Constellation plans because the hardware was already manufactured and virtually ready for launch.

Not all of those involved were sad to see the Apollo flights come to an end. They were relieved to have the actual spaceflight part of program end without an astronaut fatality other than the Apollo launchpad fire.

Next Frontier: The Space Transportation System

After the loss of the Space Shuttle *Columbia*, the CAIB described the spacecraft as "an inherently vulnerable vehicle, the safe operation of which exceeded NASA's organizational capabilities . . ." and continued:

> The increased complexity of a Shuttle designed to be all things to all people created inherently greater risks than if more realistic technical goals had been set at the start. Designing a reusable spacecraft that is cost-effective is a daunting engineering challenge; doing so on a tightly constrained budget is even more difficult.

To meet these conflicting goals, NASA had made a number of choices that added crew safety risk to the space shuttle design that was actually built. One case in point was the choice of the strap-on solid boosters to provide most of the initial thrust to get the shuttle off the launchpad and accelerate it towards orbit. NASA's design efforts in the second half of 1971 had substituted such boosters for a reusable first stage. This was one of the changes negotiated from the Nixon White House in order to control costs. The implications of this decision from a programmatic and safety viewpoint were certainly not known at the time. Solid boosters had a very high reliability rating, and the question at the time was whether such a vehicle system could be built at all, and the duration of the shuttle program was certainly not envisioned at the time to last three decades into the future. Indeed, when one recalls that the Apollo program and the Saturn launchers were conceived, developed and fully realized in well under a decade, the development time and operation for the Shuttle seems inordinately long. Most engineers and scientists would not have envisioned in the early 1970s that it would be almost 40 years (i.e., from 1972 to 2010) from the startup of the Apollo and Saturn programs until another human-rated U.S. spacecraft would be conceived, designed, tested, and commissioned for initial operational use.

Most of NASA's initial engineering design work for the shuttle focused on various liquid-fueled booster options, because that was the type of propulsion most familiar to their rocket experts, particularly at the Marshall Space Flight Center.

After basic approval to develop the space shuttle was given in early January 1972, NASA began to examine solid-fueled boosters as an alternative, fundamentally because it was thought that such boosters could be developed for $1 billion or so less than their liquid-fueled alternatives, and this gave higher assurance that the shuttle could be developed within its overall cost ceiling. The OMB staff person in charge of the NASA budget observed in January 1972: "If left to their own devices, NASA would probably select the .... [liquid-fueled] boosters." This would be "regrettable," he observed, because OMB considered the liquid-fueled booster "to be a high risk option from the standpoint of both investment cost and operating cost." Again the high reliability of the solid boosters up to this point was also a part of the consideration as well as the possibility of developing new designs if the space shuttle proved a success.

As it developed the shuttle, NASA recognized several instances of risk to crew safety during the launch phase inherent in the approved design. Most of those involved believed that launch was the riskiest part of a mission, including the possibilities of external tank rupture or explosion, solid rocket booster burn-through, major structural failure, complete loss of guidance or control, failure to ignite one solid rocket booster, loss of thrust from one solid rocket booster, main engine or solid rocket booster thrust vector control "hardover," failure to separate orbiter from external tank, nozzle failure, and premature solid rocket booster separation.

Rather than provide abort capabilities to address these possibilities, thereby adding cost to the program, the NASA approach was to judge them "highly improbable because of the shuttle design, generic reliability, redundancy, and safety margins" [11].

Another difference between the space shuttle and earlier crew-carrying spacecraft was the decision from the start of the program that once the shuttle became operational there would be no way for the crew to escape from the vehicle in an emergency situation. Instead, there had to be a way to bring the shuttle orbiter safely back to Earth, with the crew inside, under every plausible failure scenario. The initial test flights of the shuttle would have only a two-person crew, and ejection seats were provided for them. However, NASA decided that "ejection seats would not be practical for operational missions that would carry a large number of passengers who have no flight experience." This abandonment of the concept of launch-to-land escape capability was one of the more obvious departures from the safety philosophy developed from Mercury, Gemini, and even Apollo.

NASA also did not make the capability for in-orbit rescue of a shuttle crew one of the program's requirements. Early in the program, the team from the Johnson Space Center recommended that a possible requirement for in-orbit rescue "be deleted" and continued: "The rationale was that the probability of a failure that would prohibit Orbiter re-entry is sufficiently low to allow the risk to be accepted. Funding problems and schedule impact were also identified as drivers toward the deletion of this requirement." NASA also noted that "self-contained escape devices which could be carried on-board the Orbiter have been evaluated but they were determined to provide insufficient protection against the possible failures and were very costly." Instead, "the approach taken is to accept the risks [of a crew being stranded in orbit] and mitigate the risks." [12]

Challenger Accident Exposes Major Safety Issues with the Space Shuttle

The shuttle is a complex system that has lived well beyond its intended lifetime and expected time of viable and safe flight. The space shuttle program, because it first became operational in 1981, has given us remarkable achievements and enabled many spectacular results such as the deployment of the Hubble Telescope and the initial construction of the ISS. Yet this program has also given us the disastrous O-ring failures of the *Challenger* disaster in 1986, and then in February 2003 the foam shedding that damaged ceramic tiles of the *Columbia*'s TPS and ultimately resulted in the fiery deaths of the entire crew on their reentry to the atmosphere.

On 28 January 1986, the *Challenger* explosively broke apart 73 s into its climb toward orbit, killing its seven-person crew. President Ronald Reagan created the Presidential Commission on the Space Shuttle Challenger Accident, known as the Rogers Commission after its chairman, former Secretary of State William Rogers. The commission issued its report on 6 June 1986, concluding that the loss of *Challenger* was caused by the failure of the joint and seal between the two lower segments of the shuttle's right solid rocket booster.

The Rogers Commission limited its investigation to the technical cause of the *Challenger* accident. However, while the space shuttle was grounded for 32 months, NASA carried out an overall assessment and identified a number of safety issues associated with the system. As many as possible of those items, but not all, were addressed before returning the shuttle to flight. The Rogers Commission also pointed to NASA management failures that contributed to the accident and was very critical of NASA's "silent safety system." Communication failures, incomplete and misleading information, and poor management judgments led to a flawed decision to launch the shuttle in unprecedented cold weather. NASA managers, according to the commission, had required a contractor "to prove that it was not safe to launch, rather than proving it was safe." NASA's safety system was characterized by "a lack of problem reporting requirements, inadequate trend analysis, misrepresentation of criticality, and lack of [the safety program's] involvement in critical discussions."

The commission also noted another factor that NASA managers "may have forgotten—partly because of past success, partly because of their own well-nurtured image of the program—that the shuttle was still in the research and development phase."

Tragedy Strikes Again—*Columbia* Accident

The shuttle was significantly upgraded after the loss of *Challenger*, and regular missions continued for another 15 years until on 1 February 2003, on the 113th shuttle mission, the *Columbia* broke apart as it reentered the atmosphere, again with the loss of a seven-person crew. The CAIB, set up on the day of the accident, concluded in its report that it was still a research and development, not an operational, vehicle and added what the public now knew—that the Shuttle was "not inherently unsafe."

The physical cause of the *Columbia* accident was identified as "a breach in the Thermal Protection System on the leading edge of the left wing," which allowed "superheated air to ... melt the aluminum structure of the left wing," leading eventually to the breakup of the orbiter.

However, this time the investigation went further to identify the complex organizational causes of the accident. These causes, they reported, were "rooted in the Space Shuttle Program's history and culture." In a comprehensive review of the technical, management, and policy contexts of the space shuttle program, it set out 25 formal recommendations relating to the safe operation of the space shuttle in the future.

The CAIB also recommended that "because of the risks inherent in the original design of the Space Shuttle, because that design was based in many aspects on now-obsolete technologies, and because the shuttle is now an aging system but still developmental in character," the United States should "replace the shuttle as soon as possible as the primary means for transporting humans to and from Earth orbit." The design of such a replacement "should give overriding priority to crew safety."

> The design of such a replacement "should give overriding priority to crew safety."

Complexity—Thy Name Is Space Shuttle

The space shuttle flew 113 missions between 1981 and 2003, and it is undoubtedly one of the most complex machines ever built by humans, with over 2.5 million parts and 230 miles of wiring. At liftoff, it must accelerate its 4.5 million lb weight to an orbital velocity of 17,500 miles per hour in just over eight minutes. It must provide a "shirt-sleeve" living and working environment in orbit for up to seven crew members. Then on reentry, it must decelerate from orbital velocity to a landing speed of 220 miles per hour, encountering temperatures of up to 3000°F in the process.

NASA had carried out the Mercury, Gemini, and Apollo programs with the expectation that it would have the political and budgetary support required and that it could focus its efforts on mission success, with an overriding emphasis on crew safety. However, as the CAIB pointed out in their report, this has not seemed to be the case since the inception of the space shuttle program:

> At NASA's urging, the nation committed to building an amazing, if compromised, vehicle called the Space Shuttle. When the agency did this, it accepted the bargain to operate and maintain the vehicle in the safest possible way. The Board is not convinced that NASA has completely lived up to the bargain, or that Congress and the Administration have provided the funding and support necessary for NASA to do so. Since the 1970s, NASA has not been charged with carrying out a similar [to Apollo] high priority mission that would justify the expenditure of resources on a scale equivalent to those allocated for Project Apollo. The result is that the agency has found it necessary to gain the support of diverse constituencies. NASA has had to participate in the give and take of the normal political process in order to obtain the resources needed to carry out its programs. NASA has usually failed to receive budgetary support consistent with its ambitions. The result ... is an organization straining to do too much with too little. [13]

The *Challenger* and *Columbia* failures are only the headline incidents. There have also been a host of lesser problems and accidents. Great effort was made by the CAIB to identify the source of the *Columbia* accident and to set forth a clear and detailed plan to return the shuttle to flightworthiness. But in light of the great complexity of shuttle and the extremely long time of its service, the safety concern must go beyond just that of the thermal protection system.

Waivers Issue—Continuing Problem

The GW University safety review also considered—within the context of quality control and independent verification and validation (IV&V)—the problem of what appears to be an excessive and growing number of waivers that have been granted by NASA over the years in response to specifically identified problems before each shuttle launch. This is particularly key in that both shuttle accidents can be linked to the granting of waivers and quality control and verification issues—just as it was found to have been key to the Apollo I fire on the launchpad.

The *Columbia* shuttle launch records, as reviewed by the CAIB, reported that there were some 7000 waivers granted by NASA officials. Many of these waivers were minor, but others were crucial. As described earlier, a waiver was granted before the Apollo launchpad fire to allow combustible materials in the explosive pure-oxygen atmosphere of the launch capsule. Before the *Challenger* launch, several waivers were granted relating to the O-rings and the adverse weather conditions that would have prevented the ill-fated liftoff. With the *Columbia* launch, the problem of foam debris was routinely granted a waiver on the basis of "we have done so before."

The official mantra in NASA Code M after the *Columbia* accident became "Find it, Fix it, and Fly Safely,"... but the experience with the reflight of the STS (mission 114) in August 2005 proved that the problems exposed by the *Columbia* accident had yet to be fully solved and the specific foam shedding problem was far from fixed. It is our belief that more must be done. Ensuring that the new Independent Technical Authority (ITA), as recommended by the CAIB, be given full way over safety issues, including the granting of all waivers, would be a key step forward in terms of safety. Further we believe that the NASA Engineering and Space Center (NESC) must proactively address the ongoing problem with waivers and be given greater organizational coherence by bringing more competence together at one location.

> The official mantra in NASA Code M after the *Columbia* accident became "Find it, Fix it, and Fly Safely,"...

No Safe Haven

John Schwartz, a frequent reporter on NASA-related matters at the *New York Times*, wrote a newspaper article on 9 July 2004 that reported on secretly obtained internal space agency documents [14]. These internal documents, according to the Schwartz report, apparently concluded that plans to use the International Space Station as a safe haven for a shuttle crew in the case that their vehicle could not return to Earth "would carry a high risk of failure if it were ever tried." Apparently these documents were presented to the independent space shuttle review board in June 2004, but no effective response has been made (or apparently is planned to be made) to these negative safety assessments. This NASA staff report, still not publicly released, highlights that "several critical systems aboard the Space Station have no adequate backup," and thus, if they fail, life support on the ISS fails.

These critical systems include oxygen generation, carbon-dioxide removal, and waste removal systems. Further, there are reported problems associated with adequate supplies of food and water. In the non-disclosed internal report the most pessimistic assessment suggests that a stranded shuttle crew and the ISS crew (in the most conservative assessment) could survive for only about 24 days—too short a period to organize an effective rescue, except for some that might escape via the Soyuz vehicle. The more optimistic assessments, however, suggested that a stranded crew could be sustained for two to three months.

GAO and Congressional Concerns

The major independent assessments of the NASA Space Shuttle Program, conducted in recent years by the Governmental Accountability Office (GAO) and the Astronaut Safety Advisory Panel (ASAP), produced reports that contained a large number of concerns. These stated concerns related to the reduction in the space shuttle maintenance and refurbishment work force, the "graying" of the Kennedy Center work crew, increasing problems with replacement parts, the inadequacy of the aging facilities, and other issues related to shuttle management and safety.

These concerns also include postponed safety upgrades (which have been sidelined because of budgetary reduction), reductions in the workforce, as well as the budget's demands for shuttle maintenance and repair crews. Finally these reports faulted the inadequate x-ray inspections of internalized parts and wiring in the three remaining shuttles and a lack of systematic oversight to critical parts of the shuttle refurbishment process. The aging of the hundreds of miles of wiring and the fatigue factor that relates to many of the 2.5 million parts in the space shuttle alone suggest that continuing the operation of these systems for years to come represents a significant hazard.

A number of NASA spaceflight center employees, during the 2002 to 2005 time period, stated informally their ongoing concerns that employees willing to cut corners to meet deadlines and budgetary controls are those that are promoted while those that are willing to stand on principle and raise safety concerns and protest the cutting of corners are sidelined or ignored.

Senator Sam Brownback (R-Kansas), chairman of the subcommittee that oversees NASA, stated to the press in early May 2004 that "he was not convinced NASA had conducted a thorough enough assessment of whether it might be cheaper in the long run to retire shuttle now and make the switch to commercial vehicles." He went on to say: "I'm asking the question a lot of members are asking right now. Do we need to continue this or can we finish the ISS without the shuttle" [15].

Alex Roland, former NASA historian and now a history professor at Duke University, for instance, in response to the release of the CAIB report, strongly disagreed with the committee's findings that he characterized as being designed to return the shuttle to flying as soon as possible. Roland's remarks in August 2003, as reported in the *New York Times*, were as follows: "There will be a *mea culpa* from NASA, some fixes, the long term reforms will be for NASA to be done in some indefinite future." Bruce Murray, Cal Tech professor and former director of Jet Propulsion Laboratory, was even more critical in stating that the CAIB ended up "buying" NASA's program and "not exposing an analysis of alternatives to it."

William Readdy, associate administrator for human space flight, responded to these questions by saying that the use of expendable rockets such as the Atlas 5 or the Delta 4 would require twice as many expendable launches than using the shuttle as then scheduled between May 2005 and 2010. He went on to explain that there would need to be conversion costs for units already completed and readied for launch at the Kennedy Space Center and that 8 to 12 launches per year of alternative vehicles would be required. The further suggestion for the completion of the ISS by using Russian launch capacity was also discounted by the associate administrator. But despite these demurring statements by Admiral Readdy, experience to date suggests that the use of unmanned expendable launch systems coupled with the use of Soyuz vehicles might well have represented a faster, surer, and more cost-effective way to complete the ISS rather than continuing to rely on the shuttle. The savings from the shutting down of the "standing army" that supports the shuttle plus the estimated $2 billion in costs for retrofits to the three orbiters would have purchased a lot of expendable launchers and Soyuz missions and would have obviously accelerated the completion of the ISS. Too often NASA has provided critical technical analysis to Congress and the White House without the benefit of an external review by competent scientists and engineers.

Financial Constraints

Admiral Gehman, Chairman of the CAIB, in testimony to the U.S. Congress, said that NASA fiscal constraints increasingly emerged after the Apollo program and the end of the Cold War. This meant that NASA "has had to overstate its capabilities and understate the cost of doing business. I hope that Congress and the White House don't put them in that position again."

He also told Congress: "It's cost much more to operate the shuttle than anyone will ever admit." This statement was particularly telling in that NASA Administrator Griffin is currently facing a $3–6 billion shortfall in funds to complete the ISS while also developing the CRV program.

The space shuttle took some 10 years to develop, and its total cost since the 1970s has actually been measured in the tens of billions of dollars. It was developed at a time when the U.S. aerospace industry was staffed for the Cold War years, and as a nation the U.S. was ready to undertake larger global challenges than is now the case. This basic limitation needs to be recognized before moving forward into the next phase of space exploration and suggests the need for some fundamental shifts in approach to space exploration. One of the most basic of these shifts might well be that robotic exploration and unmanned expendable vehicles could lead the way in most initiatives involving the exploration of the moon, Mars, and beyond—and at lower cost and with much less risk to astronauts.

The problem is that despite these efforts to find safety issues and fix them the basic design of the space shuttle cannot be altered. There remain certain fundamental problems. These include the continued use of solid rocket boosters, lack of complete escape systems, life-support and space-suit systems, metal and other material fatigue issues, deteriorating wiring, the need for review and updating of the shuttle's outmoded information technology (IT) and communications subsystems, and concerns with regard to over a dozen other subsystems that seem to represent prime elements of risk that cannot be easily changed.

President George W. Bush in January 2004 set forth a new space vision for NASA that targeted "The Moon, Mars and Beyond." But this was not all that was asked of NASA. The full mandate was not only to return to the moon and eventually send explorers to Mars but also to bring a nearly obsolete space technology (in the form of the space shuttle) back to life, complete the ISS with another 25 to 30 shuttle missions (*Note*: This figure is now reduced to 18), and undertake a program to develop a new space exploration vehicle and go to the moon and Mars, as well as carrying out a host of other key scientific missions within an essentially flat budget. As critics have said in response to the new space exploration plans, this new agenda certainly has a certain "Alice in Wonderland" flavor to it, akin to "doing six impossible things before breakfast." This is not because the technology was too great of a challenge but because the achievement of this broad range of goals, in addition to the pursuit of space science and related research and educational goals, would require a much larger budget than could be authorized in a time when there are so many other high-priority demands on the U.S. national budget. The view that the shuttle should be retired just as soon as possible (perhaps accelerated with a reduction in the scope of the ISS) has been seen as one possible way out of the dilemma. In fact, NASA has put into play at least a part of this approach already. The short fall of perhaps $3–6 billion has already been identified, and this does not even focus on the issue of safety. Certainly a part of the pathway will be the development of new launch technology that must deliver on many fronts—safer access to orbit, greater reliability, less complexity, improved technology and materials, and greater cost effectiveness. The success of Project Constellation and indeed the future of NASA are contingent on achieving these types of goals.

At least certain things are clear. The new transportation system, which now includes a new launch system and a crew exploration vehicle, must have improved thermal protection systems, improved propulsion capabilities, complete launch-to-land crew escape capability, and other safety enhancements. The most recently announced plans for Project Constellation also includes the aspect of flexibility so that cargo and crew can be moved separately to and from space.

There are many who still believe that the usable lifetime of the shuttle can be extended six years and that the problem of foam-shedding damaging the fragile thermal protection system of the shuttle orbiter that almost reoccurred with the *Discovery* launch can indeed be solved. These advocates would still contend that such a plan of action is more reliable, safer, and even more cost effective than any other alternative such as the use of Progress 1M/Soyuz plus expendable vehicles. They believe, in short, that the space shuttle still provides the best and safest means to deploy astronauts to space and return them for some time to come. Certainly, if one is to utilize U.S. spacecraft, the shuttle remains the only astronaut-rated vehicle available for some time.

Yet even those who see a continuing role for the shuttle recognize that many steps remain to be implemented. These include another test flight to test the problem with dislodged foam and the full implementation of other CAIB-mandated changes. Even if these modifications do succeed, everyone recognizes that a space system that is now 25 years old (and designed over 30 years ago) cannot be sustained indefinitely. The predominant or at least "official" view within NASA is that it is possible to make the shuttle fleet safer and viable for another six years or so, but the doubts continue to grow in Congress, in the space community, and even inside NASA.

Applying the Lessons Learned to Project Constellation

For the first time in over 20 years, NASA is now clearly embarked on developing a new and potentially better way for access to space. The announced plans for the new launch system has had wide input from many systems planners including innovative thinkers such as those from Scaled Composites and other innovators. The strengths of the Project Constellation plans include the following specifics—with many of these elements seemingly coming from the review of the early astronaut programs that preceded the space shuttle program:

1) Develop a provision for a complete launch-to-land emergency escape capability and significant and consistent rescue elements for the entire program.

2) Develop a new launch system rather than trying to upgrade and "man rate" existing launch vehicles developed initially without the exacting standards needed for an astronaut-rated launcher.

3) Opt for simplicity of design rather than extremely complex systems wherever possible.

4) Separate launch systems to low Earth for cargo from launch systems for crew with systems only being joined together after achieving orbital speeds.

5) The crew exploration vehicle builds on many of the programs developed by NASA over the past few years and is conceived on the principle of "spiral development" so that new technologies and materials can be integrated into the system over time.

6) Use and reapply the orbiter liquid-fueled engines in the crew exploration vehicle and using and reapply the solid fuel engines from the shuttle program to lift cargo to low Earth orbit.

7) Use capsule return systems that have proven the greatest reliability for deorbit and return to the Earth surface. (The insistence on the creation of a reusable vehicle in the case of the space shuttle implied a level of reliability and safety akin to a jet airliner that was never the case.) This reusable

design demanded a level of complexity (and system parts) that ultimately served to undercut the reliability and safety of the space shuttle.

8) Recognize the fact that safety and system reliability can only be "designed in" and that quality control and testing can only lessen the possibility of system failure. (In short the Project Constellation design recognizes that safety is a fundamental design issue that transcends quality control and testing.)

These are all solid reasons why the launch system design for Project Constellation appears to be well conceived. The projected cost of the overall Project Constellation, designed to provide a number of manned missions to the moon, however, is estimated to cost $104 billion. Such a huge cost is seen as a major downside. The fact that Project Apollo was accomplished in nine years, and the shuttle was developed in a similar time frame, but Project Constellation would not deliver an astronaut to the moon until 2018 is seen as an even larger negative. These concerns are accentuated by the fact that such ambitious technological developments often tend to go over budget and take longer than first planned. The glaring example of the International Space Station is, of course, the most spectacular case in point.

NASA—Victim of Its Own Successes?

The history of the U.S. astronaut program since the early 1960s is long, distinguished, and at times even awe inspiring. The successive developments represented by the Mercury, Gemini, Apollo-Saturn V-Skylab programs followed by the space shuttle and the International Space Station program have demonstrated remarkable success over the years. It is the expectation of success and the fact that "success" is seen as the norm that now represents NASA's greatest challenge. The space shuttle was, in a sense, sold to the American people and to Congress as a sort of space truck or space aircraft freighter that would operate with enormous reliability, safety, and would eventually also be very cost effective. The space shuttle would not only deploy the Hubble Telescope, recover failed satellites from space, and carry out important space science experiments, but it would also make the construction of the International Space Station almost routine and certainly safe. At least that was how many thought the script would read as first drafted in the early 1980s. Space, however, is more difficult than that. Rocket scientists are indeed fallible.

> NASA, in some sense, has now become a victim of its past successes and the expectation that the near impossible could consistently be achieved.

Today, the reality of how hard it is to achieve safe and low-cost access to space has become clear. NASA, in some sense, has now become a victim of its past successes and the expectation that the near impossible could consistently be achieved. Today's reality includes the wisdom of international space cooperation wherever possible, the need to develop and share space safety standards, build on the practices that have enjoyed the greatest successes over the last 40 years, and recognize that performance and safety must be designed into space programs and cannot be simply grafted on to programs over time.

The particular importance of simplicity of design—as opposed to excessive complexity—is one of the most important lessons that NASA and all space programs should have learned from the space shuttle and the International Space Station. This lesson is key to moving forward in space in the decades ahead.

The creative combination of robotic and "smart" automated systems with astronaut exploration programs might represent the second most important lesson. The example of the Italian robotic project to build an observatory on the moon as presented in Chapter 10 could serve to illustrate such a pathway forward for NASA's space programs.

A third and final lesson is that when NASA undertakes space projects it is putting American prestige and the international technical standing of the United States on the line. It might well be that with the evolution of entrepreneurial talent and very considerable technical expertise in the private sector that a number of space initiatives might be pursued as competitive projects within the commercial sector with entirely new models of financial compensation. The U.S. government in this context could then oversee safety standards, but not necessarily run the programs. This would mean, among other things, that private astronauts could be commercially compensated and insured so that their families could be financially sustained in the case of a fatal accident. The experience with Space X, Space Dev, SpaceOne/Scaled Composites, and other such entrepreneurial organizations, suggests that new space initiatives could well be a faster, more cost efficient, and less prestige-threatening way to explore space in coming decades. Such projects might start out with robotic missions to build infrastructure and science projects on the moon as well as new launch systems and then go on from there. This might ultimately lead to such commercial projects as a space elevator to geostationary (GEO) orbit or higher thrust electric ion propulsion systems that could go from low Earth orbit to the moon or even Mars. The request for proposal (RFP) to contract for launch services to the ISS by NASA in December 2005 could be considered a bold step in this direction. Further this private space exploration initiative could also allow greater flexibility with regard to international cooperation.

References

1 Mullane, M., Riding Rockets—The Outrageous Tales of a Space Shuttle Astronaut, Scribners, New York, 2006.
2 Heppenheimer, T. A. The Space Shuttle Decision: NASA's Search for a Reusable Space Vehicle, NASA, Washington, DC, 1999, p. 111.
3 Gugliotta, G. "Bush's Space Plan in Danger," Washington Post, 24 Nov. 2004, pp. A1, A11.
4 Leary, W. E., "NASA Planning Return to Moon Within 13 Years," New York Times, 20 Sept. 2005, pp. A-1, A-15.

[5] Glanz, J., with Broad, W. J., "Is the Space Shuttle NASA's 1976 Dodge Dart?," *New York Times*, 27 Jan. 2004, pp. D1, D2.

[6] Logsdon, J. M., with Lear, L. J., Warren-Findley, J., Williamson, R. A., and Day, D. A. (ed.), *Exploring the Unknown: Selected Documents in the History of the U.S. Civil Space Program*, Vol. I, Organizing for Exploration, NASA, Washington, DC, 1995, p. 422.

[7] Murray, C. and Cox, C. B., *Apollo: The Race to the Moon*, Simon and Schuster, New York, 1987, pp. 262, 263.

[8] Slayton, D. K., paper, Society of Experimental Test Pilots, Oct. 1959.

[9] Courtney B., Grimwood, J., and Swenson, L., Chariots for Apollo, NASA, Washington, DC, 1979, pp. 221–222.

[10] Glenn, Senator John, "Remarks Made at the National Air and Space Exhibit Facility," Dulles, VA, 10 June 2004.

[11] Jenkins, M. V., "Shuttle Launch Abort Review," NASA, Dec. 1976.

[12] "Response to Congressional Questions," NASA official letter of response, January 12, 1976.

[13] Report of the Columbia Accident Investigation Board 2003, Washington, DC, p. 97 and p. 209, URL: www.NASA.CAIB.

[14] Schwartz, J., "NASA Rescue Plan Is Reported to Have High Risk of Failure," *New York Times*, 9 July 2004, p. A-12.

[15] Berger, B., "NASA: Finishing Station with ELVs Would Cost More, Take Longer," *Space News*, 10 May 2004, p. 8.

Additional Reading

Brooks, C. G., Grimwood, J. M., and Swenson, L. S., Jr., Chariots for Apollo: A History of Manned Lunar Spacecraft, NASA, Washington, DC, 1979.

Chaikin, A., A Man on the Moon: The Voyages of the Apollo Astronauts, Penguin Books, New York, 1998.

Hacker, B. C., and Grimwood, J. M., On the Shoulders of Titans: A History of Project Gemini, NASA, Washington, DC, 1997.

Managing the Moon Program: Lessons from Project Apollo, Monographs I, Aerospace History No. 14, NASA, Washington, DC, 1999.

Presidential Commission on the Space Shuttle Challenger Accident Report, Government Printing Office, Washington, DC, 1986.

Space Safety Report: Vulnerabilities and Risk Reduction in U.S. Human Space Flight Programs, George Washington Univ., Washington, DC, March 2005.

Swenson, L., Grimwood, J., and Alexander, C., This New Ocean: A History of Project Mercury, NASA, Washington DC, 1998.

Welsh, E. C., Executive Secretary, National Aeronautics and Space Council, "Space Rescue," Memorandum to the President, 21 May 1965.

CHAPTER 3
Reexamining the Space Shuttle's Purpose, Mission, and Technology-Based Safety Problems

"Using the Space Shuttle to launch astronauts into space makes as much sense as using an aircraft carrier for water-skiing."

—*Robert Zubrin, President of the Mars Society*

"Going ahead half-cocked and losing a third Orbiter for known defects will affect the rest of [space] history in ways that are immeasurable, and lead to the demise of NASA as we know it."

—*A Member of the* Columbia *Accident Investigation Board [anonymously attributed in a* New York Times *cover story, 7 Feb. 2005]*

Basic Limitations

The space shuttle was a decade in development from the early 1970s to the early 1980s. The total cost of developing, testing, launching, and operating this launching system since the 1970s has mounted to the tens of billions of dollars. The shuttle was developed at a time when the U.S. aerospace industry was staffed for the Cold War years and the nation was ready to undertake larger global challenges than is now the case. The first shuttle, the *Enterprise* (OV-101), was developed for atmospheric testing and never used as an operating vehicle. The *Enterprise* was followed successively by the *Columbia* (OV-102), the *Discovery* (OV-103), the *Atlantis* (OV-104), the *Challenger* (OV-105), and ultimately, after the demise of the *Challenger* in 1986, the *Endeavor* (OV-106). The *Endeavor*, on President Reagan's orders, was created from the shuttle parts that were then available.

Despite efforts by NASA and the U.S. Department of Defense, the shuttle fleet never grew to a larger size, and it is now clear after the *Columbia* accident that there will be no new shuttle craft to replace the latest launch failure. In fact, NASA, as of 6 Dec. 2005, formally initiated a program to develop the crew launch vehicle (CLV) and the crew exploration vehicle (CEV) that can ultimately go to moon and Mars but with the understanding that the first versions of these launch systems also

53

might be used to provide assured astronaut access to low Earth orbit (LEO) and the International Space Station (ISS). What is not clear is the extent to which the CLV and the CEV systems, which are being designed to go beyond LEO, will be used for ISS access. This is because NASA, as of late January 2006, formally issued an RFP to solicit proposals from U.S. aerospace industry to offer launch services to provide access to and from the space station on a contractual basis [1]. The clear implication is that NASA will let private enterprise increasingly address near-space operations and the U.S. space agency will boldly seek to explore the new horizons of true outer space.

The only thing that seems sure at this point is that the shuttle will be permanently grounded by the end of 2010 if not before. From a safety viewpoint the sooner the grounding of the shuttle is achieved the better.

The purpose of this chapter, however, is not to explore the future of crewed vehicles that might go to the moon and Mars or commercial transport to the ISS. Such issues will be examined in Chapters 8, 9, and 10. The purpose of what follows is to understand the shuttle program in some considerable depth. Thus we will examine in detail the technical aspects of the shuttle program and prove the strengths and weaknesses of the only U.S. vehicle that is "human rated."

One of the key lessons to learn from this review is that the problems with the shuttle go beyond the thermal protection system (TPS). We will learn why many experts believe that the shuttle design is too complex, too demanding to operate reliably and cost efficiently, and too difficult to efficiently refurbish for relaunch in a timely manner.

Congress and the American public were told in 1972–1973 there would be a rapid refurbishment process that could result in a two-week turnaround between launches and of course lead to a highly cost-effective space shuttle operation.

The "routine access to space" with "airline-like operations" that could support up to 60 shuttle launches per year was ultimately seen by everyone inside and outside of NASA as only an illusion. The extent to which this illusion was presented to a sympathetic Congress reflected an honest mistake, or not, and is not the purpose of this analysis. The key element to explore is the great complexity of the space shuttle system (with a huge number of some 2.5 million parts and some 30,000 parts in the TPS alone). The ultimate issue is whether the shuttle external tanks and orbiter represent a reasonable design concept going forward to support NASA's astronaut program in finishing the ISS.

The following detailed analysis of the space shuttle and its various safety issues support several main conclusions:

1) The phase-out of this program as soon as possible is really the wisest and most cost-effective way forward for NASA and the U.S. space program.

2) The problems of complexity and cost inefficiency with regard to the space shuttle were increasingly apparent by the time of the *Challenger* launch failure. This basic fact should have resulted in 1986 in strategic

shifts in the planning of the ISS to create alternative ways to lift large components to low Earth orbit (i.e., the Columbus Space Lab, the Japanese Experimental Module, the Centrifuge Accommodation Module, or the ISS gyroscopic-stabilization units). These large units should have been designed as modularized components that could have been launched by alternative expendable and unmanned vehicles and assembled in space by the Canada2arm.

3) The design by NASA or other space entities of future launch systems should learn from the shuttle experience and thus emphasize designs that a) are simpler in nature; b) provide key elements of safety such as launch-to-land full-envelope escape capability; c) separate cargo and crew; and d) otherwise emulate the best aspects of design safety that have now emerged from the commercial and entrepreneurial design sectors as represented by Space X, Space Dev, SpaceOne/Scaled Composites, etc.

4) Recognize that the overly complex design of the shuttle, as reviewed in this chapter, involves far more than just the issue of the TPS. In short, there are many other issues and components that raise safety concerns, as will be discussed next and are summarized in Table 3.1 at the end of this chapter.

5) Designing, building, and operating launch systems that are rated sufficiently high in reliability to support human operation is very expensive. When cargo, equipment, and robotic systems can be lifted into space without a crew aboard, this makes programmatic sense and removes needless risk to astronauts.

Table 3-1 Cumulative Technical Assessment: Key Space Shuttle Safety Concerns and Issues

Nature of Space Shuttle Safety Concern	Has Problem been Evident on One or More Shuttle Flight	Seriousness of Problem (1, least; 5, highest)	Areas to Explore in Terms of Possible Upgrades
Aging factor 1: wiring	Yes	4	Rewiring wherever possible.
Aging factor 2: Brittle bolts and/or welds	No	2	Replacement of bolts and enhanced X-ray of welds
Aging factor 3: Hydraulics	No	3	Updated review of hydraulics systems
Aging factor 4: Corrosion of structural elements	No	3	Retreatment of exposed elements with anticorrosives
Aging factor 5: X-ray examination cannot reveal all problems	No	3	Braking gear problem only recently diagnosed. More powerful X-ray review of entire shuttle

(continued)

Table 3-1 Cumulative Technical Assessment: Key Space Shuttle Safety
Concerns and Issues (continued)

Nature of Space Shuttle Safety Concern	Has Problem been Evident on One or More Shuttle Flight	Seriousness of Problem (1, least; 5, highest)	Areas to Explore in Terms of Possible Upgrades
Aging factor 6: Deterioration of shuttle infrastructure	Yes, (shuttle mobile platform failure)	3	Modernization of most critical facilities and equipment; extensive modernization of shuttle facilities at KSC; probably too expensive unless done as part of planning for new launch system capabilities as well. Alternative would be to create a new launch site in an area not exposed to hurricanes, less populated, etc.
TPS factor 1: Destruction of tiles at liftoff	Yes	4	CAIB recommendations are being implemented. Eliminate ramp.
TPS factor 2: Loss of tiles caused by improper installation	Yes	4	Staff training and recruitment at KSC; new bonding materials or installation techniques
TPS factor 3: Too many irregularly shaped tiles and protective layers on orbiter	Yes	4	See above.
TPS factor 4: Lack of video monitors able to see shuttle tile damage	Yes	3	Additional video cameras have now been installed and use of spy satellites now possible. Free flyer video module controlled with joy stick.
Power factor 1: Auxiliary power unit fuel	Yes	3	Less toxic fuel for APU

(continued)

Table 3-1 Cumulative Technical Assessment: Key Space Shuttle Safety Concerns and Issues (continued)

Nature of Space Shuttle Safety Concern	Has Problem been Evident on One or More Shuttle Flight	Seriousness of Problem (1, least; 5, highest)	Areas to Explore in Terms of Possible Upgrades
Power factor 2: Power reactant storage and distribution (PRSD) cryogenic leaks	Yes	3	Better seals on storage unit
Power factor 3: Fuel cell performance	Yes	3	Higher performance and less costly fuel cell (i.e., PEM)
Power factor 4: Electrical power dist. and control (EPDC) failure	Yes	3	Improve design of power system where possible
Environmental control and life-support system factor 2: Noxious gas detection	Yes	4	More redundancy in system and display signals
Environmental control and life-support system factor 3: heating and cooling	Yes	4	Redesign and more redundancy
Propulsion factor 1: SRB concerns	Yes, damage to orbiter	4	No viable shutdown capability exists for first 2 min. No short-term answer until new vehicle available.
Propulsion factor 2: OMS	Yes	4	Upgrade of OMS system
Propulsion factor 3: RCS control jets	Yes	4	Upgrade of RCS system
Escape capability factor 1: Slide pole inadequate if solid motors fail	No	4	No complete solution if solid motors used in shuttle program are continued; propulsive ejection in new manned vehicle design; also separate crew and cargo

(continued)

Table 3-1 Cumulative Technical Assessment: Key Space Shuttle Safety
Concerns and Issues (continued)

Nature of Space Shuttle Safety Concern	Has Problem been Evident on One or More Shuttle Flight	Seriousness of Problem (1, least; 5, highest)	Areas to Explore in Terms of Possible Upgrades
Escape capability factor 2: HL 20 and other escape programs canceled	Yes; could have allowed *Columbia* crew safe return	5	Explore reactivation of X-38 or upgrade of Soyuz for full crew escape capability or upgrade ATV to be able to provide capsule return to Earth
Braking gear factor	Yes	2 or 3 (but problem now solved)	Avoid similar design issues in follow-on craft
Air lock controls for shuttle docking	No, but unmanned ISS raises concern	3	More redundancy in air lock operation and control
Docking maneuver operations with ISS	No, but close calls	3	Improved instrumentation for docking; key upgrade if automated Shuttle or docking modules launched by ELVs were implemented
Software patches: Excessive no. operator errors likely	No, but close calls	3	Permanent fixes to software patches
IT or communications failures	Yes	4	Upgrade IT and comm. systems; more broadband capabilities; more auxiliary power
Debris impact with shuttle	Yes	5	Improved shuttle window strength; improved shuttle orientation; improved programs to limit new debris

(continued)

Table 3-1 Cumulative Technical Assessment: Key Space Shuttle Safety Concerns and Issues (continued)

Nature of Space Shuttle Safety Concern	Has Problem been Evident on One or More Shuttle Flight	Seriousness of Problem (1, least; 5, highest)	Areas to Explore in Terms of Possible Upgrades
Debris impact with astronaut space suits	Yes	5	Improved space-suit design; minimize EVAs and use Canadarm2 in lieu of astronaut repair and construction duties
Space-suit valve issues	Yes	4	Improved design
Health issues (e.g., bone loss and other weightlessness problems)	Yes	1	Only artificial gravity can overcome; not possible with shuttle design. This is more of an issue for the ISS.

These basic limitations—indeed shortcomings—in the space shuttle design in terms of complexity, lack of escape capability, and questionable safety practices need to be noted before we can truly move forward in the next phase of space exploration.

The analysis that follows strongly suggests that robotic exploration might need to lead the way in initiatives involving deeper space exploration of the moon, Mars, and beyond. The way to have safe havens for long-term human presence on the moon might involve much more extensive use of robotic systems that is currently envisioned in Project Constellation.

During the period 2003 through to early 2005, the George Washington University team researched the technical, management, and operational status of the space shuttle program in parallel with efforts to return this vehicle to flight. The prime focus of this analysis was on all aspects of space shuttle safety. However, this review was quite broad and looked beyond the specific issues that were the cause of the *Columbia* accident. In many ways the *Columbia* disaster and the 2003–2005 grounding of the shuttle changed almost everything. This shuttle accident not only changed the timetable, cost, and program for completing the ISS, but it also impacted space programs around the world. It apparently led the Chinese to redouble their efforts, with the successful flights of their manned Shenzhou craft in 2003, 2004, and 2005. Russia is designing new spacecraft to go both into low Earth orbit and into deeper space. Japan has now announced plans to send their own craft to the Moon by 2020 [2].

There can be no doubt that the *Columbia* accident triggered renewed efforts to understand how to achieve improved space safety on a technical level but also to improve the safety culture of NASA and space agencies around the world. This has been reflected in new safety programs and reviews of space shuttle safety, not only by NASA, but also by all organizations with international astronauts scheduled for future manifested launches. At this stage, overseas space agencies including the Japan Space Exploration Agency (JAXA), the European Space Agency (ESA), the Canadian Space Agency (CSA), and the Russian Space Agency (RSA) have recertified the shuttle for their astronauts, but only after a careful review process.

Perhaps the most significant event from a global perspective has been the creation of the new International Association for Astronaut Space Safety (IAASS), which held its first international conference in Nice, France, in October 2005. Although perhaps the prime focus of this new initiative is ISS safety, the Association will also address launch-vehicle safety standards. Despite the urging of the IAASS, the various ongoing efforts of the United States, Europe, Japan, Russia, and China to develop new space access vehicles for human crews are not necessarily coordinated in terms of design philosophies, safety standards, or functional compatibility.

Meanwhile, President Bush has set forth a new "Space Vision" that includes completing the ISS by 2010 or as soon thereafter as possible and retiring the shuttle once that mission is completed.

Our analysis has examined risk factors related to as many key systems and subsystems as possible within the limits of our resources and access to information. We also reviewed shuttle-related quality control and verification, granting of waivers, training and mission selection, and management. A wide range of vulnerabilities and risk factors were analyzed and these are set out in detail in Table 3.1 and Appendix C of this book.

Concerns About the Return to Flight by the Shuttle

Since the grounding of the shuttle as a result of the *Columbia* accident, there has been special focus on the TPS. This is because the foam shedding that damaged this system at liftoff was found by the Columbia Accident Investigation Board (CAIB) to be the primary cause of the catastrophic loss of this vehicle. The GW study on the other hand was very broad. It examined the problems associated with the TPS, but also examined many other potential vulnerabilities to the shuttle.

The safety review, beyond looking at technical reliability issues, also considered the lack of effective escape systems for the space shuttle from launch to landing and especially at critical stages of its operation at liftoff and touchdown. Within the context of quality control and independent verification and validation (IV&V), the study examined the problem of what appears to be an excessive and growing number of waivers granted by NASA over the years in response to specifically identified problems before each shuttle launch. This is particularly key in that one can link both shuttle accidents to the granting of waivers and quality control and verification issues [3]. And a growing consensus of experts has suggested that NASA space safety cannot be improved unless there is not only greater controls on the granting of waivers, but greater emphasis of solving problems rather than granting exceptions to various problems as they emerge via waivers [4].

The official mantra in NASA Code M since the *Columbia* accident has been "Find it, Fix it, and Fly Safely." The bottom line that emerged from the flight and video data after STS 114 in August 2005 is that the key problem of foam-shedding had not been fixed. Until a space shuttle Independent Technical Authority (ITA), as recommended by the CAIB, assumes full sway over safety issues, including the granting of all waivers, there appears to be danger that key problems will not be adequately fixed. The establishment of the NASA Engineering and Space Center (NESC) is a useful first step, but more needs to be done to finish the task. These management issues related to the shuttle program are addressed in greater detail in the next chapter.

The basic problem is that despite efforts to find safety problems and fix them, one cannot alter the basic design of the space shuttle and overcome inherent conceptual flaws. There remain certain fundamental problems with the shuttle such as the continued use of solid rocket boosters, lack of complete escape systems, the incredible complexity of 2.5 million parts that includes miles of wiring and other parts that are not replaced with each launch, the lack of reliable supply of replacement parts, the outmoded test equipment, and the large-scale retirement of key personnel with crucial shuttle knowledge. Further there are over a dozen other subsystems—beyond the TPS—that seemed to represent prime elements of risk that cannot be easily changed. These problems represent possible dangers to the space shuttle and suggest on a cumulative basis the desirability of obtaining a new crew launch space vehicle as soon as possible. These same problems likewise support the idea of operating the shuttle as a robotically controlled vehicle and limiting the number of flights to complete or service the ISS. Thus the decision by NASA in recent months to reduce the number of shuttle flights by 10 (i.e., from 28 to 18) is thus consistent with these findings and indeed seems to be highly prudent.

In short, we do not conclude that the refurbished shuttle fleet, now reduced to three orbiters, is unsafe at any speed, but we do feel the shuttle system in many ways represents increasingly obsolete technology and should be replaced by newer and safer launch systems at the earliest possible date.

Complexity and Too Many Parts

The space shuttle has some 2.5 million parts, and the TPS alone has 26,300 parts. Most of the parts of the TPS are unique and have to be hand fitted and glued one at a time into place by highly skilled technicians.

Table 3-2 Calculated Cumulative Risk of a Category One Failure Based on
Number of Additional Shuttle Launches

Number of Further Shuttle Flights	If a 1 in 50 Risk of Failure, %	If a 1 in 55 Risk of Failure, %	If a 1 in 60 Risk of Failure, %
20	35	33.6	32
25	40	38.1	34.3

Composite risk factor analysis for the shuttle, based on assessments provided to the CAIB, shows that probability of some critical components failing after multiple launches continues to grow over time. The cumulative risk calculations provided in Table 3.2 indicate the implications of continuing to launch the shuttle if we assume that the component risk factor is in the 1 in 50 to 1 in 60 range. One would hope that the odds would be better than this, but actual experience with the shuttle falls in this range.

The view that there are risks associated with an extended number of shuttle launches is not only the finding of the GWU team, but also of the CAIB and of other independent review panels. Today, the space shuttle is America's only human-rated vehicle launch system. Even with the upgrades recommended by the CAIB, there still remain elements of risk that include the cracks in the PAL ramp constructed to deflect exploding foam from the external tanks (detected in NASA inspections made in December 2005) as well as the many other subsystems not addressed by the accident review panel. At best the shuttle's reliability rating is statistically comparable to that of the Russian Soyuz/Progress 1M launch system, and this system has flown some 900 times compared the shuttles' 114 flights.

The following sections describe individual vulnerabilities of some concern. In addition, the results of interviews with various experienced individuals that highlight their areas of greatest concerns with regard to shuttle safety are also summarized in Appendix C. Although these views are subjective, the collective knowledge represented by those interviewed should not be ignored. The inclusion of these interview results is important because it emphasizes that there are many elements of shuttle safety review, management, and control that go beyond the famous TPS problem. Further these interviews suggest that management and safety review processes and procedures are indeed key elements to be considered. Key subjective elements of shuttle safety include management decisions on launch budget and schedule, oversight and staffing of the shuttle refurbishment effort, selection of manifested cargo for shuttle flights, granting of waivers, quality control and verification, and the work prioritization program, staffing, budgeting and mission of the NESC, as well as the influence and level of control given to the new Independent Technical Authority. Most of these safety elements involve discretionary judgments and thus can also be categorized as subjective in nature. These issues are addressed in greater depth in the next chapter.

The CAIB's final report did not ultimately conclude that the *Columbia* disaster could be laid at the feet of NASA, but rather pointed to a failure of national leadership that asked NASA to continue to do more with less. As Professor John Logsdon, a member of the CAIB said in an interview reported in January 2006 with regard to the both the Space Shuttle and the International Space Station (ISS): "NASA is attempting now to recover from 35 years that in many ways was a dead end. That was not NASA's mistake, but the country's, the national leadership." He went on to say that: "It took two disasters—the Challenger and then the Columbia—to shock the White House and Congress into trying to redirect the program" [5].

> "NASA is attempting now to recover from 35 years that in many ways was a dead end. That was not NASA's mistake, but the country's, the national leadership."

Certainly the way forward has not always been particularly clear. The value and reliability of the space shuttle has been far from widely agreed. The George Washington University research team that the author headed from 2003 to 2005 found itself torn by contradictory data and findings. On one hand top-level action within NASA seemed to suggest excellent technical management when it came to matters of safety concerns. Action was taken by top management to establish the Diaz Committee in order to enhance NASA-wide efforts to increase awareness and concerns for safety; the BST, Inc., exercise and the return-to-flight program, headed by Admiral Readdy, clearly tried very diligently to implement the findings and recommendations of the CAIB [6]. The establishment of an independent board (headed by astronauts Stafford and Covey) that has continued to monitor space shuttle safety-related progress is also clearly an important and welcome step.

In all of these contexts, NASA, in most cases, seems to be taking its responsibilities seriously indeed. The review by other overseas space agencies of space shuttle safety for their astronauts represents yet another endorsement of NASA's renewed commitment to giving safety top priority. Also the new NESC, established in the Fall of 2003, added new capability to enhance safety. It has been estimated that close to $1.75 billion in direct and indirect costs [5] was spent at NASA to ensure that the space shuttle could fly safely when the *Discovery* flew in August 2005. Beyond this amount a significant amount more has been spent since August 2005 to address the problem of the exploding foam insulation fragments that reemerged after the reflight of the shuttle in the summer of 2005. All of these steps, at least through August 2005, seemed reassuring and gave confidence in NASA's technical commitment to make the space shuttle as safe as possible. In short, it would seem on the surface that NASA should be given an A for effort, but also a much lower grade for actual results.

But the story does not end with the reassuring steps that NASA took after the *Columbia* accident and the efforts made to implement the CAIB recommendations. Confidential interviews undertaken by the GW study team with former NASA employees and astronauts, academics in the field, and others knowledgeable about NASA programs seem to reveal a different story concerning technical and program management. Here, there was a recurring indication that safety concerns—on the part of both NASA employees and shuttle-related contractors—were still being glossed over and that corners were being cut because of the special circumstance of the shuttle grounding and the huge and mounting cost associated with the delays in the ISS program. There appeared to be some evidence that safety assessments and analyses presented by competent staff within NASA were still being overlooked or pigeonholed for budgetary or other reasons and that the "broken safety culture" issues reported by the CAIB are a continuing reality at least in certain areas of the program [7].* Indeed there have been consistent reports in the press of concerns being raised by safety personnel who have spoken off the record because of fear for their jobs [7]. This issue has most recently reemerged in the context of the FBI investigation of the NASA inspector general that is discussed in Chapter 10.

This situation of budgetary cuts in key shuttle-related safety staff was alleged in the *New York Times* in its 26 December 2004 editorial about the departing NASA administrator. This editorial noted that this problem preceded the current administrator and thus by implication extends its circle of blame to congressional oversight. Indeed many of the safety concerns extend back to the Rogers Commission report after the *Challenger* accident nearly 20 years ago [8].

A disturbing number of qualified individuals (in and out of the government), however, made statements in confidential interviews that safety programs are not all that they should be and there remain reports in the press of "ups" and "downs" in addressing safety issues related both to the shuttle and in general [6,7].

Some individuals, although a small number (i.e., only 10%) of those interviewed by the GW team on a confidential basis, have gone so far as to assert that the shuttle orbiters should be immediately and permanently grounded and the ISS construction halted because of the risks presented by the ambitious launch schedule needed to complete it. These individuals with major safety concerns have also said that "to the extent that the ISS construction is continued or operated further" the program should be serviced by expendable vehicles and upgraded Soyuz vehicles rather than by space shuttle launches to the maximum extent possible and that new, higher reliability human-rated launch vehicles as well as robotically controlled heavy-lift expendable vehicles should be developed as a matter of priority to support all future space exploration programs. In some cases, but not all, those expressing such reservations are individuals strongly allied with programs favoring unmanned exploration of space (interviews undertaken by the GW University study team in 2004, see Appendix C).

There are many, many more individuals (i.e., about 90%) who were consulted but did not agree with this assessment. These persons acknowledged

---

*Data available online at http://www.nasa.gov/CAIB.

that there were concerns, but they strongly felt that the refurbished shuttle orbiters and the external tank system were highly reliable and could be safely used to complete the ISS and to repair and resupply the Hubble Telescope.

In summary, we believe that technically significant progress has been made to increase the safety of the shuttle TPS. Nevertheless in the areas of quality control and verification (what NASA calls IV&V), control of waivers, management and staffing of the refurbishment team and its equipment and facilities at Cape Kennedy could all be further strengthened. Further we believe that the NESC and the ITA for space shuttle and the ISS should be given a much more proactive mission related to the management and oversight of the subjective part of the shuttle safety program as well as the technical aspects of quality control and verification. This means, in particular, oversight and control of clear and widely known safety definitions, control of granting of waivers, and management oversight of quality control and verification. Finally we believe that NASA's approach to safety and reliability processes does not rely sufficiently on initial design, up-front and ongoing system engineering and analysis, and elimination of safety issues as opposed to testing out problems through IV&V activities. In particular the so-called "waivers" issue is of ongoing concern.

Aging Problem

There a clear concern related to the reduction in the space shuttle maintenance and refurbishment work force, the "graying" of the Kennedy Center work crew, increasing problems with replacement parts and the inadequacy of the aging facilities [9–11].

Further, a number of NASA spaceflight center employees, during the 2002 and 2003 time period, stated in the context of safety review processes their ongoing concerns that employees willing to cut corners to meet deadlines and budgetary controls are those that are promoted, whereas those that are willing to stand on principle and raise safety concerns and protest the cutting of corners are sidelined or ignored [12].

Some of those interviewed contended that staff reductions, lack of replacement of key refurbishment personnel, and other such cost savings can lead to another shuttle disaster that would likely severely cripple, if not have devastating impact on, the U.S. space research and exploration program for decades to come.

Any congressional review should start with a truly independent assessment by a competent research organization that is equipped to explore not only the basic management issues but technical program competencies as well.

The Presidential Commission on the Implementation of U.S. Space Exploration Policy in their report entitled "A Journey to Inspire, Innovate and Discover" issued a formal 60-page report that calls for many institutional changes and organization reforms. The commission concluded that

NASA and the NASA centers not only need to be restructured, reorganized, and revitalized but also challenged to create new capabilities such as new advanced research capability based on the DARPA model [13]. At present, it seems unlikely that NASA, the White House, or Congress will decide other than to rely on the shuttle as the prime vehicle to finish and service the ISS, and indeed this approach is found in the presidential budget proposed for FY 2007. Nevertheless, within this context several options still seems reasonable. These options include flying one or more of the shuttle orbiters as a robotic mission for lifting cargo to orbit. Unfortunately the option of creating, for about $2.5 billion, an entirely robotic orbiter without life-support systems has likely passed. (Although this might have been a viable option some 10 years ago, this approach today would not only be considered to cost too much but would also likely take too long to accomplish.)

Other options include either reactivating the X-38 or alternatively agreeing to an upgraded Soyuz with full escape capabilities for ISS crew, plus expanded use of the expendables and the Ariane 5/ATV launch systems for ISS support. Finally there is the option of reducing the scope of the ISS so as to limit the number of remaining shuttle flights—this option, however, is already underway. Finally NASA has also issued in December 2005 an RFP to the U.S. aerospace industry to obtain launch services to and from the ISS with such services to be provided on a contractual basis. NASA has even budgeted up to $500 million to support this effort. The problem with this option is that it would apply to services that would be available after the ISS was complete.

Next Steps Forward?

There are certainly major implications for astronaut safety as well as cost and schedule implications by continuing the ISS program construction and ISS resupply using the shuttle vs expendable launch vehicles (ELVs). These questions include the following: what if a mixed fleet of U.S. and Russian ELVs were to be used? Or a mixture of shuttle launches (either manned or unmanned) for essential cargoes plus ELVs? There must also be consideration of what would happen to the program in the event of yet another shuttle failure, given the fact that only three orbiters remain? The largest question of all is what elements of the ISS need to be completed to achieve U.S. space objectives as they apparently have now been redefined? And could international obligations with regard to the ISS be changed or renegotiated to achieve expanded experimental goals but with cost savings for Japan, Europe, Canada, and Russia?

New human-rated launch systems that have much lower risk factors than the refurbished but aging space shuttle orbiters can ever achieve are clearly needed. The Rogers and Paine Commissions in 1986 explained why the shuttle needed to be replaced with newer and safer launch capability by no later than 2001. This lack of a new human-rated space vehicle remains a central and unanswered topic in U.S. space policy. This unanswered question is vital to the past, present, and future of astronaut safety. It transcends concerns of safety and goes to the very heart of what should be NASA's priorities in the next 20 years. A subsidiary question is why none of the various NASA X-Programs designed to develop new human-rated vehicles and costing billions of dollars did not succeed over a period that now exceeds over a decade? In other words, if NASA (with necessary congressional appropriations and White House support) had devoted more sustained and more carefully managed resources to these programs, as opposed to always giving top priority to the full completion of the ISS and sustaining the shuttle, would the U.S. astronaut program now be able to achieve safe access to space and thus not be completely dependent on the Russian Progress/Soyuz program?

The CAIB report summed up this concern when it stated: "It is the view of the Board that the previous attempts to develop a replacement vehicle for the aging shuttle represent a failure of national leadership" [14]. Certainly it is true that undertaking what might be called "grand projects" on the part of a government within a democracy, especially if they are of long duration, are always difficult. The success of the Apollo Lunar Program is more likely representative of the exception (peculiar to the Cold War era) rather than the rule. The inability to develop a follow-on to the shuttle is perhaps a failure of national leadership. In particular it seems to be a failure of complex national governmental processes not being able to set long-term goals. This is often the expected result when there are competing priorities mixed together with shifting budgets and priorities that vary not only year to year but sometimes even month to month [14].

It is simply not possible to answer such questions, but just the asking of these questions suggests current vulnerabilities for both the space shuttle and the ISS (in terms of both technical and management concerns). The bottom line is that the U.S. manned space program is now dependent on Russian vehicles, and if there should be a major Russian failure the ISS would be in considerable difficulty.

Assessing Shuttle Vulnerability

A comprehensive and accurate assessment of the current vulnerabilities and possible threats to space shuttle safety is difficult to develop. This is because there are so many thousands of failure modes in a vehicle that has some 2.5 million parts in its makeup with a huge number of hand-fitted parts in the TPS alone. The chart provided in Table 3.1 summarizes at least some of the most important issues and concerns. Appendix C provides even greater detail and a summary of the results of interviews that were carried out during 2004 with many knowledgeable individuals in the field. The results are presented in summary form in Appendix C to avoid duplication of comments and in such a way as to protect the identity of individual comments.

An estimated $1.75 billion was spent on safety upgrades to return the shuttle to flight by midyear 2005, and many millions additional after the problems with exploding foam were shown to still be present with the reflight launch in August 2005. This extensive NASA program to get the shuttle flying again was initially premised on a 28-flight manifest to complete the ISS and service its operations and to resupply the Hubble. Now that the flight manifest has shrunk to 18, the wisdom of taking the shuttle reflight route can only come back into question. One cannot help but wonder if moving to use a combination of expendable rockets to build the ISS plus using other vehicles to ferry astronauts to and from the ISS might have been wiser, less costly and safer. Had the shuttle been grounded in 2003 and the CEV program began immediately, a great deal of progress could have been made by now not only on the new vehicles but on finishing the ISS.

In Appendix C we provide quotes or paraphrases from extensive interviews conducted by the GW University team concerning shuttle and astronaut safety. Those interviewed noted some of the issues and concerns already outlined, but they did not particularly highlight or emphasize as a group such concerns as debris and micrometeorites, shuttle docking, aging-related issues, life-support systems, radiation, or terrorist attack.

Space Launch Crisis

In a June 1999 letter to the White House, NASA Administrator Daniel Goldin declared that the nation faced a "space launch crisis." He then reported on a NASA review of shuttle safety that indicated the budget for shuttle upgrades in Fiscal Year 2000 was "inadequate to accommodate upgrades necessary to yield significant safety improvements" [15]. Yet only modest budgetary increases ensued after these urgent pleas.

On 23 September 1999, space shuttle safety hearings were held before the House Science Committee's Subcommittee on Space and Aeronautics. These hearings were called to allow the subcommittee to be briefed on recent events in the space shuttle program that had raised safety concerns. STS-93 problems prompted this hearing. U.S. House Subcommittee Chair Representative Rohrabacher applauded NASA's decision to halt flights, thoroughly investigate, and fix the problems associated with bad wiring, which has since been found in all four space shuttles. Rohrabacher repeated a long-standing personal concern that budget cuts and contract milestone incentives might be having an impact upon maintaining a sufficient level of safety assurance in the space shuttle program. Despite Rohrabacher's comments, monies for major refurbishment for the shuttle were not forthcoming.

After malfunctions during STS-93 in July 1999, NASA Administrator Daniel Goldin established a Shuttle Independent Assessment Team (SIAT) chaired by Harry McDonald, director of NASA Ames Research Center. Among the team's findings, reported in March 2000, were the following:

1) SIAT had a major concern that "safety of the Space Shuttle Program is being eroded." The major factor leading to this concern "is the reduction in allocated resources and appropriate staf.... There are important

technical areas that are one-deep." Also, SIAT felt "strongly that work-force augmentation must be realized principally with NASA personnel rather than with contractor personnel." Despite these findings, the money for shuttle refurbishment shrank, and the recruitment and training of a new workforce to replace the aging workforce at Kennedy Space Center did not occur.

2) The SIAT was concerned that the "Space Shuttle Program (SSP) must rigorously guard against the tendency to accept risk solely because of prior success." Yet it would appear that prior success allowed conditions just noted to continue without remedial action.

3) The SIAT was very concerned with what it perceived as "Risk Management process erosion created by the desire to reduce costs...."

4) The Shuttle Independent Assessment Team report also stated that the shuttle "clearly cannot be thought of as operational in the usual sense. Extensive maintenance, major amounts of specialized labor and a high degree of skill and expertise will always be required." However, "the workforce has received a conflicting message due to the emphasis on achieving cost and staff reductions, and the pressures placed on increasing scheduled flights as a result of the Space Station" [16].

Senator John McCain, R-Arizona, requested a GAO study in August 1999, a few weeks after the STS-93 mishap. The subsequent report in August 2000 from the GAO, a congressional investigative body, stated: "Workforce reductions are jeopardizing NASA's ability to safely support the Shuttle's planned flight rate. Reduced to 1,800 employees, the Shuttle program has many unfilled positions and current employees (show) signs of overwork and fatigue." The GAO report noted that serious staffing challenges will remain in the future, as the shuttle program has more than twice as many workers over 60 years of age than under 30. Even after the *Columbia* accident these issues have still not been redressed as the return-to-flight activities have focused on the primary recommendations that involved making the shuttle fleet less vulnerable to TPS failure, but no substantive redress to the Kennedy Space Center (KSC) staffing and training issues appears to have been made [9].

If anything, the current situation at of the start of 2006 has eroded further. Many professionals and technicians assigned to the shuttle program have been eagerly seeking reassignment to the forward-looking and intellectually more exciting Constellation Program to undertake renewed exploration of the moon. This process has eroded even further the support staff and "standing army" of personnel whose responsibility is to oversee the refurbishment and safety of the three remaining shuttle orbiters.

At its March 2001 meeting, NASA's Space Flight Advisory Committee offered the advice that "the Space Shuttle Program must make larger, more substantial safety upgrades than currently planned...a budget on the order of three times the budget currently allotted for improving the Shuttle systems" was needed [17].

The following sections summarize *the many* safety and reliability problems found with the space shuttle—some modest and others of much more major concern. In addition to this summary of vulnerabilities, further details from the GW study can be found in Appendix C at the back of this book.

Vulnerabilities Caused by Age

A number of studies and congressional testimonies related to the aging issue and shuttle safety date from at least 1999. This concern with aging has only accelerated with new data developed in the context of the *Columbia* accident review. There are problems related not only to the aging of the shuttle orbiters but also serious concerns related to the infrastructure and equipment that support the shuttle program as well. These studies have raised serious questions about the effect of age on the reliability of the program. These reviews and key documents underline the extent to which the shuttle program could now be considered obsolescent as a result of the wear and tear of time and the difficulty of sustaining highly trained NASA maintenance and refurbishment staff technicians over long periods of time, in addition to the many outmoded design features of the shuttle. Elements such as hydraulics, wiring, brittle bolts, gearing systems, and even structural elements subject to salt-water corrosion are all components within the space shuttle orbiter that must be considered risk factors caused by aging.

The combination of age and obsolescence, when considered together with a reduced NASA and contractor workforce for maintenance and refurbishment and reduced funding for the shuttle program, combine to raise serious questions as to whether program safety remains in jeopardy despite the estimated nearly $2 billion in expenditures associated with the return-to-flight activities that NASA has undertaken in response to the CAIB report as well as in reaction to the shuttle reflight in August 2005 that led to the program being grounded again. In short, aging concerns will only continue to increase as the currently planned 18 further flights of the shuttle continue through 2010.

In April 2002, Richard Blomberg, former chair of the Astronaut Safety Advisory Panel (ASAP)—an independent review group to NASA—testified before the House Subcommittee on Space and Aeronautics, raising his concerns about an aging shuttle fleet:

1) "In all of the years of my involvement, I have never been as concerned for Space Shuttle safety as I am right now. That concern is not for the present flight or the next or perhaps the one after that. In fact, one of the roots of my concern is that nobody will know for sure when the safety margin has been eroded too far. All of my instincts, however, suggest that the current approach is planting the seeds for future danger."

2) Blomberg said that, because of budget shortfalls, many already planned and engineered improvements to the space shuttle system have had to be deferred or eliminated. Some of these would directly reduce

flight risk. Others would improve operability or the launch reliability of the system and are therefore related to safety.

3) "Moreover, the current plans and budgets are not adequate even to retain the present Space Shuttle risk levels over the entire likely service life of the system," Blomberg stated.

4) "Unfortunately, as systems continue to age, they tend to change. Some of these changes are predictable. Others, however, are subtle and often unpredictable. As components and subsystems age beyond their design lives, they may fail more often and with new and unanticipated failure modes. Thus, the well-established characterization of the system is no longer fully valid. The Aerospace Safety Advisory Panel believes that the Space Shuttle is heading in this direction."

"The problems that arise with an aging complex system can be exacerbated if critical skills are lost. Even with the best documentation and succession planning, some expertise is lost as experienced personnel retire. In the case of the Space Shuttle, repeated Government and contractor hiring freezes during its operating life have led to a lack of depth in critical skills. Thus, it is reasonable to assume that the ability of the Space Shuttle workforce to anticipate new problems and to mount innovative efforts to maintain safety will inevitably diminish" [18].

All aerospace and electronic systems are known to have an increased rate of failure with age. Studies made of failure rates in electronic equipment have shown that the reliability of components decays over time. It is also known that the rate of failures increases as the device nears the end of its life, as predicted by mean time-to-failure calculations. This concept of system failure is sometimes referred to as a "bathtub curve" because certain "shakeout" failure modes tend to occur early in a system lifetime and then failure modes as a result of aging emerge again near the end of a system's operation. During most of the useful life of the equipment, however, the rate of failure tends to remain constant and at a low level.

Predictions of failure can be made for typical systems using well-known reliability models. However, systems such as the space shuttle, which are subjected to extreme and variable environmental conditions, make the science of reliability prediction much more difficult. Moreover, the constant retrofitting and changes to the space shuttle, although extending its utility and life, further complicates these reliability predictions.

Concerns with aging of the space shuttle also apply to the maintenance of the shuttle program ground infrastructure (i.e., buildings, launch gantries, etc.). This is particularly true because many of these facilities date back to Project Apollo and thus even predate the start of the shuttle program construction. Figure 3.1 depicts the age of the shuttle's infrastructure as of 2000. Most ground infrastructure was not built for such a protracted lifespan. Maintaining infrastructure has been particularly difficult at the Kennedy Space Center because at this location the Space Shuttle is constantly exposed to a "humid salt-water" environment. CAIB

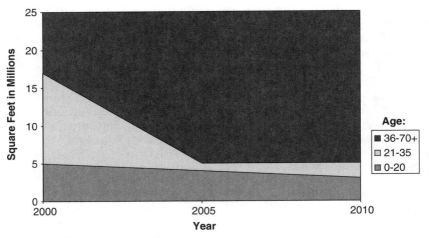

Figure 3-1   Age of the space shuttle infrastructure. (Source: Connie Milton to Space Flight Advisory Council, 2000.)

investigators identified deteriorating infrastructure associated with launchpads, the vehicle assembly building, and the crawler transporter.[†]

The problem of skill loss and institutional memory continues to worsen as many of the skilled workers on the shuttle have sought and obtained transfer to Project Constellation. If the shuttle program is to continue another six years, recruitment and training of new personnel before retirement of key personnel occurs is essential. Further adequate budgetary resources, facilities, and training capabilities must be provided. NASA personnel, in short, need more support to do their jobs adequately. It is likely to remain a problem as long as the high-maintenance shuttle remains in operation. On the other hand, if the scope of the ISS could be reduced and the shuttle program could be phased out earlier, this could lead to substantial cost savings that could be reinvested in new programs.

Vulnerabilities Caused by Retrofit

Since the shuttle's first flight in 1982, the space shuttle program has developed and incorporated many modifications to improve performance and safety. These include a superlightweight external tank, cockpit display enhancements, and main engine safety and reliability improvements. In 1994, however, NASA for the most part stopped approving

---

[†]Data available online at http://www.nasa.gov/CAIB.

additional shuttle upgrades!! It was thus 12 years ago—a time that translates to several generations of technology in a high-tech world— that NASA stopped making major improvements to the shuttle. This was because NASA leadership foresaw the "imminent replacement" of the shuttle with another reusable launch vehicle. NASA now believes that it will have to maintain the current shuttle fleet until at least the end of the decade if not beyond. Accordingly, it established in 2001 a development office to identify and prioritize upgrades [10]. A fully up-to-date report on such upgrades has still not been acquired by the review team, and thus this also remains an area of concern with regard to shuttle safety.

NASA upgrades have been intended not only to reduce risk of failure but also to extend its serviceable lifetime. Logistics support mandates that parts be ordered in a timely manner, so as to not jeopardize human life or launch schedules. Many space shuttle parts have very long lead times and involve manufacturers who might even have gone out of business. Failure to plan ahead for adequate logistics could lead to cannibalization or even grounding of the space shuttle. With the post-*Challenger* creation of the *Endeavor* orbiter (OV-106) in 1986 from parts that were then available, the problem of parts was at that time already beginning to occur. This was some two decades ago, and the problem has increased exponentially since that time.

Plans to retrofit the space shuttle have been delayed at times by the shortage of specialized workers, including those in the fields of mechanical engineering, computer software, and software assurance engineering. The workforce demographics at NASA today indicate an aging and retiring workforce to support the shuttle. Further stress among the workers has been evidenced by forfeited leave, absence from training courses, and counseling sessions.

Vulnerabilities at the Gantry and at Liftoff

There are many critical elements leading up to and including liftoff of the space shuttle. These steps include operations at the gantry, countdown to liftoff, and the actual liftoff. The shuttle program has suffered from degradation of the ground infrastructure, as reported in the CAIB report, previous reviews from Congress, and the GAO and other reports, as noted elsewhere in this report [19].

In 2002, the NASA Office of Inspector General reported safety and logistics problems associated with the ground-support equipment (GSE). Safety problems with lifting devices and equipment at the Stennis Space Center were also reported by the Inspector General's office. Unfortunately the demands of the return-to-flight program for the Shuttle, budgetary restrictions for all NASA programs, and the demands of repair of the vehicle assembly building from hurricane damage in 2004 and 2005 have allowed little money for infrastructure upgrades in the past three years.

Vulnerabilities from Liftoff Through Orbital Insertion

The process of placing the shuttle into orbit begins when the main engines and the solid rocket boosters (SRBs) ignite on the launchpad. The sequence of events to follow places the shuttle at an appropriate altitude and attitude for orbital insertion. At an altitude of 48 km above the Earth, the SRBs separate from the shuttle. The external tanks are then jettisoned shortly after the main engines of the shuttle shut down. The orbital maneuvering system (OMS) then takes over to achieve the final step in the process of orbital insertion. The OMS engine is located on the aft portion of the shuttle. This engine is responsible for the orbital insertion, and once in orbit the reaction control system (RCS) is used to make adjustments on the three axes of rotation (roll, pitch, and yaw). The RCS is made up of 14 thrusters located on the nose of the vehicle and can be fired in various combinations to make the desired attitude adjustments.

Clearly one of the most critical elements at launch has been the susceptibility of the space shuttle to tile damage. These problems are in part caused by the design and installation of the tiles themselves. In a 1994 report on tile vulnerability, one conclusion was that "it was clear at the onset of the study that some management problems affected the quality of the tile work." During some operations, it was found that a few tiles had no primary bond with the shuttle; they were held in place only by the friction of the gap fillers.‡

This report recommended "that NASA inspect the bond of the most risk-critical tiles and reinforce the insulation of the external systems (external tank and solid rocket boosters) that could damage the high risk tiles if it de-bonds at takeoff." Only a small percentage of the tiles constitute high risk. Damage to those tiles during launch has always been a significant concern. As observed in the 1994 report, "de-bonding of insulation on the external tank (an event of minor concern) could damage critical tiles on the Shuttle, eventually causing the loss of the vehicle and crew." Unfortunately, this statement proved to be prophetic in the case of *Columbia*'s last mission. The corrective actions in this respect, however, have been fully set forth in the CAIB report and addressed in depth in the return-to-flight program.‡

The other critical element is the escape capability for the astronauts at the point of liftoff. Currently the astronauts only have the option of a slide escape system, which is very likely to represent too slow of an exit path in case of a large-scale explosion of the rocket fuel. The design of the shuttle does not allow for an explosive ejector system that would allow egress with a much higher chance of survival.

Ironically the Apollo astronauts in the 1960s had such a capability to blast off to safety with a 20-g thrust escape pod. This feature, as noted

---

‡Data available online at http://www.spacedaily.com/news/fischbeckshuttle.pdf.

earlier, was eliminated for budgetary reasons and on the assumption that the shuttle was "so safe" that an escape capability was not needed. This is typical of the logic that has prompted former astronaut Mike Mullane to speak out in his recent book to describe the shuttle as dangerous vehicle because it has no escape capability [20].

Currently only the design and operation of a totally new personal launch system would solve this problem of complete mission escape capabilities. (This is one of many reasons why the Rogers' commission and various reports on safety that followed have urged the development of a new manned launch capability to replace the shuttle.) Fortunately this is now a design feature for the CEV and also the design plans to separate the crew launch vehicle that will use orbiter liquid fuel motors from the cargo vehicle that will use solid rocket boosters.

Because there is no viable escape capability for the space shuttle during launch for the first few minutes of launch and limited options for repair of the shuttle in orbit, there are limited safety options to explore except for better planning for new vehicles. The current safety options related to the shuttle come down to such alternatives as robotically controlling the shuttle orbiter, use of expendable vehicles to complete much of the ISS, and/or reducing the scope of the fully deployed ISS.

Liftoff Through Orbital Insertion

Vulnerabilities during this stage include two malfunctions that occurred on STS-93 during the orientation process. This resulted in an improper orbital insertion and resultant safety hazards. Further upgrades to the orbital maneuvering system (OMS) and reaction control system (RCS) would be desirable, primarily with respect to the propellants used, to achieve more efficient operation and maintenance of the shuttle. More importantly such changes would reduce the safety risks associated with these two of the shuttle's attitude control subsystems [21].

One of the critical elements in the telemetry, command, and control of the space shuttle during its launch into low Earth orbit is the advanced tracking and data relay satellite systems (ATDRSS) network. This network allows real-time communications from the shuttle during launch and after deployment in LEO orbit via a network of geosynchronous-based satellites and is key to the safe operation of the shuttle as well as the ISS. The ATDRSS system has increased bandwidth and enhanced performance, but there are several questions about the extent to which further redundancy as well as security precautions against terrorist or hacker attacks against the system would be advisable in terms of systems upgrade or third-generation designs for the next system. An increasing number of shuttle and ISS operations are being automated and often require continuous telemetry command and control operations to make continuous real-time communications with NASA ground control, which increases the importance of noninterrupted links being sustained.

Vulnerabilities Through On-Station Operations

Many of the critical phases during a shuttle mission are automated processes controlled by the onboard computers, which can be taken over by the crew and executed manually if it is deemed necessary. The docking of the shuttle to the ISS, however, is only initially computer controlled, as the final step of mating the two is currently a completely crew-controlled operation. The launch of the shuttle is also carefully timed in order to place the shuttle on a direct course for the ISS as it orbits the Earth. Two vulnerabilities exist during the docking of the shuttle with the ISS. The first vulnerability is the possibility of a docking anomaly caused by control mechanisms or if being manually docked as a result of pilot error. The second key concern is a launch anomaly that could place the shuttle in an improper orbit that would not allow or make much more difficult the proper mating with the ISS. Software malfunctions, either onboard the ISS or on the shuttle, could also complicate the proper mating between the two systems. Beyond the vulnerabilities related to the mating process, the delivery of cargo payload also represents issues of vulnerability.

Docking Between the Shuttle and the ISS

When the shuttle is nearly 2000 ft (or about 600 m) from the ISS, the commander moves to a flight station in the rear of the crew cabin and takes control of the vehicle. Through careful manipulation of the shuttle's thrusters (and only those thrusters facing away from the ISS solar arrays to avoid damaging them), the commander must mate the two surfaces within an error of 3 in. to allow the seal on the shuttle and ISS docking rings to form an airtight seal.[§]

Mission specialist Mary Ellen Weber who has docked with the ISS aboard *Atlantis* said, "I don't know if most people realize how complex an effort this is," when referring to the docking process.[§] Pilots train for over a year in NASA simulators, and human pilots control an enormous amount of government aerospace operations. Although risks are involved, pilots trained by NASA and other government agencies are extremely well qualified to manage these risks and accomplish their mission's objective. Nevertheless an improved laser guidance and alignment system designed for close-quarter maneuvers and improved vernier thruster system could certainly be designed for a new personal space launch system as would undoubtedly be the case with the crew exploration vehicle. If the shuttle were to be converted to complete robotic control, the docking process would likely be the area where the greatest attention would need to be directed.

[§]Data available online at http://www.space.com/missionlaunches/missions/sts101_docking_dodont_000421.htm.

Vulnerabilities in Orbital Flight and EVAs

There are several vulnerabilities for the space shuttle during orbital flight. One of these safety concerns in low-Earth orbit is orbital debris. This includes both meteorites and man-made objects in space. There are, of course, also concerns with regard to relevant shuttle subsystem failure such as failure of life-support systems, control thrusters, etc. during orbital flight, but these are addressed elsewhere.

Another possible hazard of great significance is that of radiation. Shuttle missions because they are of short duration and only involve low-Earth-orbit missions below the protective Van Allen belts do not expose the crew to radiation hazards that are greater than previous space missions conducted near the Earth. In fact risks from radiation are reduced compared to the Apollo missions, especially those that went to the moon, where radiation levels can be extremely high during solar storms. Further, measurement techniques are greatly refined over those used in earlier missions, and so risk levels can be instantly know. All shuttle crew members thus wear dosimeters, and dosages are monitored on an ongoing basis [22]. Risk factors related to radiation, cosmic rays, or other such hazards are addressed in Chapter 5 and Appendix D, which review the safety of the ISS where astronauts have extended stays in space and encounter much higher risk levels. In many ways the orbital debris and micrometeorite hazard is not only the most significant factor for shuttle and ISS crew members but also one that is increasing over time.

Vulnerabilities of Space Suits

Space suits, from their earliest designs to those envisioned for Mars, provide environmental protection, reliability, and redundancy. However, vulnerabilities of space suits are considered small compared to other concerns covered in this report. Details regarding U.S. and Russian space suits are addressed in Appendix C. Nevertheless better suits are being designed for the ISS and especially for extended stays on the moon as a part of Project Constellation.

Review of Shuttle Thermal Protection System

The thermal protection system (TPS) is arguably the most important and most vulnerable element of the space shuttle system design. For the completion of a shuttle mission, the TPS is as crucial as other systems such as the avionics, structure, and propulsion because of its vital function of protecting the shuttle from temperatures as low as $-250°F$ in orbit to heat temperatures close to 3000°F during reentry. The crew's safety relies on the ability of the TPS to withstand such temperature ranges. Failure in any area can result in complete disintegration of the shuttle as seen in the *Columbia* disaster of February 2003.

The TPS consists of approximately 24,000 tiles and 2300 flexible insulation blankets that thermally insulate each orbiter. These materials come in a variety of sizes, shapes, thicknesses, and materials. Table 3.3 outlines the approximate temperature capabilities and location on the shuttle of the different materials used in the TPS.

The tiles that make up the TPS are delicate and have to be protected from the stresses on the shuttle's structure during flight. During launch, the shuttle's overall structure bends and shifts from the aerodynamic forces, vibration and acceleration. The vulnerability of the TPS is not only a result of the complexity of the system but also the maintenance and refurbishment process that is required to restore its reliability after each orbiter flight. Each of the 24,000 tiles as well as the insulation blanket system must be manually checked to see if it is cracked or damaged.

NASA researchers are developing a new adaptable, robust, metallic, operable, reusable (ARMOR) TPS, as a potential system for future NASA spacecraft. The ARMOR TPS promises a greater level of safety as it has similar thermal capabilities to ceramic tiles and it reduces the amount of maintenance required to keep the TPS intact. ARMOR panels are larger than the ceramic tiles, do not require waterproofing, and attach directly to the underlying structure by means of mechanical fasteners. This reduces the complexity of the TPS because it is easier to inspect/replace the smaller

Table 3-3   Materials Used in TPS Systems, Capabilities and Locations

Material	Maximum Surface Temperature, °F	Location on Shuttle
Felt reusable surface insulation (FRSI) blankets	350–700	Payload bay doors and inboard sections of upper wing surface
Low-temperature reusable surface insulation (LRSI)	700–1200	Upper surface of fuselage around cockpit
Advanced flexible reusable surface insulation (AFRSI)	700–1200	Majority of upper surface of shuttle
High-temperature reusable surface insulation (HRSI)	1200–2300	Lower surface, edges of vertical stabilizer, and around forward windows
Fibrous refractory composite insulation (FRCI)	1200–2300	Penetrations and leading-edge areas
Toughened unipiece fibrous insulation (TUFI)	1200–2300	Base heat shield (around engines) and upper body flap
Reinforced carbon-carbon (RCC)	2300–2960	Nose cone and wing leading edges

quantity of panels. At present however these panels still weigh more than current tiles, and there are no plans to use this technology on the space shuttle. Further, because the design of the CEV and CRV have gone away from reusable systems like the shuttle and taken on the retro design of the Apollo program, this work on long-lasting metallic thermal shields is largely being put off to future systems. Indeed systems of this type might be first applied to the new Russian reusable launch system.

In-Orbit Repair

In the wake of the *Columbia* disaster, in-orbit repair of the shuttle TPS has become a major focus in returning the shuttle to flight status. The future of the shuttle program is thought to rely partially on the ability to inspect and repair the TPS, both in orbit and when docked at the ISS. The first step in this process is obviously developing reliable techniques for inspecting the TPS for damage, gaining access to all possible damage sites, and perfecting tools and materials needed to patch over cracked, erode, or missing tiles. The CAIB addressed the subject of inspection and repair of the shuttle's thermal protection system in some depth.

There are now various ways that the shuttle can be examined for damage. The use of spy satellites or other imaging systems to view shuttles in orbit could help assess damage before attempting reentry. Further cameras have been installed at various parts of the shuttle systems so that the behavior of any exploding foam fragments can be monitored at liftoff. These new cameras indeed clearly showed the large piece of foam material that just missed the orbiter on the occasion of the reflight test in August 2005.

If any or all of such methods had been adopted on the 2003 flight, the extent of damage to *Columbia*'s leading edge might have been accurately assessed and possible alternative plans made for the return of the crew. The remote manipulator system (RMS) has been used in the past to obtain an external view of the shuttle by having a camera attached to the end and steered to see certain parts of the vehicle. Unfortunately *Columbia* was without the RMS during its critical last mission, and, even if it had been installed, its ability to view out-of-the-way locations, such as the underside of the wing, was restricted. The use of astronauts' EVA is another option to inspect and repair the shuttle in orbit, but this was not done either. To date, only the repair of minor cracks seems to have been clearly addressed, and work continues to be able to develop a capability to repair more extensive damage on orbit [6].

Vulnerabilities During Reentry

The *Columbia* disaster on STS-107 took place during the reentry of the shuttle. The CAIB reported the physical cause of the accident as follows: a piece of insulating foam, which came from the left bipod ramp of the external tank, struck the carbon-carbon panels of the left wing of the shuttle. This resulted in a breach of the TPS that allowed superheated air to penetrate and melt the aluminum structure of the left wing leading to the breakup of the shuttle.¶ This disaster took place during reentry, but the events that led to the breach of the TPS took place 81.9 s after liftoff. This underscores the possibility that the vulnerabilities that exist during any phase of a shuttle mission can originate much earlier in the mission.

There are studies underway to address the issue of deorbiting and safety. One set of studies involves the development of new materials such as metal thermal protection systems (like the ARMOR system noted earlier). These new passive thermal protection systems would be safer and easier to work with as larger modular units than the ceramic tile systems used on the shuttle. The other set of studies is exploring if there could be ways to allow reductions in speeds other than through atmosphere braking. Certainly the huge temperature differentials that are involved in deorbiting space systems in one of the largest safety hazards associated with astronaut space safety.

Vulnerabilities at Touchdown and the Shuttle Braking System

The most perilous part of the shuttle's return to Earth is caused by extreme heating to temperatures in the range of 2000 to 3000°F created by friction against the atmosphere, but these risks extend to the period after orbital reentry for a lifting body without active control capability. These risk elements include atmospheric conditions during reentry and landing, the parachute system, and the active braking capability. It was found in the case of the shuttle orbiter braking system that the gearing system was installed backwards and in such a way that there could have been a category one failure. Even more remarkably, this situation continued undetected for a considerable time as a result of not X-raying and examining these images in detail [23].

Fuel Tank Vulnerabilities

The space transportation system design includes solid-fuel rockets plus liquid-hydrogen- and oxygen-driven motors. The solid rocket system was initially chosen because of its reliability, but these systems once ignited cannot be turned off or shut down. Further, there have been many changes and consolidations in the suppliers of solid fuel rockets over the last 40 years. With the most recent consolidations, only two suppliers of solid-fuel rockets remain in the United States.

Although it is not now possible to eliminate the SRBs from the shuttle, the design process for the CEV has wisely decided to adapt these boosters for the launch of cargo, but use the liquid-fuel motors from the

---

¶Data available online at http://www.nasa.gov/CAIB (p. 49).

shuttle to support the launch of the crew. After the cargo is safely launched into orbit, then crew and cargo systems can be united for missions to the moon or Mars. This is critical to providing a full-envelope escape capability for astronauts. The details of the design for the launcher systems are described and pictured in Chapter 8.

Escape System Capabilities

Early designs of the space shuttle assumed that it would be operational much like a commercial airliner, so that a shuttle crew escape system was considered unnecessary. From the initial design stages, however, the shuttle was designed to provide a complete rescue capability for stranded astronauts. This included sufficient cabin space to allow the rescue up to seven stranded members of the crew. Because rapid response of the rescuing vehicle is essential for a rescue mission, it was initially thought that it might be able to launch a second shuttle within 24 hours of notification. In the popular image presented to the public in such media as the James Bond movie *Moonraker*, this concept of rapid liftoff and ultrareliable shuttle operation was widely accepted.

> In the popular image presented to the public in such media as the James Bond movie *Moonraker*, this concept of rapid liftoff and ultrareliable shuttle operation was widely accepted.

Rescue of stranded astronauts in space is still a possibility and can be accomplished via the docking of two space shuttles with crew transfer accomplished in a pressure-controlled environment, or if docking is not possible, transfer is done using extravehicular mobility units (EMU) [18].

But even from the first test flights, NASA has been exploring other crew escape options. Crew ejection seats, crew extraction systems, and a crew compartment/capsule escape system have been considered. Although crew escape systems have been discussed and studied continuously since the shuttle's early design phases, only two systems have been incorporated: one for the developmental test flights and the second current system installed after the *Challenger* accident. Both designs have extremely limited capabilities, and neither has ever been used during a mission.**

Vulnerabilities in the Electrical Power System and Environmental Control and Life-Support System

The ability for astronauts to survive and operate the space shuttle during a mission is the result of the electrical power system (EPS) and the environmental control and life-support system (ECLSS). These systems

---

**Data available online at http://www.nasa.gov/CAIB.

provide the flight crew with a habitable environment and the power required to complete their mission. They have proved highly reliable in the past, but failure could result in lack of power, water, temperature control, or breathable air within the shuttle, which could have devastating consequences.

A failure in a fuel cell led to the emergency return of Apollo 13 to Earth as a result of an inadequate oxygen supply. Most recently, in early September 2004, the main oxygen generator for the ISS failed because of a blockage in the generator lines. Clearly, careful review of oxygen generator safety needs to be maintained although the shuttle system is different from the Russian-designed system onboard the ISS. A new U.S.-designed oxygen generator is indeed planned to be installed on the ISS on the next shuttle launch, but the oxygen generators for the shuttle are to remain unchanged [24].

Propulsion

The propulsion system of the shuttle comprises the space shuttle main engines (SSME), solid rocket boosters (SRB), the orbital maneuvering system (OMS), and the reaction control system (RCS). The three SSMEs and two SRBs are used to launch the shuttle into low Earth orbit before the OMS inserts the shuttle into the correct orbit.

Although there are specific safety vulnerabilities of serious concern with regard to the SSMEs or the SRBs, the combination of these systems on the space shuttle remains of concern because of its impact on a functional escape system. Further, NASA should provide a full list of all retrofits and upgrades that are to be made prior to the next shuttle launch (including all aspects of the propulsion system) as well as indication of the schedule of or plan for all deferred safety operations such as those just discussed. There is some concern because the high level of focus on the TPS issues and problems might have resulted in some other key safety retrofits involving the propulsion system not being completed.

Computer and Software Vulnerability

The space shuttle is a fly-by-wire vehicle with redundant computer systems and extremely sophisticated software capable of entirely controlling the shuttle during many—if not all—phases of a mission. The computer system and its backups can control most operations and rocket and thruster firings, for example, during reentry and ascent. The critical element of mission operation where fly by wire is currently not available is during docking and separation operations.

Five general-purpose computers (GPCs) control the shuttle's data-processing system. These computers vote to determine if one has failed and provide redundancy in case of a failure. Four of the five computers run the primary avionics software set (PASS), and the fifth is a backup flight system (BFS) capable of performing most of the important functions of PASS. Two magnetic tape mass memory units (MMU) store the large amounts of data produced during a mission, and a computer data bus network allows for serial digital communication to systems on the shuttle and back to the GPCs.[††]

PASS is composed of the operating system software and the application software, which is capable of controlling the shuttle and is divided into operation sequences that control different phases of the mission. The application software is divided into overlays and loaded from the MMUs when the phase of flight it controls is reached. The software is written in high-order assembly language (HAL/S), which is a language specifically designed for real-time flight-control software [25].

From this brief description of the flight computers, it can be seen that there is enormous complexity to this system, and the software controlling it is a source of vulnerability for shuttle missions.

The NESC and the new independent technical authority, when implemented, should oversee the IV&V of the shuttle software and avionics. They should also assume responsibility for the conduct of a study to explore the feasibility of a completely robotically controlled space shuttle orbiter so that operations could take place without astronauts aboard.

Communications Subsystem Vulnerability

The shuttle's communications system is made up of the following primary subsystems: S-Band system, Ku-Band and UHF system, payload communications system, and an audio system. As described in more detail in Appendix C, these subsystems are vulnerable to hardware failures.

The upgrade of communications, radar, and inertial guidance systems is of great strategic importance to the safety of current and future launch systems. NASA should also explore new and more efficient ways of flight-qualifying advanced systems so that they can fly on the shuttle or follow-on systems in a timely manner, which is a key safety objective. Perhaps most significantly, upgrade of shuttle avionics so that one or more shuttle orbiters can completely fly by wire, including docking operations, should be explored and implemented to the maximum extent possible.

Computer and Communications Security

The number of cyber attacks has grown considerably over the past few years. This affects the shuttle because it is a vehicle largely controlled by computers. The intended interference with either the software onboard the vehicle or the software controlling various ground monitoring and command activities poses a risk to the safe operation of the shuttle.

[††]Data available online at http://science.ksc.nasa.gov/shuttle/technology/ sts-newsref/stsref-toc.html.

Although the safety of the astronauts has not been compromised to date, past incidents serve to highlight that the security of the systems on the ground communicating with the shuttle, as well as the shuttle's system itself, requires high-level security measures to ensure uninterrupted communications.

Space Navigation Systems and Global-Positioning-System Applications

Because of the intrinsic worldwide coverage of the global positioning system (GPS), it is logical to implement GPS-based tracking and navigation architecture in order to support human spaceflight. However, experience with GPS in this arena is somewhat limited and lacks the sort of high-accuracy performance in space that is available in the terrestrial environment. Basically, there are only two GPS-based navigation systems with a history in NASA crew-based spaceflight; they are the Rockwell International miniature airborne GPS receiver/shuttle (MAGR/S) and the Honeywell space integrated GPS inertial (SIGI) system, detailed in Appendix C.

Potential Terrorists Threats

The first concern with regard to protecting the shuttle against terrorist attacks logically focuses on physical assaults on the spacecraft at the time of launch, landing, transport across the country on its especially adapted 747 transport vehicle, or even within the shuttle maintenance facilities. Although there is a reasonable level of security maintained in shuttle-related facilities at all times and the takeoff and landing facilities at the Kennedy Space Center and Edwards Air Force Base are not easily accessible, the level of security could nevertheless be further increased. Even one individual with a rocket-propelled launcher could attack and potentially destroy a shuttle or render it unable to fly.

It would appear desirable for further physical security and protection of the remaining shuttle fleet to be studied and implemented as soon as possible. This would include direct physical attacks at any possible location as well as attempts to jam its controls or use radio surges to destroy the shuttle's electronic or power systems by wider perimeter attacks.

There is perhaps an even greater danger that a shuttle could be attacked via digital assaults against its communications or navigational systems. This might involve the shuttle's tracking telemetry, command and monitoring (TTC&M) system that provides vital ground-based commands, by interfering with voice or video communications with the shuttle crew, or electronically interfering with onboard computer systems during liftoff, landing, or other parts of its flight. Also an attack against the advanced TDRSS could prove fatal to a shuttle mission.‡‡

---

‡‡Data available online at http://www.cnn.com/2000/TECH/space/07/03/nasa.hacker.02/[cited 3 July 2000].

Conclusion

There are still vulnerabilities in the shuttle that add up to the conclusion that the risk of a catastrophic category one failure on any single mission might well be in the range of one in 50 to one in 60. The analysis presented in Table 3.1 and Appendix C suggests that dangers are more significant and diverse than just protecting the TPS, which the CAIB report focused on so thoroughly. This focus on the TPS was quite reasonable because the mission of the CAIB was to find the cause of failure that cost seven brave astronauts their lives. Astronaut Mullane has now courageously come forward and explained why the astronaut corps is reluctant to speak out about safety concerns at NASA and why he feels the shuttle needs to be replaced by a much safer launch system that at least affords the crew a possibility of escape when an accident occurs.

The call by Mike Mullane for improved NASA astronaut safety practices is nevertheless no more than a call to return to past practices. The idea of an escape capability was key element in the history of the U.S. space program up through Apollo—strongly endorsed and observed by scientists, engineers, and astronauts alike. In some ways, Professor Logsdon's suggestion that the last 35 years of space exploration might have been largely lost by putting most of NASA's resources into a basket labeled the "Shuttle and the International Space Station" resonates with many space enthusiasts. Those who heard President Kennedy's charge to undertake the Apollo program in 1961 and then witnessed the moon landing in 1969 just eight years later sometimes wonder what might have been. One must look forward, however, and not rue the past. New and bold programs are now possible that build on the abilities of private entrepreneurs, new technologies, international cooperation, and innovative thinking. Clearly now is a time for a new beginning. Grounding of the shuttle, with thanks for its yeoman service is, simply put, a very good idea. This must be done just as soon as possible, in order to step forward into a new space age.

References

1 "NASA Issues an RFP for Launch Transportation to the International Space Station," *Astro News*, 8 Dec. 2005.
2 "News Analysis: What Space Shuttle Columbia Disaster Brings to Human Spaceflight," *People's Daily*, 6 Feb. 2003.
3 Astronaut John Glenn, "Remarks made at the National Air and Space Exhibit Facility," Dulles, VA, 10 June 2004.
4 Kelly, J., and Halverson, T., "NASA Must Reduce Safety Waivers," *New York Times*, 10 May 2004, p. A11.
5 Wilford, J. N., "Space Program Disasters Help Chart Its Future," *New York Times*, 24 Jan. 2006, p. D4.
6 Leary, W. E., "NASA Notes Some Progress in Making Shuttle Safer," *New York Times*, 27 Aug. 2004, p. A14.
7 Zabarenko, D., "Are NASA's Human Shuttle Flights Worth the Risk," *Reuters*, 15 Sept. 2003, pp. 10–11.

[8] "NASA's Chief Bails out," *New York Times*, Washington Week in Review, 26 Dec. 2004, p. 8.

[9] General Accounting Office Report, "Review of Space Shuttle Safety" Washington, DC, Aug. 2000.

[10] General Accounting Office Report, "Space Shuttle Safety," Washington, DC, 6 Sept. 2001.

[11] Astronaut Safety Advisory Panel, Washington, DC, Report, 2002.

[12] General Accounting Office Testimony Before the Subcommittee on Science, "Space Shuttle Safety" Technology and Space, Committee on Commerce, Science and Transportation, U.S. Senate, September 10, 2003.

[13] Presidential Commission on the Implementation of U.S. Space Exploration Policy, "A Journey to Inspire, Innovate, and Discover," Report of the Presidential Commission Washington, DC, June 2004.

[14] "NASA: Snapshot of a Bureaucracy," NASA 2004 Budget Request, *Popular Science*, Feb. 2004, pp. 23–26.

[15] Letter from Daniel Goldin to Jacob Lew, Director, Office of Management and Budget, "NASA Budget for FY2000" 6 July 1999.

[16] NASA, Space Shuttle Independent Assessment Team, "Report to the Associate Administrator, Office of Space Flight, October-December 1999," Washington, DC, 7 March 2000; also CAIB document CTF017-0169.

[17] Space Flight Advisory Committee, Meeting Report, NASA Office of Space Flight, Washington, DC, 1–2 May 2001, p.7; also CAIB document CTF017-0034.

[18] Richard Blomberg Statement, Former Chair, Aerospace Safety Advisory Panel, Before the House Subcommittee on Space and Aeronautics, 18 April 2002; URL: http://www.space.com/missionlaunches/sts107_fleet_030201.html.

[19] "Summary of Space Shuttle/Safety-Related Products from the NASA Office of Inspector General," NASA Oversight of United Space Alliance's Safety Procedures at the John F. Kennedy Space Center (IG-02-018, 24 June 2002); URL: http://www.hq.nasa.gov/office/oig/hq/ig-02-018r.pdf.

[20] Mullane, M., *Riding Rockets: The Outrageous Tales of a Space Shuttle Astronaut*, Scribners, New York, 2006.

[21] "Report to the Associate Administrator, Office of Space Flight, October-December 1999," Washington, DC, 7 March 2000; also CAIB document CTF017-0169.

[22] Schulze, N. R., and Prichard, R. P. "Occupant Safety in the Space Shuttle," NASA Headquarters, Feb. 1978.

[23] Dunn, M., "Shuttle Gears Were Installed Backward: Error Could Have Had Disastrous Consequences," Washington Post, 23 March 2004, p. 13.

[24] Leary, W. E., "Oxygen Generator on Space Station Fails," *New York Times*, 10 Sept. 2004, p. A22.

[25] The Aeronautics and Space Engineering Board, "An Assessment of Space Shuttle Flight Software Development Processes," National Academy of Engineering, Washington, DC, 2001, 1992–2000, pp. 1–15.

Additional Reading

Government Reports, Government Testimony, and Conference Reports

Aerospace Safety Advisory Panel (ASAP), Annual Report, Washington, DC, 2002.

General Accounting Office (GAO), "Space Program: Space Debris a Potential Threat to Space Station, and Shuttle," Report to Congress," GAO/IMTEC-90-18, Washington, DC, April 1990.

General Accounting Office (GAO), Testimony Before the Subcommittee on Science, Technology and Space, Committee on Commerce, Science and Transportation, U.S. Senate, Washington, DC, Sept. 2001.

Robert Frosch Memorandum, "Examination of the Shuttle Program," NASA, Washington, DC, 18 Aug 1980.

"NASA's Implementation Plan for Space Shuttle", NASA Report, NASA-SP 1928 Washington, DC, 26 April 2004.

Presidential Commission on the Space Shuttle Challenger Accident, Governmental Printing Office, Washington, DC, 6 June 1986.

"Space Shuttle Safety," Hearings before the House Science Committee's Subcommittee on Space and Aeronautics, 23 Sept. 1999.

XVIII Congress of the Association of Space Explorers, "Learning from Space— Enriching World Culture," Tokyo, Japan, Oct. 2003.

Publications and Articles

Berger, B., "Moon-Mars Panel Recommends Sweeping Changes for NASA," *Space News*, 14 June 2004, pp. 1, 3.

Berger, B., "NASA: Finishing Station with ELVs Would Cost More, Take Longer," *Space News*, 10 May 2004, p. 8.

Blumenthal, J. L., "After the Challenger: Evolution of a Redesign," *Elastomerics*, Vol. 120, No. 7, 1988, pp. 10–16.

Booth, W., "Starship Private Enterprise," *Washington Post*, 22 June 2004, pp. A1, A8.

"The Bush Space Plan Leaves a Gap," *The Guardian*, 15 Jan. 2004, p. 1.

"Chicken Littles and Ostriches at NASA," *New York Times*, 27 Sept. 2003, p. A-26.

David, L., "NASA's Aging Shuttle Fleet Called to Question," *Space.com* [cited Feb. 2003].

David, L., "NASA Releases Shuttle Return to Flight Plan," *Space.com* [cited March 2003].

David, L., "Shuttle Heat Shields Have Flawed History," *Space.com* [cited Feb. 2003].

Glanz, J., and Schwartz, J., "Dogged Engineer's Effort to Assess Shuttle Damage," *New York Times*, 26 Sept. 2003, p. A-1.

Leusner, J., Spear, K., and Shaw, G.K., "NASA Avoids Pinning Blame for Columbia," *The Orlando Sentinel*, 15 Sept. 2003, p. A1.

"NASA Leadership Rated Poor in Worker Survey," *Washington Post*, 11 Dec. 2003, p. A37.

Neal, V., "Three, Four, or More: How Many Orbiters in the Space Shuttle Fleet Are Necessary?," *Space Times*, Vol. 42, No. 3, 2003, pp. 4–7.

Overbye, D., "At NASA, Science Sharply Changes Its Course," *New York Times*, 18 April 2004.

Pelton, J. N., "Why Space? The Top 10 Reasons," *Space News*, 8 Sept. 2003, p. 13.

Roland, A., "Twenty Years Later, NASA Caught in a Shuttle Trap," *Florida Today*, 8 April 2001.

Sanger, D. E., "Report on Loss of Shuttle Focuses on NASA Blunders and Issues Somber Warning," *New York Times*, 23 Aug. 2003, p. A-1.

Sawyer, K., and Planin, E., "In Broad Indictment of Practices Shuttle Panel Says Safety Suffered," *Washington Post*, 27 Aug. 2003, p. A-16.

Schwartz, J., and Wald, M. L., "Complacency Seen," *New York Times*, 27 Aug. 2003, pp. A1, A17.

Singer, J., "Pratt & Whitney Facility Closure Leaves Two US Solid Rocket Motor Companies," *Space News*, 17 May 2004, p. 1, 3.

Smith, R. J., "NASA Culture, Columbia Probers Still Miles Apart," *Washington Post*, 22 Aug. 2003, p. A-3.

Stein, R., "Miscommunication, Bungling Halted Bid for Shuttle Photos," *Washington Post*, 27 Aug. 2003, p. A-15.

Tumlinson, R. N., "Scuttle the Shuttle: Part One—The Problem," *Space News*, 15 Sept. 2003, p. 13.

Wald, M.L., "Decision Near on Licensing for Private Space Flights," *Washington Post*, 10 Feb. 2004, p. C-2.

Weiss, R., "NASA's Underlying Woes: Fading Support and Science," *Washington Post*, 27 Aug. 2003, p. A-14.

CHAPTER 4
Review of the Management and Institutional Issues

"The granting of various waivers can be traced back to be major contributor factors in every NASA accident where Astronauts have lost their life."

—*John Glenn, National Air and Space Museum Seminar, 10 June 2004*

"...the Soviets had lost men in space: the three Soyuz pilots on re-entry that the world knew about, and a number of others known only by rumors......He wondered....if NASA had been too cautious? With fewer safety precautions the United States could have reached the Moon a little sooner, done a could deal more exploring, learned more—and yes created a martyr or two."

—*Larry Niven and Jerry Pournelle, Lucifer's Hammer (1977)*
—*A novel about a comet hitting planet Earth*

Fixing NASA's Management and Safety Culture

There is more to NASA's manned flight and safety programs than technical issues; management and institutional issues are equally if not more important. Astronaut accidents have in all cases been tracked backed to issues of waivers being granted that should not have been approved. (See Figure 4.1). Management, institutional issues, and a "safety culture" are part and parcel of NASA's manned space programs, and all of these factors impact the integrity of its performance.

When the George Washington University study reviewed the strengths and weaknesses of NASA astronaut launch systems, it considered the following management and safety culture issues and information: 1) the overall effectiveness of NASA's organizational management and safety culture [largely as reported by the Diaz Committee, by Behavior Science Technology BST, Inc., and the multivolume report of the *Columbia* Accident Investigation Board (CAIB)]; 2) the ability and willingness of NASA management at critical times to override the concerns and reservations of NASA safety officers; 3) the problems of sometime inconsistent congressional and executive branch oversight, particularly when it comes to safety, performance, schedule, and budgetary issues [1].

The CAIB's final report did not ultimately conclude that the *Columbia* disaster could be laid at the feet of NASA, but rather pointed to a failure of "national leadership"—a leadership that consistently asked NASA to

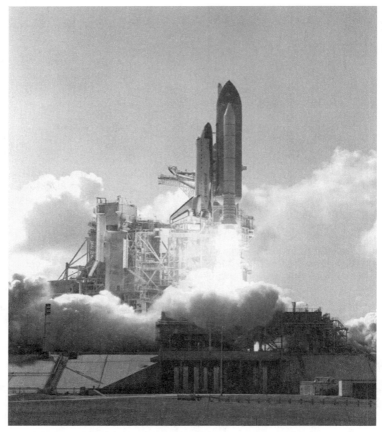

Figure 4-1   Failures of *Columbia* and *Challenger* can be traced to waivers (photo courtesy of NASA).

continue to do more with less and never made difficult choices of focus and priorities.

Diaz Committee Report on Implementation of the CAIB Recommendations

On 1 February 2003, the day Space Shuttle *Columbia* was lost, Sean O'Keefe, in accordance with NASA policy, rapidly assembled a CAIB to investigate and analyze the causes of the accident. The findings of the CAIB were released in August 2003. The CAIB report consisted of recommendations, observations, and findings (R-O-Fs). These R-O-Fs were aimed not only at technical concerns and issues but also at NASA's organization and culture.[*]

---

[*]Data available online at http://www.nasa.gov/CAIB.

Following the release of the CAIB report, the return-to-flight team and the continuing-flight team were convened and charged with developing implementation plans to respond to the technical CAIB recommendations, observations and findings for the space shuttle program and the International Space Station, respectively. However, NASA recognized that a significant value of the CAIB report was in its identification of organizational causes of the accident. Further, NASA understood that this was an organization-wide issue that must be considered in all areas of NASA's operations (not only the human spaceflight program). Thus the "Diaz team" (named after its team's leader, Al Diaz, then director of the Goddard Space Flight Center) was assembled. The team's goal was to identify and analyze those points that have agency-wide application.[†]

The team's official charter was as follows:

1) Identify those R-O-Fs from the CAIB report that might apply across the agency.
2) Identify a set of actions and suggested leadership for those actions.
3) Include the "One NASA" team concept in all activities.
4) Summarize results in a report to the NASA deputy administrator.

The team began by identifying 85 recommendations, observations or findings from the CAIB report that had agency-wide value and developing 40 recommended actions to address these points. (In a number of cases, actions addressed more than one point in the CAIB report.) To gain information and perspective from NASA employees and its contractors, the team recommended the Safety and Mission Success Week. The purpose of this week-long review was to allow employees to discuss the relevance of the CAIB report and determine what can be done to address the impact of the report within each unit. The NASA headquarters and centers then summarized the widespread themes from each work unit's discussion and provided them to the Diaz team. The team found that its initial identification of key points with agency-wide implications was largely consistent with those issues identified by NASA employees during the Safety and Mission Success Week.

Based on the team's analysis, and the Safety and Mission Success Week feedback, seven broad categories were identified in the Diaz report that would classify each of the 85 R-O-Fs. The Diaz report was organized into chapters that addressed each of these seven categories as follows.

Leadership

The team recognized that an overall theme of the CAIB report was the need for an improvement in NASA leadership practices. Three observations

---

[†]Data available online at http://www.nasa.gov/pdf/55691main_Diaz_020204.pdf.

and 14 findings were identified from the CAIB report in this category, and the team developed seven actions to satisfy them.

The team recommended that NASA leadership should begin an aggressive effort to change its leadership patterns as currently observed within the organization. The team recommended following the eight stages approach cited in Jon Kotter's book *Leading Change*. These eight stages emphasized the establishment of a sense of urgency to improve leadership practices and most importantly that change be based on a common framework.

The Diaz team developed a goal for this category that it believed would enhance the probability of success. This goal is stated as follows: "The Agency should assess whether program management and budget formulation processes are adequate to assure there is an appropriate balance of requirements, resources, and risk to ensure safety and mission success."‡

Learning

The CAIB report specifically stated that NASA did not demonstrate the characteristics of a learning organization. Learning is the category that the team identified with the widest applicability across the organization. One recommendation and four findings were identified to apply to this category from the CAIB report.

The feedback generated during the Safety and Mission Success Week as well as an analysis of past NASA missions provided strategies for "learning" what should consistently apply across the organization. The team recognized that steps were already underway to ensure that knowledge is not lost as a result of retirements in the face of an aging workforce. However, the team recommended that more be done to understand what is the knowledge architecture of NASA. In addition, the team recommended that NASA personnel must achieve a higher level of competency and readiness to manage the complex situations that arise in the aerospace systems they manage. To further this point, the team recommended that NASA ensure that its technical tools, information systems, and knowledge repositories are up to date and readily and broadly available to personnel.

The CAIB report had noted that NASA training did not always simulate actual operations during shuttle operations (Fig. 4.2).

The team identified this as having organization-wide applicability. This was reinforced by the feedback from Safety and Mission Success Week, where NASA personnel agreed that increased training resources are necessary to facilitate learning. It was also identified that increased training was necessary to ensure the proper use of NASA's technical tools. This is exemplified in the CAIB report, where it notes that the simulation

---

‡Data available online at http://www.nasa.gov/pdf/55691main_Diaz_020204.pdf.

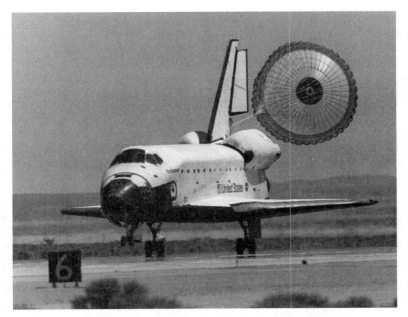

Figure 4-2   One of the findings in the CAIB is that simulations did not necessarily mirror actual shuttle operations (graphics courtesy of NASA).

of the debris impact was performed by an inexperienced team using an inappropriate modeling tool for the size of the impact.§

The team recommended more apprenticeships and hands-on work. The consolidation of the disparate NASA databases using the Internet would also increase the coherence and ease of distribution of knowledge across the organization. Encouragement for personnel to increase their certification levels to ensure technological currency is also recommended. Many of these preceding recommendations are in place within the agency, but a comprehensive analysis is required to determine which areas need improvements.

The goal developed by the team for the learning category is as follows: "The Agency should identify an appropriate approach for the future development of a knowledge management system and infrastructure to assure knowledge retention and lessons learned."¶ (*Note*: The GW team endorsed this approach and suggested that the knowledge management software tools which are developed should include historical information that can be

§Data available online at http://www.NASA.gov/CAIB.
¶Data available online at http://www.nasa.gov/pdf/55691main_Diaz_020204.pdf.

made available to NASA personnel on all relevant and related programs, including the history of the Mercury, Gemini, Apollo, Skylab, shuttle, and International Space Station, and in a rapidly searchable format.)

Intra-Agency Communications

The CAIB report describes communication within the agency as being dispersed as a result of informal networks and hierarchies that have formed. These information networks and complex hierarchies represent a barrier to the clear flow of information within NASA. Two actions for implementation were developed in this category based on feedback from the Safety and Mission Success Week and five findings from the CAIB report. These actions are intended to develop a communication culture that will facilitate anomaly resolution, follow a clear process of organization communications, and utilize a set of formal communications and reporting policies.

The team also recommended a communication culture change whereby all viewpoints are considered. It was determined by the team that the existing culture is one where "minority views" are discouraged and considered to be career limiting. The feedback from the Safety and Mission Success Week confirmed this problem as an issue. The same feedback indicated that rank and file personnel reported a sense that they could not participate in decision making processes.[**]

The team stated that leaders should actively encourage a diversity of viewpoints and that the structure of the organization should ensure that decisions are based solely on facts, rather than subjective feelings and relationships. The success of the change in NASA communication culture will be measured by employee's feedback. The goal stated in this category is as follows: "The Agency should continue the dialog that it began with the NASA workforce during Safety and Mission Success Week."[**] (*Author's note*: There is, however, little evidence that there is a concerted continuing effort within NASA to follow up on these issues of communications, diversity of viewpoint, and greater openness in decision-making processes and setting of priorities.)

Processes and Rules

The CAIB report made it clear that NASA did not follow its own rules. The Diaz report states: "One of the findings [in the CAIB Report] directly stated that NASA did not follow its own rules on evaluating foam-shedding from the external tank." The team reports that the CAIB found that managers did not follow the established protocols, while requiring engineers to follow strict protocols. In addition, if managers did follow established

---

[**]Data available online at http://www.nasa.gov/pdf/55691main_Diaz_020204.pdf.

rules, those rules often turned out to be the most bureaucratic and in some cases actually hindered communication.

The team determined that agency-wide processes and their application across the agency were needed. Both the CAIB report and employee feedback validated this. The goal developed in this category is: "The Agency should conduct a review of its approach to maintaining and managing rules."[++]

Technical Capabilities

The CAIB report discussed the eroding technical capabilities of an agency that was once considered cutting edge. This is caused in part by the aging workforce of experienced engineers, the lack of availability of analytical tools and simulation models, and the misapplication of these tools when they are used. The CAIB report noted the need for an accurate physics-based computer to model the thermal protection system. The Diaz team identified this need as one that had agency-wide applicability. The team stated in their report: "it is clear that all NASA programs need validated models and analytical tools to assess the state of their systems and components." The team also determined that managers must know the capabilities and limitations of these tools to ensure they are not misapplied.[++]

The team identified an agency-wide need for the technical capability to maintain documentation, databases, and knowledge management systems to support technical decision making in a uniform manner across the organization. This need was validated by the responses received during Safety and Mission Success Week. The goal developed in this category is the following: "The Agency should develop guidelines and metrics for assessing and maintaining its core competencies, including those associated with in-house work."[++] (*Author's note*: The findings with regard to simulation models and databases are clearly sound. The blanket application of this finding would, however, add considerable staff, overhead, and cost to current NASA programs. Thus the corollary to this recommendation might be for NASA to focus on specific goals related to launch systems and launch safety, space sciences, space applications, etc. and revamp and streamline each center so that it has focus on a clear mission. This would mean "streamlined" staff competencies would be precisely targeted to achieve its defined prime objectives. It is the further perspective from the GW University study that NASA staff and officials might also seek ways to draw further on the innovative thinking of entrepreneurial organizations in seeking new approaches to safety in launch systems and then seek to institutionalize key results once proven to be effective.)

[++]Data available online at http://www.nasa.gov/pdf/55691main_Diaz_020204.pdf.

Organizational Structure

The CAIB report recommended the creation of an independent technical and engineering authority for the space shuttle program; in addition, the CAIB report recommended that the NASA Headquarters Office of Safety and Mission Assurance should have direct authority over the safety organization of the shuttle program. The team identified this recommendation as having agency-wide application. Independent technical authorities for each of the NASA programs will ensure that technical standards are being met within each program. This will ensure appropriate checks and balances across the organization.

The team also discussed the overall NASA organizational structure and highlighted the need for a structure that implements NASA's policies, but minimizes the real or perceived barriers. A full cost-accounting system would also allow for the proper allocation of resources to those assigned capabilities that are in balance with schedules as well as technical and strategic considerations.

The goal developed for this category is as follows: "The Agency should complete its current NASA-wide assessment and establish an independent technical authority for the Shuttle."‡‡

Risk Management

The major risk management theme identified by the team is the need for uniform standards and assessment methodologies across all programs. The CAIB documents the discrepancy in micrometeoroid and orbital debris standards between the ISS and the space shuttle programs. The management tool employed to monitor deadlines was also addressed as having agency-wide applicability in terms of potential safety implications. This was clearly verified by employee feedback. Deadlines must be evaluated with a risk management perspective in order to ensure that safety will not be compromised in order to meet deadlines in all NASA programs.

Another point of discussion was the allocation of resources. The team recommended an analysis of independent organizations and units within NASA to ensure they are properly resourced.

The CAIB report states that a lack of uniformity in management process, too stringent deadlines, and resource constraints led to an enormous increase in the amount of risk in space shuttle operations. The measures needed to reduce this risk have agency-wide applicability.

The goal developed in this category is as follows: "The Agency should identify a set of risk management processes and tools which can be

---

‡‡Data available online at http://www.nasa.gov/pdf/55691main_Diaz_020204.pdf.

applied across all programs which recognize the diversity with respect to risk tolerance."§§

Impact and Scope of Diaz Report Findings

The Diaz team defined the seven categories just discussed and recommended a systematic approach to a cultural change within NASA for each of these categories. Clearly, if fully implemented, these recommendations could help the NASA organization become "more responsive" and better prepared for the "promising opportunities of the American space program's future."§§

The 85 R-O-Fs identified by the team, as well as the 40 actions assigned to each of them, can be found in the Diaz team matrix as provided in that report. What appears missing from this process is the designation of a high-level person to oversee the full implementation of these recommendations. Subsequent to this report there have been press interviews with NASA engineers who remain skeptical of the changes and have indicated that there remains no high-level accountability among NASA officials for major errors of judgment. Further the processes subsequently developed seem to have largely assumed a continuation of "business as usual" as practiced within a large U.S. governmental agency and did not look to outside sources of innovation in terms of enhanced safety practices [2]. The objective of NASA seriously becoming a "learning" organization, especially at the management level, still seems to be far from being realized some three years after the Diaz report was rendered.

> Subsequent to this report there have been press interviews with NASA engineers who remain skeptical of the changes and have indicated that there remains no high-level accountability among NASA officials for major errors of judgment.

Shuttle Return to Flight

NASA very publicly accepted the CAIB report findings and immediately embarked on an extensive return-to-flight program that involved extensive use of human resources. A total expense budget for the return-to-flight initiative grew from an initial estimate of about $1 billion to a projected total of direct and indirect costs of about $1.75 billion as of the time of the STS 114 flight in August 2005. Now these costs have mounted to over $2 billion in the pursuit of making the STS 115 flight as safe as possible when this launch is achieved sometime in 2006. Of the nearly 30 different recommendations handed down by the CAIB, it determined that

---

§§Data available online at http://www.nasa.gov/pdf/55691main_Diaz_020204.pdf.

at least 15 specific requirements needed to be met before the shuttle could be certified as being safe to resume flight. Other actions and recommendations handed down by the CAIB reflected ongoing longer-term efforts to improve the safety of the overall human spaceflight program.

Table 4.1 outlines the 15 specific recommendations for return to flight in a clear-cut tabular form.

The bottom line on these CAIB recommended changes is that three out of 15 of the most critical safety upgrades (namely, recommendations 1, 3, and 5) have not be achieved and recommendation 13 has only been

Table 4-1 Status of Shuttle Return-to-Flight Implementation of CAIB Recommendations as of Late Summer 2004

Methodology	Discussion
	1) *Eliminate all external tank foam shedding with emphasis on area where bipod struts attach.*
Problem	Immediate cause of *Columbia* accident
Solution	Add heaters to the bipod strut connector and eliminate or redesign foam ramps
Status	Completed, however, problem still continues. July 2005 flight-demonstrated a continuation of the "foam-shedding problem. Further, as of late 2005 potentially dangerous cracks were found in the PAL ramps designed to help with the foam-shedding problem, and there is now thought of eliminating the ramps altogether. This would lead to an additional six months delay.
	2) *Test and qualify bolt catchers.*
Problem	Containers that catch bolts are inadequate. Flying metal could damage shuttle.
Solution	New bolt catcher redesigned with better energy absorber
Status	Completed
	3) *Increase the orbiter's ability to sustain minor debris damage by improving impact resistance of TPS materials.*
Problem	Orbiter's TPS is fragile and susceptible to damage.
Solution	Redesign, refabricate, or upgrade vulnerable areas. Add instruments and sensors to detect damage to the TPS.
Status	Work in this area is ongoing and not completed. Stafford–Covey panel minority report indicates The that this problem has been addressed by revising requirements and thus "defining" it away rather than truly addressing this issue.

(continued)

Table 4-1   Status of Shuttle Return-to-Flight Implementation of CAIB
Recommendations as of Late Summer 2004 (continued)

Methodology	Discussion
	4) *Inspect all reinforced carbon parts for structural integrity.*
Problem	Parts critical to surviving reentry were not properly inspected between missions.
Solution	Introduction of nondestructive testing
Status	Thermography, contact ultrasonics, eddy current, and radiography were selected as the most promising techniques to be used for on-vehicle inspection. These methods are being implemented.
	5) *Capability to inspect and make emergency repairs to TPS for all missions.*
Problem	No in-orbit capability to inspect/repair TPS damage
Solution	Define damage thresholds where repair is required, and develop full in-orbit inspection and repair capability.
Status	One of the most challenging and extensive return-to-flight tasks. Techniques are undergoing development and testing. Non-ISS mission techniques are still being developed. Capability not yet fully developed; those that exist only apply to minor cracks and damage.
	6) *Arrange with Defense Department to require imaging of each shuttle in orbit.*
Problem	"Spy" satellites with high-resolution cameras should have taken photos of *Columbia.*
Solution	Reach agreement with the National Geo-spatial Intelligence Agency.
Status	An agreement has been reached. NASA personnel are receiving training and security clearances.
	7) *Get high-resolution images of external tank after it separates.*
Problem	Insufficient spacecraft images to determine if damage has occurred
Solution	Install digital cameras and transmit images to Earth.
Status	A new high-resolution digital camera will be utilized in the Orbiter umbilical well. Testing of handheld crew cameras completed and system implemented. Demonstrated on reflight mission in August 2005 of the STS 114 were successful. This imaging clearly showed that significant foam-shedding problem still remained.

(*continued*)

Table 4-1   Status of Shuttle Return-to-Flight Implementation of CAIB
Recommendations as of Late Summer 2004 (continued)

Methodology	Discussion
	8) *Get high-resolution images of the underside of the wing's leading edges and forward sections of the wing's carbon panels.*
Problem	Insufficient images of spacecraft to determine if damage has occurred
Solution	Install digital cameras and transmit images to Earth.
Status	Cameras installed and new capability completed. Demonstrated on reflight mission in August 2005.
	9) *Upgrade cameras to provide at least three useful views of the shuttle from liftoff to solid rocket booster separation.*
Problem	Inadequate launch images
Solution	Add, replace, and fix launch cameras, and ensure they are operational before each launch.
Status	Additional cameras are being added, with existing cameras being refurbished. Initially launches will occur during daylight for extra visibility. This capability showed the narrow margin that the foam missed the orbiter on the reflight mission in August 2005. Further improvements are being investigated.
	10) *Shoot and digitalize closeout photos of all critical parts that differ from engineering drawings.*
Problem	Engineering drawings do not reflect equipment changes.
Solution	Improved cameras and new software to index images
Status	Completed
	11) *Require at least two employees at all final closeouts and intertank hand spraying.*
Problem	Lack of observation and documentation—particularly hand spraying insulation on external tank
Solution	Train employees and develop standards.
Status	A TPS verification team has been established to implement a material processing plan. The return-to-flight task group has advised NASA to expand its response to include review of closeout for all flight hardware.
	12) *Kennedy Space Center workers must return to the industry-standard definition of "foreign object debris"*
Problem	Term for debris found around processing of flight hardware changed to reinforce the serious safety implications.
Solution	Training and enforcement

(*continued*)

Table 4-1 Status of Shuttle Return-to-Flight Implementation of CAIB Recommendations as of Late Summer 2004 (continued)

Methodology	Discussion
Status	All debris will now be categorized as "foreign object debris" that is perceived as more dangerous than the previous "processing debris" term. Training and surveillance will be ongoing. Task completed.

13) *Make a realistic flight schedule. Evaluate deadlines regularly to ensure that risks taken to meet the schedule are recognized, understood, and acceptable.*

Problem	Unrealistic schedule pressures created unsafe environment
Solution	Routine risk assessment and more room for changes. Make schedule and risks indicator data available in real time.
Status	A computerized manifesting capability is under development to more effectively manage the schedule margin, launch constraints, and manifest flexibility. Still be developed. This is a function in which the NESC and the new ITA should have increased operational role.

14) *Train the mission management team (MMT) to face a wide variety of potential crew and vehicle safety problems.*

Problem	Questionable decisions surrounding the *Columbia* accident
Solution	Extensive training with emphasis on encouraging dissenting views
Status	A review of MMT processes has been undertaken and training plan developed. Training plan completed in February 2004. Training was ongoing until return-to-flight STS-114 and continues.

15) *Prepare a detailed plan to create an independent technical engineering authority, independent safety program, and reorganized space shuttle integration office.*

Problem	NASA's organization with lack of true safety over ride authority
Solution	Extensive reorganization and change in NASA's "culture"
Status	NESC established and reorganization of NASA announced. The establishment of a new independent technical authority has also been completed, but duties and responsibilities are still to be refined.

partially implemented as well. The minority report of the Stafford–Covey oversight committee for the shuttle reflight program is sharply critical of this lack of results, especially after a great deal of time and money had been spent to achieve these goals.

Another important area that remains a concern is the extensive use of waivers for the space shuttle program. This was considered to be a major problem by the CAIB and the GW research team in that it exposed the large number of vulnerabilities that existed in the space shuttle program. As noted in the opening quote to this chapter, former Senator and astronaut John Glenn believes the "waivers" process led to not only the *Columbia* accident but was the root cause of the other astronaut disasters as well [3].

Under the waivers process, if a defective system were found on the space shuttle, NASA could either redesign the system to meet requirements or redefine the requirement. If fixing the problem could involve a lengthy or costly redesign, an engineer could recommend the acceptance of a certain element of risk, thereby allowing the shuttle to fly with a known defect under what is known as a waiver.

As noted in the CAIB, NASA launched the Space Shuttle *Columbia* with a rather incredible number of "5800 waivers, 1672 of those involving critical parts that could have caused the destruction of the orbiter." This critical parts list included 652 waivers on the *Columbia* Orbiter itself, 312 on the main engines and 163 on the external fuel tank.¶¶ This large number of waivers, in and of itself, does not seem to be reasonable. At the time of the *Challenger* accident in 1986, NASA admitted flying with 829 waivers on critical systems. One of those waivers was related to the rubber seals on the booster rocket, later found to be the cause of the *Challenger* disaster. This continuing problem with the granting of waivers suggests that the lessons of the *Challenger* were never completely learned. The ongoing references to a "broken safety culture" within NASA ultimately come back to such issues as the high number of waivers granted by NASA management—often by overruling safety officers.

In the event that a shuttle is damaged during flight and a sufficient repair job cannot be completed in orbit, a second shuttle could be required to perform a rescue mission. The return-to-flight task group stated in its report that in the very short time frame between the launch of the first vehicle and the requirement for a rescue flight no significant changes could reasonably be made to the second vehicle.

This means that it would be difficult to add additional rescue hardware or make vehicle modifications to respond to problems encountered in the first launch.

Not having sufficient time to make needed changes to the rescue vehicle or the cargo could add significant risk to the rescue flight crew or to crew transfer. The whole process would be under acute schedule pressure, and undoubtedly many safety and operations waivers would be required [4].

¶¶Data available online at www.nasa.gov/CAIB.

Return-to-Flight Costs

During fiscal year (FY) 2003, NASA incurred direct costs of $93.5 million initiating return-to-flight actions based on the CAIB report and internal assessments. For FY 2004, $265 million of return-to-flight activities were identified and increased even more for 2005. The costs identified in NASA's official implementation plan for return to flight, however, are only the direct costs and do not include the indirect costs, including those of maintaining a standing army of 1800 skilled personnel that must be retained to support the shuttle program regardless whether it is flying or not [4].

As indicated earlier, the costs (direct and indirect) through the flight of the STS-114 have been placed at around $1.75 billion and now have soared to over $2 billion in preparation for STS-115. In fact, if the shuttle program were to be ended and the orbiters permanently grounded, there would likely be substantial savings that could be realized by reassigning personnel to other functions or closing down facilities that only support the shuttle program. These savings, however, cannot be realized until the completion of the shuttle mission.

NASA Engineering and Safety Center

One of the most tangible steps that NASA has taken to reassert the primacy of its core commitment to safety as a value has been to create the NASA Engineering and Safety Center (NESC). The creation of NESC was approved as a new unit on 1 August 2003, and it was formally brought into being under its first Director Ralph Roe on 1 November 2003. NESC resides at the Langley Research Center and has an extensive technical staff of some 30 scientists and engineers that reside in the office of the director, the business management and support office, the systems engineering office, the NESC chief engineers office, and a discipline engineering office. The stated purpose of NESC, as stated on the official NASA web site: www.NASA.NESC.gov, is "to provide technical expertise for engineering and safety and mission assurance review or audits, perform independent engineering and safety and mission assurance, trend analysis, provide system engineering review of program management practices and processes, and facilitate or lead mishap investigations."

The structure of the office is very much of a "distributed matrix" with the NESC chief engineer's office staffed by 10 engineers from each of the NASA centers. These engineers, however, continue to reside at their own centers. Further, the disciplines engineering office has engineers that stay at the various NASA centers and are available on call. Initially, the specific disciplines covered by NESC include software; fluids/life support/thermal; structures; materials; human factors; mechanical systems; flight science; power and avionics; and propulsion. There is also the possibility of adding additional capability in other disciplines as needed. At this point most of the key disciplines appear to be covered, although systems engineering, engineering management, telecommunications and IT, systems integration and test, safety engineering and statistical analysis, robotics, stabilization, and medical systems appear NOT to be covered. Also some of the combinations of expertise seem linked to individual skills rather than system requirements.

There is a question as to whether the NESC can or will have a pro-active capability or be merely reactive to problems. The NESC thus has two restrictions of concern. It is essentially a scientific and engineering entity without clearly apparent management and process capability. It is geographically distributed around the United States in a number of states. There is also a seeming assumption that problems related to safety management, safety testing and evaluation, and safety engineering will all stem from technical issues or concerns. Problems related to management, process and independent validation and verification (IV&V) techniques, however, do not necessarily become known through technical tests or some form of quantitative failure. The distributed organization approach strongly suggests that "teams" will be pulled together as problems or the need for audits arises. Thus the NESC, at least as structured, appears to be envisioned as reactive in nature rather than a proactive entity that is constantly seeking safety improvements.

On the other hand, the report of the independent consulting firm of Bio Systems Technology, Inc. (BST) entitled "Assessment Plan for Organizational Change at NASA" seems to suggest strongly that many of the problems of safety actually stem from the NASA organization, management, and safety-related practices. In particular, the problem that is highlighted in the BST report is the need for management to be completely open to all concerns about safety and to see that these concerns are addressed [5]. Thus what seems to be missing from the NESC organizational structure are people with skills in engineering management, systems and safety engineers, and people who would actively go out and "shake the trees" not only within NASA but within contractor plants to find out if communications problems exist and to learn where safety concerns might not be fully addressed.

This function might, in fact, be very much like that of an ombudsman office that finds out where issues and concerns exist. It seems that the NESC could be more productive if it could operate on a proactive basis rather than being a technical review group that addresses issues after they have become problems, which are identified only through a long and detailed audit process. The types of talents that one might look for in this part of an NESC organization would be most like that of a good journalist rather than a classic engineer. Although review of "program management practices and processes" is a part of the NESC mandate, it seems not to be highlighted in the structure of the center as it has been organized, or in the personnel recruited to date. Finally there is also a question as to how the NESC activity relates to the efforts of the NASA inspector general's office that is about eight times larger in size. The inspector general's (IG) charge is to investigate not only financial issues but organizational violations including safety issues.

It might very well be that it is intended for the NESC to play a proactive role in discovering safety-related issues and problems and work closely in tandem with the NASA IG's office, but none of this is clearly revealed by a review of its organization structure. It is of great importance to note that for such a proactive role on the part of NESC to be successfully prosecuted requires it to have great autonomy so that its efforts are not easily "sidelined." The CAIB report, in a number of cases, documents in a number of cases this sidelining of safety officers.

Independent review of the quality of space program and safety analysis carried out over the years has shown that if the NESC is not able to report independently, both to the highest levels of NASA and to other oversight bodies, its effectiveness can and likely will be compromised. In particular, the idea that the NESC would be located within a new and "empowered" independent technical authority for the shuttle and the ISS seems to be of critical importance to future astronaut safety. Further the NASA inspector general's office, which now includes some 200 people, would also appear to need strong new leadership to investigate both safety practices and mismanagement issues and a mandate to work with the NESC to carry out such a mission.

Changing the NASA Culture

One of the major findings by the CAIB was that NASA's culture and history were as much to blame for the *Columbia* disaster as any technical fault. Further, there was the even more general conclusion of the CAIB that there was a fault of national leadership that transcended NASA's ability to operate effectively when lacking sufficient congressional and presidential support and reasonable guidance. The CAIB concluded that there needed to be a cultural change within the agency to place renewed emphasis on and attention to safety. As a result, Bio Systems Technology, Inc., was selected as an independent consultant and tasked with assessing the current safety climate and culture norms within NASA. Further it was tasked with developing an implementation plan to introduce new behaviors that would 1) eliminate barriers to a safety culture and mindset; 2) facilitate collaboration, integration, and alignment of the NASA workforce in support of a "strong safety and mission success" culture; and 3) align with, but not duplicate, current initiatives already underway in the agency such as "One NASA" and "Return to Flight."

The result of the BST effort was a comprehensive, nearly 150-page report entitled "Assessment Plan for Organizational Change at NASA," rendered to NASA on 15 March 2004 and posted in full on the NASA Web site shortly thereafter [5].

For BST, Inc., to identify areas for improvement and develop an implementation plan, they first had to understand the culture and climate at NASA. They approached this with the belief that their efforts could help strengthen the positive aspects of the existing culture and at the same time address the issues raised in the CAIB report. The resultant assessment reached by BST was based on a review of the Diaz report and previous culture surveys, a survey of NASA employees agency wide, and a program of interviews with employees.

The CAIB report addressed organizational causes as a critical contributor to the *Columbia* accident and made specific recommendations for a number of structural changes to the NASA organization and identified a number of gaps in leadership practices important to safety. BST's review of the CAIB report identified many examples of these gaps in leadership with regard to safety issues, such as 1) failing to follow NASA's own procedures; 2) requiring people to prove existence of a problem rather than proactively seeking the solution to problems; and 3) creating a perception that schedule pressure was a critical driver of the program.

As described earlier, in late 2003 the Diaz team (led by Goddard Center Director Al Diaz) conducted a detailed review of the CAIB report to determine which recommendations, observations, and findings in the report had agency-wide applicability to NASA and to develop measures to address each one. The Diaz report focused on the organizational causes identified in the CAIB report but did not do a broad, in-depth assessment of the cultural changes needed to address the organizational issues. BST's review of the CAIB and Diaz team reports was a key step toward improving NASA's safety culture, but more than study safety problems must be done.

Previous culture surveys conducted at NASA were reviewed by BST. Then a specially modified version of the BST Safety Climate and Culture Survey was conducted in depth at all 11 NASA locations. The survey provided a wealth of valuable data to assist in the development of a plan for cultural change within the agency. The BST report indicates that there are three themes that emerge from their analysis of the survey data:

1) Overall, NASA has strong work-group level teamwork and communications. (Certainly, the fact that in 2003 NASA received the top rating among U.S. Federal agencies as a good place to work is indicative of such good working relationships.)

2) Overall NASA still needs to promote new opportunities in upward communications about safety as well as to improve employee perceptions about the extent to which the organization cares about employee input.

3) Overall there is little variation among NASA locations and offices in terms of values and concerns about safety.

Interviews were conducted with more than 120 people that helped to provide context for the survey results. BST found a strong sense of dedication and commitment to the agency's work but did uncover frustration about a number of things, including lack of communication between centers and NASA headquarters; impeded upward communications; variability in the leadership and management skill level; the need for inclusion of primary contractors in the cultural change as they are a key part or the overall NASA culture; and confusion over the overlapping nature and wide variety of initiatives such as Return to Flight, NASA One, Freedom to Manage, the Diaz Report, the Clarity team and efforts to integrate the new national vision for space exploration into the agency.

The BST report noted that NASA has identified and espoused its core values to be "safety, people, excellence, and integrity," but that these core values have yet to be fully institutionalized and can be overridden by factors such as budget constraints and schedule demands. BST examined these core values and came to the following conclusions:

1) *Safety* is something to which NASA personnel are strongly committed in concept, but nevertheless they still lack a culture that is fully supportive of safety. Open communication is not yet the norm, and people do not feel fully comfortable with raising safety concerns to management.

2) *People* do not feel respected or appreciated by the organization. As a result, the strong commitment people feel to their technical work does not transfer to a strong commitment to the organization. People in support functions frequently do not understand or appreciate their connection to the agency's mission, and people in technical positions do not fully value the contribution of support functions to their success.

3) *Excellence* is a treasured value when it comes to technical work, but is not seen by many NASA personnel as imperative for other aspects of the organization's functioning (such as management skills, supporting administrative functions, and creating an environment that encourages excellence in communications).

4) *Integrity* is generally understood and manifested in people's work. However there appear to be pockets where the management chain has (possibly unintentionally) sent signals that the raising of issues (including safety issues) is not welcome. This is inconsistent with an organization that truly values integrity [5].

Approach to Cultural Change at NASA

NASA has the objective of transforming the organizational culture within the next three years to help drive a commitment to excellence within the agency. The BST report states: "In order to achieve cultural change of this magnitude across a large, decentralized, geographically dispersed agency, perseverance and strong support from senior agency leadership will be required. Cultural effects are systemic and enterprise-wide; accordingly cultural transformation requires a systemic, enterprise-wide approach" [5]. The report goes on to conclude the following:

> Senior management alignment, focus, openness, teamwork and discipline will be required in ways that have perhaps never before been fully contemplated. Changes will be required in many deeply-embedded organizational systems and processes. Leadership attitudes, beliefs and behaviors will need to change in very significant ways, and sound management practices will be more important that ever. While it may seem daunting, culture change is possible, and the actions such as those outlined above will have the effect of creating the organizational conditions wherein the preferred culture will emerge, gain momentum, and ultimately flourish [5].

In summary, the BST report states: "Safety is something to which NASA personnel are strongly committed in concept, but NASA has not yet created a culture that is fully supportive of safety. Open communications is not yet the norm, and people do not feel fully comfortable with raising safety concerns to management" [5]. BST's report noted that NASA's core values of "safety, people, excellence, integrity" have yet to be fully institutionalized, and the NASA implementation plan envisions three years to accomplish its goals in this area. In short, factors such as budget constraints, schedule demands, and other such administrative and management matters can and often have overridden the primacy of these core values. As long as conventional governmental oversight processes pertain to NASA and other high technology agencies, there remains a strong likelihood that schedules and budgets will continue to override safety.

New NASA Priorities in Terms of Budgetary and Financial Planning

NASA's current planning priorities, as defined by the George W. Bush administration, can be seen in the proposed budget for 2005 to 2009. Figure 4.3 shows a proposed huge increase in new vehicle development and robotics totaling around $15 billion for FYs 2004–2009. In addition, another $6 billion plus was also proposed for exploration of the moon and Mars for the 2004–2009 period.

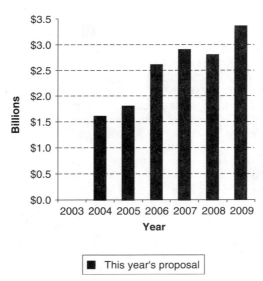

Figure 4-3 Proposed new five-year plan for new developments to support the new space vision (Source: *New York Times* new analysis).

Because the stated objective was to initiate these new programs largely on a pay-as-you-go basis with only about $1 billion a year in new funding, there is increasing recognition within NASA and Congress that realization of these new objectives will likely only be accomplished by reducing existing and planned programs.

This has led to the exceptional budgetary flexibility given to NASA to reallocate resources within future budgets. These five-year budgetary planning documents are an indication of where shifts in budgets will occur—that is to say, solar-system exploration (other than Mars), as seen in Fig. 4.4, followed by sun–Earth connections, the Earth study and observation, and in study of the universe.

Projected cuts in the study of sun–Earth connections were estimated to be around 15% or about $0.75 billion in reductions over a five-year period starting with FY 2005. The cuts in Earth study and observation were projected to be around 3% or $0.5 billion in reductions over the same five-year period. And for the study of the evolution of the universe, the cuts were projected to be around 1.5% or about $0.25 billion in reductions over the same time frame.

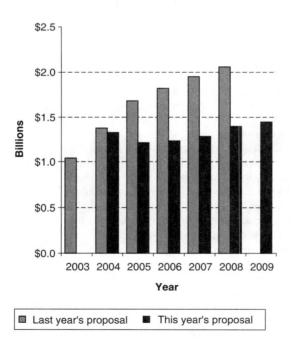

SOLAR SYSTEM EXPLORATION

Figure 4-4 Proposed cuts in solar-system exploration—around 30% or about $3 billion in reductions over the five-year period (starting with FY 2005) (Source: *New York Times* news analysis).

In addition to these cutbacks, research related to the practical or commercial applications of space such as satellite telecommunications, solar-power satellites, remote sensing, geospatial applications, and other forms of space commercialization are funded virtually not at all, in sharp contrast to the other major space agencies of the world that devote 5 to 30% of their budgets to these practical areas that are often seen of greater interest to the man or woman in the street.

The great emphasis on new initiatives in the proposed NASA budget for 2005–2009 is clearly on robotics and new vehicles (just above $15 billion over the next five years). The NASA budget for FY 2005–2006 is not only geared toward the definition and the design of the crew exploration vehicle but has been revised to add $300 million to this effort. This work will involve the definition of the critical safety elements as well. The extent to which safety factors such as crew-escape capability are built into the system specifications will have a critical impact on future safety performance. And indeed a full-envelope escape capability has now become a critical aspect of the specifications for the crew exploration vehicle and all future vehicles designed to carry crew [6].

Space Shuttle Program and the President's New Vision for Space Exploration

Historical shifts in national policies—whether they are related to the environment, strategic goals, or space exploration and applications—are never easy to detect in the heat of the moment and the crush of presidential politics. The NASA 2005 budget was largely defined within the scope of President George W. Bush's announcement in January 2004 of his new space objectives in a document entitled "A Renewed Spirit of Discovery: The President's Vision for U.S. Space Exploration." This "new space vision" has now been further amplified by the report of the Commission on the Implementation of the U.S. Space Exploration Policy, known informally as the Aldridge commission, by calling on NASA to reorganize its centers to achieve the new NASA goals and objectives, expand international cooperation, increase privatization of NASA programs, and strengthen space-related educational programs.

Certainly this redefinition of NASA goals has many implications. This new space vision sets forth specific objectives for a new manned space vehicle that now more or less coincides with the planned dates for the phase out of the shuttle and completion of the space station. The current form of the new space vision emphasizes the call for enhanced synergy between robotic and manned exploration missions. It also announces goals and objectives for the ISS, the exploration of the moon and Mars, other lesser targets and processes for moving forward with space exploration, prizes for college and university research achievements, and in effect reduction of many other space activities such as space applications and education.

It is clear that these new goals, if they continue into the future, have many implications for the future direction of manned space programs and thereby implications for astronaut safety. These goals include the following:

1) The first goal is integrated planning and execution of human and robotic space exploration programs to enhance astronaut safety, be more cost effective, and likely advance the space exploration agenda in the coming decade. (*Note*: If one or more of the shuttle orbiters were converted to robotic operation, this would also serve to increase astronaut safety.)

2) Proceeding to implement the recommendations of the CAIB and returning the shuttle to flight capability with the maximum assurance of safe human flight conditions is the second goal. (*Note*: This does not necessarily mean that NASA needs to proceed with as many shuttle flights as first planned prior to the *Columbia* accident. Clearly the fewer the launches of the space shuttle before it is phased out the lesser the chances of a category one failure and hence a reduction of the risk to astronauts. Currently it seems that the number of remaining space shuttle flights will be reduced from 28 down to 18.)

3) The third goal involves proceeding to develop a new crew launch vehicle (CLV) and a crew exploration vehicle (CEV) as well as solid rocket booster to lift lunar exploration equipment to the moon surface (as will be discussed in Chapter 8).

4) Further there are the visionaries who believe that NASA should also be concentrating on developing innovative new launch systems. These new manned space vehicles might utilize ion engines, nuclear energy, tether-based launch systems, or other new approaches that if taken seriously could ultimately be more cost effective and safer than conventional chemical-fueled rockets.

5) Finally there are those who believe that there is a fundamental imbalance in NASA objectives and that far more emphasis should be placed on space applications and systems to benefit people here on Earth such as environmental problems, global warming, rather than on space exploration. This would mean that the NASA organization and its budgets should be rescaled to more pressing needs on Earth, with exploration goals for the moon and Mars deferred for many years into the future. Such an approach to astronaut safety would thus be premised on reducing astronaut and manned space programs expenditures by relying on robotic systems and other economies that might come from a more entrepreneurial-type initiative. These are key issues here that go beyond safety but nevertheless deserve national debate and ultimate resolution. These issues will require some specific consideration of the international dimensions of future space exploration programs because the U.S. approach pursued by NASA today is singularly different than the other space agencies around the world.

NASA, as described in the five-point program in Chapter 10, is in need of a fresh approach in many areas of its program definition, strategic planning and focus to become more effective, win new public support, achieve enhanced astronaut safety, and produce more bang for the buck. NASA Administrator Michael Griffin who has tried to refocus NASA on new goals and achieve economies and greater agility through more entrepreneurial approaches has found this is not easily done.

Institutional Adjustments?

A number of the people surveyed by the GW team suggested a need for more than a new space vision. They suggested a need for NASA to be reshaped or reconstituted. They also indicated their views that the aerospace industry has been overly consolidated and large corporations that have emerged might also contribute to safety problems by, in effect, slowing down the innovation and design process and contributing to the creation of overly complex designs.

Organizations such as Space X, Scaled Composites, Bigelow Aerospace, and Space Dev among others sincerely seem to believe that entrepreneurial talent and innovation need new support and encouragement by the new NASA. Entrepreneurs can often come up with unique and outside-of-the-box solutions. In contrast, very large aerospace organizations sometimes tend toward building systems that are complex, expensive, and difficult to deploy except over a protracted period of time. In short, some critical observers of the U.S. space program urge institutional, managerial, and entrepreneurial reform of NASA programs to make them better, more cost efficient, and through simplification potentially safer. Large and sophisticated aerospace organizations are needed to implement advanced systems, but smaller entrepreneurial organizations, might help in the design of new systems that allow breakthrough advances but on shoestring budgets.

In terms of space safety, the President's space vision clearly supported the full implementation of the CAIB recommendations before the return of the shuttle to flight. The space vision also advanced the idea that the space shuttle program should be ended as soon as practicable because its design is almost impossible to modify in a fundamental way to increase safety. The President's space vision for this reason recognized that the space shuttle needed to be replaced with a safer manned flight vehicle as soon as practical.

The President's space vision was reported by some analysts to have been significantly shaped by representatives from large aerospace companies. Regardless of whether this analysis is correct, most of the recommendations do support larger, big project space missions that favor the largest aerospace companies [7].

To finance these larger projects, cuts will be made in space astronomy, space science (solar and planetary studies), and other smaller projects for university grants and educational undertakings. Further, space applications such as communications, navigation, etc. have for some time been largely eliminated from NASA active programs and remote sensing reduced in scope [8].

Presidential Commission on Implementation of U.S. Space Exploration Policy

As described earlier, when President George W. Bush announced his new space vision in January 2004 he also set up a Presidential Commission on the Implementation of U.S. Space Exploration Policy that became known as The Commission on the Moon, Mars and Beyond, or alternatively as the Aldridge commission after its Chairman Pete Aldridge. After months of hearings and consideration of voluminous documentation, the commission came up with a number of findings and recommendations that can be broadly grouped into themes that include the following components [9]:

1) *Space education*: The need for improved space education to inspire young people to pursue space exploration as a career and to strengthen the U.S. basic research capabilities to help sustain American high-tech industries was discussed. (*Author's note*: The budget demands of Project Constellation and those of the shuttle program and ISS are such that NASA is currently reducing its educational programs.)

2) *Transformation of NASA*: The need to modernize and restructure NASA so that it is suitably organized to carry out its new missions was highlighted. In particular the suggestion was made to transform NASA centers to be more flexible so that they can serve NASA and other government agencies and to revise their status so that they could assume the same "private research status as Federally Financed Research & Development Centers (FFRDCs)," similar to the Jet Propulsion Laboratory as an adjunct, to California Institute of Technology. There was also the suggestion that other U.S. government agencies, including the Department of Defense, could be more involved in the new space vision and that the renewal of the equivalent of a National Space Council (to be designated a Space Exploration Steering Council and preferably reporting to the Vice President) should be formed with a view to providing high-level and longer-term guidance to a space program that would not be subject to year-to-year vagaries of funding. Clearly improved management and better fiscal controls are needed in light of the reports of the NASA inspector general and others about serious budgetary problems in administering NASA that were disclosed in December 2004 [8]. (*Author's note*: Despite the fact there has been some reorganization, none of the basic restructuring of NASA recommended by the commission has taken place, and the centers status remains the same.)

3) *International cooperation*: This finding stressed the fact that there were many opportunities for new types and forms of international cooperation, and in light of the high cost of space exploration international cooperation could not only add talent and expertise but also help to spread the cost of longer-term space objectives. (*Author's note*: The international dimensions of Project Constellation remain to be defined, and other space explorations programs by other countries proceed in apparent competition with the U.S. initiatives.)

4) *Research*: As analyst Frank Fietzen, Jr., stated in his assessment of the report [10], the commission essentially concluded that "the agency should award competitively bid contracts with private and non-profit organizations, limiting its own role in management and operations." Indeed the report rather radically states that NASA should restrict its role "to only those areas where there is irrefutable demonstration that only government can perform the proposed activity" [11].

If this approach were followed literally, the size of NASA would presumably be reduced greatly in size, and NASA would be left with little or no independent research and analysis role. In short, NASA would become essentially just a contracting agency rather than a scientific organization. Such a radical shift, if literally implemented, would likely undercut astronaut safety and contribute to a "science and engineering vacuum" within the U.S. government that would be highly counterproductive.

(*Author's note*: A more moderate shift, especially if it allowed stronger participation by entrepreneurial organizations and smaller research institutes and universities, would seem desirable. Also, if at least some additional NASA centers were moved to FFRDC status and at the same time these centers were given more specific research and programmatic focus, such changes might well produce benefits in terms of cost savings, clearer goal orientation, and less overlap of function between the various centers.)

Indeed the experience demonstrated by such entities as Scaled Composites, Space Dev, Space X, Bigelow Aerospace, and even the Space Elevator enterprise, strongly suggests that some aspects of new research and design (R&D) related to manned spaceflight and exploration might be carried out more effectively as private entrepreneurial efforts. This is not only because of outside-of-the-box thinking but also because risk and even potential loss of life can be compensated for and covered by legal waivers more effectively in the private sector than in governmental programs. Further, test operations involving private entities do not necessarily carry national prestige on its shoulders.

Such possible adjustments to NASA's space exploration and safety practices, in this more moderate vein (see Table 4.2), are seen more as a fine tuning of NASA practices, however, rather than as a dramatic change of course that the Aldridge commission would seem to imply. A radical shift that would take most development activities to the private sector would seem unwise for safety as well as other reasons. Because no specific actions to implement the Aldridge commission have been taken to date, this does not seem to be a danger.

It is unfortunate that the new presidential vision of 2004 did not give rise to any major reforms in the NASA organization structure or specific goal setting for the various centers that could have had lasting impact on the U.S. space program.

Table 4-2 Key Space Shuttle Safety Concerns and Issues: Cumulative Management and Environmental Assessment

Nature of Management Concern	Element of Risk	Importance (1, least; 5, high)	Areas to Explore in Terms of Possible Upgrades
Structure, role, and mission of ITA and NASA Engineering and Safety Center	NESC is highly distributed among all the NASA centers. Its role seems to be largely restricted to reacting to problems.	4	Giving ITA and NESC specific proactive tasks related to shuttle infrastructure, quality control and IV&V processes, retrofit priorities, etc. Also develop clearer definitions of astronaut safety in quantitative terms.
Extremely high number of waivers granted for each shuttle launch	Waivers have had direct impact on both shuttle accidents.	5	Giving ITA approval authority for all waivers. Instill a culture of safety that leads to correcting problems rather than granting waivers. Develop safer and less complex human-rated launch system that can limit extensive waivers.
Significant number of manifested shuttle launches to complete ISS	Each shuttle launch raises risk of another category 1 failure.	5	If the number of shuttle launches can be reduced, then the chance of another catastrophe could also be reduced. Use of unmanned vehicles (i.e., robotic shuttle operation) for cargo missions could reduce potential loss of astronaut lives further.

(continued)

Table 4-2　Key Space Shuttle Safety Concerns and Issues: Cumulative Management and Environmental Assessment (continued)

Nature of Management Concern	Element of Risk	Importance (1, least; 5, high)	Areas to Explore in Terms of Possible Upgrades
Possible accelerated development of new U.S. human-rated vehicle or contract for private launcher access to the ISS	Some reduction in scope of ISS and less shuttle launches could allow earlier start on new U.S. vehicle.	5	Explore improved TPC and new escape capabilities for new launch system. Assist private industry to develop manned access to the ISS. (*Note:* NASA has assigned $500 million to such an effort and issued an RFP to this effect in Dec. 2005.)
Pattern of override of many concerns of safety program officers by NASA shuttle management officers	Evidence of this type of problem hard to verify because many issues not available in external record.	3	Implement new ITA with full authority and final sign off over all safety issues, waivers, and safety definitions.
Lack of clear and comprehensive identification of new safety upgrades and retrofit designs for shuttle	The likely continuation of the shuttle program for a number of years means that deferred safety upgrades should all be reassessed.	4	Explore new priority listing of all current and pending shuttle safety upgrades and retrofits that will be a part of the new computerized status reporting system.
Improved management control of shuttle	Need for full implementation of new risk, budget and scheduling system by NASA management after CAIB recommendations fully in place.	3	Fully implement new computerized system that gives real-time status of all aspects of shuttle and safety enhancements. This must flag most critical safety issues/constraints. Training for the effective use of this system.

Recruitment of new engineers to replace retiring staff needed for refurbishment of space shuttle	The retirement of shuttle staff represents a major recruitment and training issue.		A huge amount will be spent on the return to flight of the shuttle, but the NASA personnel for refurbishment of shuttle 2005 through 2010/2012 needs competent new staff and major budgetary support.
Introduction of knowledge management system to ensure institutional memory for remainder of shuttle program	Issue is not only recruitment of new staff but knowledge transfer process.	4	The highly specialized nature of shuttle and its huge number of parts, plus difficulty of supply of key parts, etc. might require a new active knowledge management system to span potentially the next six years or more. NASA is currently working in this direction in response to CAIB rec. 13.
Clarification of corporate and NASA roles	Examine new possibilities set forth in this report.	4	Clarification of role of NASA and industry; new recruitment, knowledge transfer, waivers, and modernization programs.
Follow through on the Diaz committee and BST, Inc., report	As memory of *Columbia* accident fades, so too will be the lessons learned from the BST report and Diaz committee.	3	Continued commitment to new safety culture must be seen from top down and bottom up. Work with IAASS, other space agencies. Create on sustained basis more open NASA culture.

(continued)

Table 4-2 Key Space Shuttle Safety Concerns and Issues: Cumulative Management and Environmental Assessment (continued)

Nature of Management Concern	Element of Risk	Importance (1, least; 5, high)	Areas to Explore in Terms of Possible Upgrades
Need for upgrade of maintenance and retrofit facilities and equipment at KSC	Out-of-date test equipment, obsolete facilities, transporter, gantry	3	Comprehensive safety report on all primary launch support equipment prior to the next shuttle launch
Concern about NASA structural handbook be updated in context of aging and corrosive factors	Aging factors, corrosion and structural concerns need to be examined in synergistic fashion.	3	Review and update NASA structural handbook in context of other aging factors and examination of all pressure vessels, corrosive concerns, and primer inspections.
Concern about shuttle safety upgrades that have been deferred or not fully implemented	Now that Shuttle is expected to operate a number of additional years, some safety upgrades are more important.	4	Request for fully up-to-date report on all such deferred or partially implemented upgrades from NASA office charged with this responsibility
Transfer of all safety and QC functions to Shuttle ITA and NESC	Current system allows mission officials to sign forms to override safety officer concerns.	4	Restructure safety and QC function to achieve high-level accountability within ITA and the NESC.
Terrorist attack at liftoff, on systems control, jamming, active debris assault	Hacker attack on STS. Indicates need for better security	2	Improved security; more coding

The commission's report was entirely premised on the broad scope of President George W. Bush's space vision and had no particular focus on space safety *per se*. The blueprint already declared by the President was "taken in all of its points," as the prescribed way forward. Thus the entire report assumed that NASA would be focused on returning the shuttle to flight status, completing the space station, developing new launch capability in order to explore the moon (using both astronauts and robotic devices), and then going on to explore Mars.

There appeared to be little opportunity for the commission to address questions about the safety implications of returning the shuttle to flight or completing the ISS, nor likewise any opportunity to raise questions about the fundamental purposes of the ISS or whether it was truly needed to carry out life sciences work needed to go to the moon or whether it might have a role as a space port as the Russian Federated Space Agency (Roskosmos) has suggested. Thus, although there were many interesting aspects of the commission's report, such as the reorganization of NASA and its centers and international participation, the bottom line is that it did not have strong implications for space safety, other than to support strongly the concept of combining manned and robotic missions for both the moon and Mars missions. Further, it has ultimately had very little impact on NASA's planning at all [9].

References

1   Pelton, J. N., Smith, D., Helm, N., MacDoran, P., and Caughran, P., "Space Safety Report: Vulnerabilities and Risk Reduction in US Human Space Flight Programs," Space and Advanced Communications Research Inst., George Washington Univ., Washington, DC, 2005, URL: www.spacesafety.org.
2   Kelly, J., and Halvorson, T., "NASA Must Reduce Safety Waivers," *New York Times*, 10 May 2004, p. A 11.
3   Astronaut John Glenn, Remarks at the Smithsonian Air and Space Exhibit Facility, Dulles, VA, 10 June 2004.
4   "NASA's Implementation Plan for Space Shuttle Return to Flight and Beyond," NASA Report, NASA SP-2318, 2004, Washington, DC, p. 54.
5   "Assessment Plan for Organizational Change at NASA," BST, Inc., Houston, TX, 2004.
6   Overbye, D., "NASA's CEV Development Program," *New York Times*, 18 April 2004.
7   Wayne, L., "Pentagon Brass and Military Contractors' Gold," *Washington Post*, 15 Nov. 2005, B-1.
8   "NASA's Chief Bails Out," *New York Times*, 26 Dec., Washington Week in Review, 2004, p. 8.
9   "A Journey to Inspire, Innovate and Discover," Report of the Presidential Commission on the Implementation of United States' Space Exploration Policy, Washington, DC, June 2004, URL: www.space.com.
10 Leary, W. and Schwartz, J., "NASA Is Urged to Add Task for Industry," *New York Times*, p. A–12.
11 Fietzen, F., Jr., "Roadmap for Re-Inventing NASA," *Aerospace America*, Sept. 2004, Vol. 42, Issue 9, pp. 32–39.

Additional Reading

Kotter, J., *Leading Change*, Harvard Business School Press, Cambridge, MA, 1996.

NASA Office of Space Flight, Space Flight Advisory Committee, Meeting Report, 1–2 May 2001, p. 7; also CAIB Document CTF017-0034.

"Status Report on Space Shuttle," NASA, 18 April 2002.

"Summary of Space Shuttle/Safety-Related Products from the NASA Office of Inspector General, NASA," Jan. 2004, URL: http://www.space.com/missionlaunches/ sts107_fleet_030201.html.

CHAPTER 5
International Space Station– Status and Vulnerabilities

"It is awe inspiring to see the International Space Station passing
overhead in its nightly travels."

—*Former astronaut and Senator John Glenn, Smithsonian Air and Space
Museum, 10 June 2004.*

"... the space station, which has been occupied
since 2000, is itself troubled, with its crew scaled back from
three people to two after the loss of Columbia. Crucial systems
like the oxygen generator have malfunctioned repeatedly, and
supplies are dwindling without the freight-hauling capacity
of the shuttle."

—*John Schwartz*, New York Times, 7 *February 2005*

Problems with the International Space Station: Are There New Answers?

This chapter addresses the current doleful status of the International
Space Station (ISS). There are problems everywhere one might look.
Safety concerns abound for this megaproject that is now a decade behind
schedule and billions of dollars over budget. The meter is whirring away
regardless of whether one is counting time, money, or even safety problems. The "progress" made on the ISS in the past few years has consisted
mainly of delaying or scrapping components of this once grand space
science project that has, in essence, not aged gracefully. Nor is the problem just that of finishing the ISS and ferrying crew to and from low Earth
orbit. Only a deal signed with the Russian Federal Space Agency in
December 2006 that guarantees the United States a seat on the Soyuz for
an American astronaut allows a continued U.S. presence on the ISS [1].

The problem is, of course, more than time or money or even American
prestige. The real issue is whether the ISS can be viably sustained for the
longer term. If problems with the gyro system, the oxygen generator, etc.
cannot be solved, the ability to sustain the ISS for the longer term comes
into question.

A summary of the major findings and recommendations concerning
ISS safety is provided in two charts at the end of this chapter. The first of
these charts (Table 5.1) indicates major technical findings and recommendations while the second (Table 5.2) provides findings and recommendations with regard to major management, quality control, and operational
issues. More detailed research material that explains in detail the various

Table 5-1 Technical Safety Issues Related to the ISS

Risk Element	Potential Upgrade	Benefit	Cost Implications
Lack of an up-to-date comprehensive listing of upgrades pending or incomplete for the ISS and especially a listing of safety upgrades	Prioritized and computer-based listing of all potential upgrades of ISS power systems, oxygen generator, air monitoring system, shielding, wiring, external surface decharging system, gyro system, debris avoidance, etc. available to NESC/ITA	Clear understanding of priority of upgrades in terms of schedule and assigned urgency	It would be desirable for each upgrade to be listed with projected cost, schedule to complete and current status.
ISS orbital stabilization and debris avoidance	1) Implement ATV systems. (Each ATV has 6-month boost capability.) 2) Amend legislation so that NASA can purchase Soyuz from Russia.	1) Could boost the ISS and also allow maneuver to avoid debris 2) Soyuz needed as backup to ATV and especially to serve as an ISS escape vehicle.	1) Cost of ATV program essentially paid by ESA that will launch ATVs on Ariane 5 2) Cost of Soyuz to be negotiated with Russia. 3) Consider Soyuz upgrade for full crew
NASA upgrade capability to inventory medium-sized and non-metallic debris	More stringent controls on new space debris; improved space-based GPS capabilities	Reduce risk of catastrophic loss of ISS or crucial subsystem; improved space tracking/surveillance systems	Variable. Most could be done without new systems or capabilities.
Minimize number and duration of EVAs by ISS crew	Increased use of robotics and Canadarm2/MSS (i.e., Canada Hand) to complete construction and repairs	Highest risk to astronauts aboard is exposure during EVAs.	This involves minimal cost if robotics and Canadarm2 and Canada Hand are used to full advantage.

Upgrade the ISS environmental control and life-support systems (ECLSS)	The current ECLSS could be improved to add noxious gas monitoring systems with distributed microsensors and add new oxygen supply and CO_2 reduction systems. (*Note:* New O_2 generator planned for STS-115).	Atmospheric hazards constitute risk especially for larger crews, and upgrades could prevent need to evacuate the ISS or loss of life.	Distributed micro-sensors could likely be added at modest cost. CO_2 and O_2 systems would require significant cost to develop and install, but new O_2 system on next shuttle launch.
Health-support systems	Current onboard health systems and space suits need upgrades to support longer-duration stays on ISS. Expanded use of Russian space suits might be explored. New health systems using nano-technology also possible.	Improved health-support systems could prevent emergency evacuation of ISS and cost of additional shuttle mission or possible loss of ISS.	If expanded use of Russian space suits possible, this could minimize cost. New medical nano-technology and expanded exercise systems could be added at modest cost.
Expanded escape capability	Additional Soyuz systems availability as escape vehicles would raise safety levels, especially if revised version with full crew capability were available. Congressional authorization is necessary.	The Soyuz is most reliable and cost-effective solution. Canceled H-20 and X-38 programs probably cannot be reactivated in time to help.	Soyuz is most likely to be lowest-cost emergency escape system. Lack of option can adversely impact cost of procurement from Russia.

(continued)

Table 5-1 Technical Safety Issues Related to the ISS (continued)

Risk Element	Potential Upgrade	Benefit	Cost Implications
Operational software upgrades	The number of "work around" and "flash" programming procedures in the software used to operate the ISS and shuttle in orbit is now viewed as a safety issue. A permanent "fix" and rewrite of software would limit the chances of erroneous commands.	Reduce the possibility of false commands or instrument readouts that might lead to some system failure or other problems.	Cost of rewrite of software would be substantial, but such a risk reduction is important and would be less than the cost of a major system failure.
Added radiation protection and shielding against debris	The amount of exposure to radiation is high for astronauts who are on extended missions. Limited options exist, but leaded protection sleep suits and reconfiguration of ISS living quarters might be considered. Also additional shielding against debris would add further security.	Enhanced protection of astronauts against radiation sickness and bodily damage as well as better protection against debris	Cost of enhanced radiation protection systems would not be high. Reconfiguration of ISS living quarters would need study to establish cost as would better shielding against debris for living areas and key ISS equipment
Upgraded "smart" sensors to predict subsystem failure	Change out and upgrade of microsensors that can detect problems with environmental control, power systems, air leaks, etc.	These upgrades could allow detection of problems before they are serious.	Cost of microsensors and nanotechnology "swarms" would be small. Can supplement existing sensors.

Lack of clear unified listing of upgrades to ISS still not undertaken or completed	A listing of all pending upgrades to oxygen generators, air monitoring system, microsensors, power system, and gyro system is requested along with status and cost estimates.	A clear status report on all pending health and safety upgrades would allow prioritization of action.	Each upgrade should include an estimate of cost and schedule for accomplishing needed actions.
Lack of a unified international approach to ISS risk management and emergency operations	Creation of a transnational authority to provide for unified control of the ISS safety systems and escape and evacuation procedures with special powers during an operational crisis	Greater coordination and allocation of resources among the international partners	The costs of such a coordinative mechanism should be minimal.
Independent safety oversight and control for the ISS by the NESC and by the independent technical authority	NASA has no truly "independent" safety review. Independent ITA might provide improved safety standards review.	Independent review authority would likely reduce number of safety waivers granted and improve ISS safety.	Cost would be minimal, especially if ITA and NESC functions were merged.
Increase Minimum crew size to maintain safe operation	Guarantee crew sufficient to maintain ISS operation while two astronauts are on EVA	Ensure that astronauts on EVA could make emergency return to ISS	Up to two Soyuz escape vehicles and shuttle must be reliably reactivated.
Greater reliance on free-flyer test modules	The idea that all in-orbit testing would have to be based on the ISS is not necessarily cost efficient. Free flyers such as the Spartan could offer effective, cost-efficient, and possibly safer ways to conduct certain space experiments.	Benefit would be to allow more experiments to be conducted with many being lower in cost and higher in safety.	Cost of free flyers vary, but the Spartan is now developed and available.

Table 5.2 Management, Quality Control and Operational Issues Related to ISS Safety (continued)

Risk Element	Potential Upgrade	Benefit	Cost Implications
Improved standards for inspection of checklist of key elements for QC (i.e., IV&V) after deployment on ISS	As recommended in NASA review process, systematic review of wiring, external perimeter of ISS. Added video surveillance capability would be of assistance.	This will allow the safety of the ISS to be constantly evaluated over time.	Cost would be minimal, but this depends on scope of checklist.
Operation of ISS by remote control without crew members aboard	Consider in depth the safety and scientific implications of remote operation of the ISS without crew aboard, and prepare a detailed report on this subject.	Understand the safety and risk factors involved with remote ISS fly-by-wire operations and upgrade comm. and command encryption.	Minimal and could lead to significant cost savings
Comprehensive review of all potential terrorist threats to ISS operations	Review of the four major terrorist threat concerns discussed in the following text	Enhanced protection and improved security against a terrorist attack on ISS	Various actions would have varying costs, but none are high and indeed are small against possible loss of $100-billion asset.
Systematic screening and computerized control of all materials launched to the ISS	This would create a systematic way of controlling all materials launched to ISS and help inventory control.	Prevention of terrorist attack on ISS	Minimal and could help control inventory costs

issues and problems found with
regard to ISS safety is provided in
Appendix D. In general, the design
and deployment of the ISS is not a
happy story. It is in many ways a saga
of opportunities lost.

> In general, the design and
> deployment of the ISS is not a
> happy story. It is in many ways a
> saga of opportunities lost.

This chapter seeks to highlight
perceived risks associated with the ISS as well as to set forth possible
improvements that can be made to ISS safety. These possible improvements involve providing greater backup, replacement of key life-support
equipment and sensors, updating wiring and aging components,
improved operating procedures and quality control, and fail-safe measures that would help to ensure greater safety for the ISS for the duration
of its mission life. The reliance on the shuttle to construct and maintain
the ISS as the priority mode of access has been, at best, a disappointment.
The continued insistence by NASA that this is the most economical and
efficient way to complete and maintain the ISS for the future is really
increasingly difficult to support. Senator Sam Brownback (R. Kansas)
questioned this approach some two years ago, and his questions seem
even more pertinent today [2]. The clear and obvious "negatives" with
regard to the use of fully crewed shuttles to finish the ISS include the
nearly seven years of down time that followed from the *Challenger* and
Columbia accidents, the $2-billion investment of research, workforce, and
equipment directed toward getting the shuttle flying again and the highly
disappointing results as demonstrated with the STS-114 flight in August
2005. More recently, in December 2005 cracks were found in the PAL ramp
that was supposed to help solve the shuttle's takeoff debris problem.
Instead there might be an additional four months' delay to remove the
ramps [3]. Then there is the detailed critique of the NASA safety and
reflight program for the shuttle, as contained in the minority report of the
Covey–Stafford panel that argues that three of the critical fixes recommended by the CAIB have not been achieved [4]. In short, the use of the
Soyuz, expendable rockets, and perhaps the operation of the shuttle as an
automated cargo lifter can represent a better, wiser, and safer approach to
finishing, maintaining, and operating the ISS. One more failure of a shuttle mission with a full crew aboard would be devastating to NASA's
ongoing operations.

We hope, therefore, that the findings and recommendations contained
in the two referenced charts and in the appendices will be considered by
NASA and other government entities in formulating ISS policy and in
establishing funding priorities.

It is recognized that implementation of some of the safety improvements with regard to the ISS might not be possible. Yet perhaps some of
the observations and findings can be constructively applied to the future
program and especially be found useful in the planning and execution of
Project Constellation. This inability on the part of NASA to act could
be for a variety of programmatic, financial, or technical reasons.
Nevertheless, these tough issues cannot be simply forgotten as the United

This not to say that the ISS is not a valuable space resource and that efforts to derive new scientific discoveries and practical industrial applications should be somehow terminated. Rather it is to say that the program could have been done smarter and better and at lower cost with greater safety and executed with greater flexibility and efficiency.

States seeks to embark on new space initiatives. The shuttle and the ISS will be a critical part of NASA's programs for the next five years or more, and these multibillion projects cannot be simply hidden behind a screen like the Wizard of Oz.

This not to say that the ISS is not a valuable space resource and that efforts to derive new scientific discoveries and practical industrial applications should be somehow terminated. Rather it is to say that the program could have been done smarter and better and at lower cost with greater safety and executed with greater flexibility and efficiency. It is, of course, always easy to be the Monday morning quarterback with 20/20 hindsight, but many of the mistakes that related to the space station are apparent to even those who designed the ISS.

In short, the prime objective today is not to critique the ISS, but rather to maximize its safety, lower risk factors, and improve the utility of this major space asset. It is beyond the scope of this book to assess the considerable quality or high value of the extensive research program that the ISS is expected to carry out in years to come. The object is to better understand where the ISS could be made safer and its objectives achieved with less risk to NASA and especially to ISS astronauts. Indeed the major role of the ISS over time might be that of a sort of stellar "bus terminal" that will allow low-Earth-orbit vehicles to interconnect with vehicles going to the moon and beyond—at least this is the vision of the ISS most recently expressed by America's international partners from Russia and Europe (see Fig. 5.1).

Many of the safety issues or concerns with regard to the ISS involve not only technical or hardware issues but also management, quality control, or operational issues, as shown in Table 5.2.

Overview of the International Space Station: Historical Perspective

To fully understand the ISS goals, objectives, risk levels, and its overall scientific mission, it is important to first put the project into a historical perspective, beginning with a review of earlier efforts to place larger-scale structures into low Earth orbit.

In 1923, the early space pioneer, Hermann Oberth, described a space center in lower space where humans could conduct research and prepare for journeys further out to the moon and Mars. Arthur C. Clarke and Werner von Braun both wrote about the usefulness of space stations in the 1950s. In 1961, Yuri Gagarin was the first human to fly in space, and just eight years later Americans walked on the moon. At the time there was not only talk by leading individuals such as Wehrner von Braun of launching

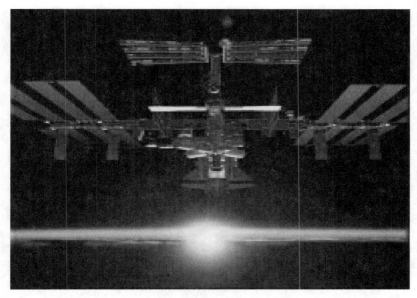

Figure 5-1 Artist rendering of the fully complete International Space Station (graphics courtesy of NASA).

truly large space stations but even of establishing permanent colonies on the moon. In 1971, the Soviet Union launched *Salyut* 1, the first space station. This project was followed two years later by Skylab (Fig. 5.2).

U.S. Skylab

The United States launched Skylab in 1973, and three different crews from the United States rotated onboard this "first American space station" before it was deorbited.

The primary goals of these fledgling space-station programs were to investigate the possibilities for living creatures (human and animal) to exist in the environment of space for extended durations, to carry out experiments in outer space, and to explore the health issues related to low to zero gravity, radiation, and other similar concerns.

Skylab experienced launch difficulties with the premature opening of the meteoroid/sun shield and the subsequent damage to one of the solar arrays. Crew members had to conduct extravehicular activities (EVAs) to address these problems. The ability of the Skylab crews to work on a damaged space-station exterior was seen as key to being able to deploy larger and more complex structures in space. It was believed with this experience that a crew member could now be called on to help deploy stations of the future.

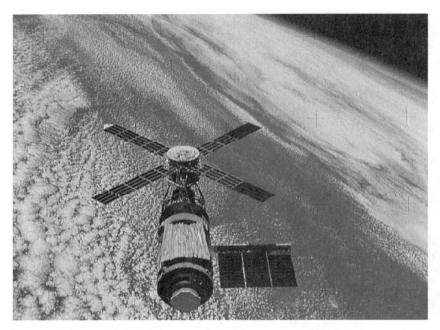

Figure 5-2   Photo of Skylab in space (graphic courtesy of NASA).

Russian Mir

The Soviet Union followed their first orbital Space Station *Salyut* with the launch in 1986 of a longer-term mission—the modular space station called Mir (Fig. 5.3). This space station demonstrated the ability for crew members to stay in orbit for durations of a year or longer and provided a stable, reliable vehicle in which to conduct research. When Russian astronauts returned from stays in orbit that lasted for more than a year, they were not able, at least for some time, to stand because of the atrophied muscles and the lack of a gravitational environment for such an extended period of time.

In 1992, U.S. and Russian leaders agreed to a cooperative space program that would include shared missions between the U.S. shuttle and the Russian Mir. The initial agreement was soon extended to have as many as 10 joint extensions of the shuttle with the Mir. The first shuttle/Mir docking took place in 1995 with exchanges of crews and the transfer of scientific equipment and research modules. A highlight of this first docking was when the Mir crew moved temporarily to their Soyuz spacecraft and moved a short distance away to video the Space Shuttle *Atlantis* and Mir separating. Americans continued to be long-term residents of the Mir. Early in 1997, astronaut Jerry Linenger used a Russian spacesuit to conduct a five-hour walk during which he installed a monitor and retrieved panels from the surface of the Mir. In addition, the Mir

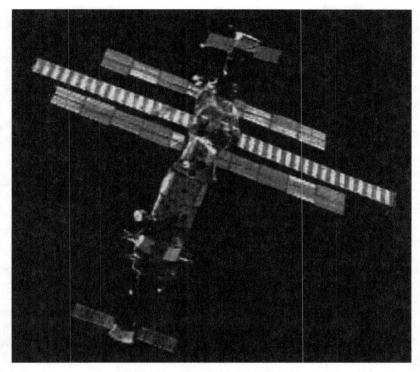

Figure 5-3 Russian Space Station Mir (graphic courtesy of NASA).

crew members used their Soyuz vehicle to leave the Mir from one docking location, fly around the Mir doing a visual inspection of their home
station, and then redocking in a new location.

This second extravehicular activity especially demonstrated the ability
of a shuttle and a station to work together to conduct visual inspections of
each other for safety and research purposes. However, astronaut Linenger's
stay on Mir was not always easy. During his mission, the Mir experienced
the worst fire to date in space. The crew was changing an oxygen-generating
canister when the chemical inside, which uses heat to make the oxygen,
began to burn. The crew members responded immediately, and with a concerted effort, amid a hot fire and heavy smoke, were able to stop the fire in
less than two minutes. Fortunately, the crew experienced no injuries, and
there was no major damage to the Mir operations. Later in 1997, during a
period when astronaut Mike Foale had replaced Linenger, the Mir experienced a second severe accident when a Russian unmanned Progress resupply vehicle hit the Mir station during a redocking system test. One of the
Mir modules (Spektr) suffered a rupture and lost all pressure.

The damage to the Spektr module and a nearby solar array resulted in
a loss of electrical power and attitude control, causing the Mir to tumble

slowly along its orbit. Again, fortunately, there were no injuries to the crew, and the damage was sufficiently controlled to allow the Mir to continue its mission. Later, the crew was able to conduct an EVA to inspect the exterior damage to the Russian station. After the docking accident, there was a serious safety and risk assessment dialog between the Russians and the Americans.

This dialogue clearly showed that the United States tended to take a more conservative and carefully programmed approach when it comes to matters of human safety. The Russian Federation Space Agency on the other hand appeared to be willing to tolerate a higher level of risk and situational response. This approach was apparently a result of their significantly reduced space budget and proven Russian ability to respond to crisis conditions in "real time." The shuttle/Mir program ended the following year.

Space-Station Vulnerabilities and Risk Reduction

The safety issues for the ISS and the shuttle are integrally intertwined. This interconnection between the two programs include the following:

1) *The primary reason for returning the shuttle to flight is essentially to construct and deploy the remainder of the ISS infrastructure and to ferry crew to and from the station.* Virtually all of the remaining flights of the shuttle support this purpose in terms of construction, resupply, and/or experimentation. The only other space activity not related to the ISS is to service the Hubble Telescope, which has been included anew in the Presidential budget proposal for FY 2007.

2) *Shuttle and ISS safety issues become closely interrelated when the shuttle mission involves docking with the space station.* There are several obvious major risk categories associated with shuttle missions, namely, launch into orbit, deorbit, and landing. When the shuttle mission is to the ISS, however, there are additional risk elements associated with the docking, tandem operations between the shuttle and the ISS, and finally shuttle departure. Most safety reviews have focused on either the launch or the deorbit phases of shuttle missions. This is quite logical because all previous catastrophic accidents have occurred at these phases. There are, however, clear risk factors associated with the ISS–shuttle tandem operations that start with the docking operations and continue through the departure stages of the mission. These issues deserve careful review and analysis. Indeed, as noted earlier, there was a major accident for the Russia Mir station that involved the Progress vehicle when it undocked.

On 3 March 2004 NASA released an 84-page report detailing the steps it had taken in the wake of the *Columbia* disaster to make the operation of the ISS itself safer. This report candidly concedes there is clearly room for improvement, including the need for more and better inspections of space-station wiring, equipment and outside surfaces, docking, improved shielding against orbiting debris, and more complete monitoring of problems. The details presented in the remainder of this section confirm that many serious safety concerns do exist, with or without the shuttle in docked position [5].

3) *There are programmatic questions concerning both the space shuttle and the ISS. (These include issues of technological obsolescence as both of these programs have stretched out years longer than originally intended.)* A large-scale space station was planned to be fully deployed in 1991/1992 when first announced by President Reagan. Then when the project was international-ized and became the International Space Station the objective was to finish it by 1994. (The 1994 date for completion was in the Paine commission report in 1986 that warned of the program, cost, and safety dangers of pro-longing the program and its completion date.) Now, rather incredibly, the estimated completion date for the ISS has been extended to 2010 or per-haps later. There are obvious questions as to whether the space shuttle or the ISS are still programmatically valid and safe given the rate of technical innovation in the past 20 years. Extensive program extensions, launch delays, and a host of production and testing problems have devoured a string of projected completion dates with a seemingly insatiable appetite.

4) The completion and servicing of the ISS is the prime reason driving the return to flight of the space shuttle. *This raises many questions related to human space safety and at many different levels. Most fundamentally there is a question as to whether this is still a rea-sonable major goal for the U.S. space pro-gram for the next six years, not only in terms of safety but also in terms of research and exploration goals. Thus* there are questions not only with regard to the adequacy of ISS safety at the level of mechanical design and operational and management proce-dures but also whether there are safer alternatives to the completion of the full-scale ISS such as scaling down the project. In fact, if there are cur-rently no compelling reasons to return the shuttle to flight except to com-plete and service the ISS, the question obviously arises whether this is an appropriate set of alternative goals for the United States as well as its space allies that could be accomplished other than continuing to try to upgrade the shuttle to meet human flight conditions?

The shuttle and the ISS are thus now directly interrelated and pro-grams that many space experts have directly or indirectly questioned. Further, some of the vulnerabilities concerning the shuttle, already exam-ined in Chapter 3, clearly relate to the ISS as well. These concerns include radiation, debris, micrometeoroids, shuttle docking with the ISS, and need for and risk of various EVAs.

Putting ISS Design for Safety and Effectiveness into Context

Clearly NASA, ever since the start of manned space exploration, has given priority to safety and especially to the needs of coping with the hazards represented by radiation, the cold, the vacuum, and the near-zero gravity of outer space. These safety needs have limited the approaches that could be prudently employed in building a space station for human habitation and has fueled some scientists' conviction that it makes sense to send robots and machines that are immune to the needs of life-support systems into space to explore the unknown wherever and whenever possible.

There are certainly many questions that leap to the fore if one looks at the ISS from a broader overview perspective. These broad-brush questions include not only what is to be accomplished with the ISS and how can it be made safer, but also how to design and build better and safer space systems for the longer-term future? These questions range from design and engineering changes to basic issues such as whether the current operation of the ISS with just two crew members can be considered safe [6].

The ISS Memoranda of Understanding signed by NASA with the international partners says nothing, specifically or generally, about safety responsibilities and roles for certification of commercial hardware and services. Key safety experts from the European Space Agency have suggested the creation of a unified ISS Safety Authority, and discussion of this subject is addressed further in Chapter 7 [7].

Concerns addressed in the *Columbia* Accident Investigation Board (CAIB) report, especially in recommendations R7.5-1 and R7.5-2, suggest that lack of safety control and standardization was an area of astronaut safety concern.* Certainly there are astronaut safety concerns with the ISS today at many levels.

For instance, NASA decided to dispatch a new crew to the ISS after formally taking into account serious concerns expressed by safety officers. With the breakdown of the oxygen generator onboard in early September 2004 and the need for an emergency EVA by both of the remaining crew members onboard to repair the gyro stabilization system, it seems clear that safety margins onboard the ISS today are extremely thin and that these earlier warnings were indeed valid [6] and that U.S. and Russian perspectives as to the stringency of safety precautions to be observed on the ISS are not always in complete agreement [8].

NASA has defended ISS safety in a series of hearings and press forums over the past few years, going back to the early 2000s. This was responding to a stinging rebuke by safety experts and even astronauts who have suggested that the inattention to safety and the granting of waivers that doomed the Space Shuttle *Columbia* will continue to plague the orbital platform as well. Ed Lu, an astronaut aboard the station, was quoted in a Reuters interview saying: "Of course, the culture at NASA is the same culture that is involved in the Space Shuttle and space station, so probably some of the lessons learned there will apply to the station."†

We will shortly return to the specifics of ISS safety concerns which astronaut Lu's remarks only seem to imply. These concerns relate, among

---

*Data available online at http://www.nasa.gov/CAIB.
†Data available online at http://www.cnn.cdm/2003/TECH/Space/10/24/ Station.Safety. [cited 24 Oct. 2003].

other things, to environmental control systems, leak detectors, monitoring of noxious gases, gyro-stabilization systems, wiring issues, oxygen generators, GPS navigational capabilities, video monitors, communications and information systems, health-support systems, software issues, and fly-by-wire operations (i.e., total ground control of the ISS) when only two astronauts are onboard the ISS and both must do an emergency space walk.‡

These types of problems have been of ongoing concern, not only in terms of ISS operations, but translating lessons learned to the design of future space systems. As NASA turns its attention to Project Constellation it should indeed focus on translating ISS safety issues into ways to design for longer-term missions to the moon and Mars. Thus the questions become how to design better systems for the future that are safer, more cost effective, and with better defined research or survival goals? With the latest technology, could smaller and more viable low-Earth-orbit systems be deployed and sustained, while proceeding to create a permanent lunar colony? Are their better sites for extended space experimentation such as one of the Lagrangian points (e.g., L2), which provide low-thrust access to anywhere in the solar system? There have even been proposals to create a private international consortium to undertake the creation of a permanent international lunar colony, perhaps based on the model of Intelsat, that could undertake the long-term lunar project and thus free NASA to concentrate on exploratory roles. Long-time NASA employee and lunar expert Wendell Mendell has led the way in exploring such options for the future [9]. The private lunar colony approach not only represents a safety issue but also presents both financial planning and budgetary issues and opportunities. Certainly, the model for safety becomes much different if a private international entity undertakes this role as opposed to this massive longer-term undertaking being the sole responsibility of NASA.

Review of ISS System Management Including Minimum Crew Size

The design and management of the ISS has been an issue of some controversy for over a decade within the U.S. Congress and by many space science critics. Cost overruns, safety concerns, substantial schedule delays, the grounding of the shuttle after the *Columbia* accident, the stresses and strains of international partnerships, software problems, slow leaks of air, gyroscopic problems, and disputes over contractor support contracts are just some of the issues that have plagued the ISS. This has led to questions about its scope and purpose and the value of the experimental and exploratory aims of the ISS, even among some of its supporters in scientific and legislative circles. Today, the ISS is to be completed in 2010 at the earliest. Proper management and control processes need to be examined to make sure that safety risks are minimized as efforts to cut costs are sought by NASA, OMB, and Congress as well as by the international partners involved.

---

‡Data available online at http://www.cnn.cdm/2003/TECH/Space/10/24/Station.Safety. [cited 24 Oct. 2003].

Most recently there have been questions about the size of the ISS crew needed to maintain its safe operation and to conduct viable experiments of sufficient scale to justify its multibillion investment—as well as the lives lost in the *Challenger* and *Columbia* accidents. The status of the ISS will likely not be clear until well after the ISS partners meet in 2006 to review revised plans for the station deployment in coming months. The *Washington Post* summed up the current approach to the ISS management and operation as follows:

> The Bush plan decrees that the Shuttles will operate again only for the limited purpose of completing construction of the space station. This is a job that NASA officials plan, according to aerospace industry insiders, to streamline by eliminating as many of the existing requirements and commitments as possible—those that do not feed the new vision of exploring the solar system. This includes consultations with the international Partners in the space station, which will be afforded a kind of "escape clause" enabling them to scrap some previous commitments, an industry representative said [10].

Astronaut John Glenn, in a speech at the new Smithsonian National Air and Space Museum facility near Dulles Airport in June 2004, strongly questioned NASA's current plans for ISS operation and management and especially the cutback of experiments. He asked what was the logic of large-scale reduction of earlier scheduled ISS testing and experimentation programs when this was the reason why the nearly $100-billion asset was put in orbit in the first place? He stated that a crew of two could barely maintain the ISS in operation and would have virtually no time for experimentation. He also questioned the logic of going to the moon if Mars was the objective because 85% of the propulsive force needed to go Mars was needed to go to the Moon [11].

NASA, in its 2005 budget, sought $800 million in new funding for its new "Moon, Mars and Beyond" mission but has also sought to free up an additional $450 million in 2005 by eliminating space-station research not tied to the new exploration vision, as well as by postponing several science satellite projects and freezing certain research and development spending. Although NASA was one of only a few agencies not to have its budget cut, it did not receive the sizable new authorizations it desired either [12]. The White House proposal for 2007 contains funds for shuttle flights, a repair and servicing mission to the Hubble, ISS operations, and an aggressive continuation of Project Constellation. Congressional approval will be needed to sustain this nearly $17 billion budget.

Beyond the clarification of NASA's management and strategic policy with regard to the ISS, the further issue of what is a safe and viable number of astronauts or cosmonauts to operate the ISS also remains very much in question. The survey carried out by the GWU study team showed a strong majority of respondents believed that the minimal crew should be three and that a larger crew of four to five was really needed to achieve a strong experimental program. As a result of the ISS partners' meeting in 2005, it was agreed that a minimum staff of four astronauts would support ISS operations as soon as shuttle operations are restored [13].

In February 2004, NASA released a 172-page internal audit that noted a number of problems with ISS safety issues that ranged from limited to inadequately trained ground control staff, wiring issues, software issues related to ISS control, and operation to management concerns. Although the report "offered no examples of any breakdowns or other problems that are not being adequately tracked," it suggested that a detailed and critical analysis of trends "is seriously lacking" and that there was a lack of trained staff to project future safety or operational hazards [14].

These expressed concerns became more tangible when there was debate between the U.S. and Russian partners as to whether an EVA or spacewalk was necessary to carry out a number of tasks. Such an operation requires that ground controllers take over the operation of the ISS and that both crew members exit the ISS to provide backup to each other. Although some 50 such EVAs have been successfully completed by Russian cosmonauts while onboard the Mir, this had never been done in U.S. space programs or with the much larger and complex ISS. A NASA engineer and health expert was quoted off the record as questioning the safety of the current situation by suggesting that space agency officials are "...considering the station to be in a contingency mode because we only have a two-man crew, therefore we can rewrite all the previous safety rules that would be violated to allow the EVA to proceed." This same individual suggested that he viewed what was happening as "risk creep" [15].

Russian ground controllers oversaw the operation while the astronauts undertook the spacewalk. It involved the collection of science experiments from the exterior of the ISS and preparing the ISS for docking with the European Space Agency's automated transfer vehicle (ATV) and the Russian Progress freighters.

The risks associated with two astronauts being outside the ISS on an EVA while automated control is provided from the ground are certainly not inconsequential. Risks identified by NASA operators include the following: 1) possible loss of the ISS orientation in space (in part because several internal systems must be shut down during the EVA, including the vernier jets that maintain orientation, which must be shut down during the EVA to protect the astronauts from contamination); 2) loss of power (in part a consequence of loss of orientation); 3) loss of control of onboard power, heating or cooling (again part a consequence of loss of orientation); 4) possible inability to repressurize the air lock; 5) possible onboard fire without astronauts being able to respond to this occurrence; 6) possible loss of air pressure caused by puncture without astronauts being able to respond to this occurrence; and 7) catastrophic failure of the astronaut space suits.

It is recommended, therefore, that NASA reevaluate the risks associated with full robotic control of the ISS without crew members being aboard and publish a report on this subject prior to authorizing another operation of this type.

Escape Systems and Strategies

Escaping from and especially abandoning the space station is considered a last resort for NASA and the ISS partners. Studies have shown that there is a 50% chance the station would be destroyed within a year if there were no crew onboard to rectify problems, although there has been ever-increasing knowledge about how to operate the ISS remotely with no crew aboard for short-duration EVAs. NASA managers have stated that they will not hesitate to order the evacuation of the crew if they are at risk, but doing so could result in the loss of the $100-billion station if this were to be of a long duration.§

The main circumstances that NASA has identified that would warrant the crew evacuating the station include medical emergencies that require evacuation within 24 hours as a result of serious injury or illness of a crew member, station emergencies that require immediate evacuation as a result of structural and/or life-support failure, and logistics interruptions that require a planned evacuation as a result of a resupply failure.

If a problem or emergency arises on the ISS, the crew onboard first has to comprehend the situation and identify the necessary actions to be taken. As long as the crew is not in immediate risk, all options are considered before evacuation of the station. During a medical emergency, it will first be determined if the crew member can be successfully treated onboard, or if a station emergency arises the crew will determine if they can fix the problem or isolate the problematic area.¶ This decision-making process was displayed in the case of the Russian Mir station in June 1997, when a Progress spacecraft collided with the Mir space station. The collision caused a leak in the Spektr module, which subsequently lost air pressure and had to be sealed off from the rest of the station. This action saved the station and allowed operations to continue.**

If a crew determines that an evacuation is necessary, they would collect and don the suits they would wear for reentry via the Soyuz vehicle, gather any injured or incapacitated crew members, and then assemble and move to the crew escape vehicle for evacuation. Considerations that could affect the evacuation and increase the risk to the crew include the following:

1) The first consideration is if the evacuation route to the lifeboat is inaccessible. A fire aboard Mir in February 1997 blocked access to the Soyuz escape vehicle, which luckily was ultimately not required.

2) Next is the ability of a seriously injured crew member to put on a space suit and navigate their way on to the crew return vehicle.

---

§Data available online at http://www.space.com/missionlaunches/ft_station_disaster_040607.html [cited 7 June 2004].
¶Data available online at http://aeromedical.org/Articles/PDF_files/ISS_Crew_Rescue.pdf.
**Data available online at http://www.pbs.org/newshour/bb/science/jan-june97/mir_6-25.html.

3) The third condition to consider is the psychological state of the crew. A prolonged time in the space environment might affect the ability of the crew to work efficiently in a life-threatening situation.

4) The last consideration is the ease and efficiency of navigating to the escape lifeboat.

Presently the only escape option for the crew of the ISS is to evacuate with the use of the Soyuz lifeboat, and that has certain limitations. Only if an upgraded Soyuz with expanded crew-carrying capability were ordered from Russia, under new enabling legislation from Congress, could a full crew be accommodated.[††]

Although the Soyuz has shown its reliability as a crew-transport spacecraft in recent years, it is not the ideal vehicle for an evacuation role. The bell-shaped reentry module measures less than 2.3 m in both diameter and length, limiting the room and comfort levels for the escaping crew. An evacuation caused by a medical emergency could be difficult, as the sick or injured crew member would have to wear a space suit during reentry and sit in an uncomfortable cramped position. There is also no medical equipment onboard for resuscitation, defibrillation, or administering drugs.[‡‡]

The reentry profile of the Soyuz is also fixed and might require the spacecraft to spend more time in orbit before reentry. The capsule design also contributes to a rougher reentry and harder landing that could be a concern when returning injured crew members.

The X-38 crew return vehicle (CRV), developed between 1995 and 2002, would have supplied a greater escape capacity than the current Soyuz. This craft was designed to be capable of carrying seven crew members. The X-38 would have provided a more comfortable ride and was more suitable for transporting injured astronauts. The X-38's lifting-body design and steerable parafoil would have allowed the CRV to land practically any-where, providing easier access to medical facilities for injured crew members. Fully automated controls would have allowed the vehicle to be controlled by flight controllers on Earth, negating the reduced performance by crew members experiencing psychological or physical difficulties. The X-38 program was cancelled in April 2002 because of budget cuts.

The evacuation of the ISS would be a major safety risk to the crew and could result in the loss of the station. Although it can be statistically predicted when a medical or station emergency might cause an evacuation, in reality it could happen at any time. Although the Soyuz can accommodate the evacuation of the crew, it is a 30-year-old design and not entirely suited in this role. The use of the Soyuz will have to continue as the ISS lifeboat, however, until NASA or one of the ISS partners can develop a

---

[††]Data available online at http://spaceflight.nasa.gov/station/assembly/ elements/soyuz/index.html [cited 18 June 2003].

[‡‡]Data available online at http://www.exn.ca.

The use of the Soyuz will have to continue as the ISS lifeboat, however, until NASA or one of the ISS partners can develop a functioning crew return vehicle (or crew exploration vehicle) that can serve this function.

functioning crew return vehicle (or crew exploration vehicle) that can serve this function. The contract that was negotiated by NASA with the Russian Federal Space Agency in December 2005 for the supply of additional Soyuz/Progress spacecraft likely means the end of any consideration of a U.S. crew return vehicle capability until the CEV system is available in 2012 or so [16].

This new agreement with Russia became possible when NASA was empowered by new U.S. legislation signed in 2005 to reach a new agreement with the Russian Federal Space Agency (i.e., Roskosmos) for the purchase of additional Soyuz vehicles rather than the "barter" arrangements that had been used previously with regard to the construction of the ISS. This legislation, in particular, granted NASA an exception to the Iran Nonproliferation Act of 2000 that prevents the purchase of equipment from Russia because of nuclear-related trade between Russia and Iran. The new legislation, signed into law in midyear 2005, now allows NASA to purchase Soyuz craft outright. Thus it seems that the ISS will be dependent on the Soyuz as the escape lifeboat for the foreseeable future.§§

As discussed in the *Guardian* newspaper of the United Kingdom on 15 January 2004, "The Bush plan could leave a gap of up to five years between the retirement of the shuttle and before the launch of the CEV, leaving NASA with no manned craft for that period." This has now been overtaken by events because of pressure in the U.S. Senate, and thus the target date to develop a CEV and CRV capable of flying astronauts to the ISS has been moved up to a target date of year end 2012. Thus Russian space vehicles will, for some time to come, represent the only means for human flight to and from the ISS as long as the shuttle fleet remains grounded. (*Author's note:* the European ATV and the Japanese HTV only provide ascent and not descent capability, except for trash disposal. Although these craft could be upgraded to human flight capabilities to and from the ISS, there are no current plans to do so, and even if such steps were undertaken this capability would likely not be available before 2012. In a strategic sense this gives Russia enormous influence over the ISS and its use and also impacts the overall strategic balance in U.S. and Russia relationships.)¶¶,***

The multination participation in the ISS has proceeded from the outset with the understanding that the United States would not fund the

§§Data available online at http://washingtontimes.com/up-breaking/ 20040421-121152-9548r.htm [cited 21 April 2004].
¶¶Data available online at http://www.cnn.com/2003/TECH/space/10124/ station.safety/ [cited 24 Oct. 2003].
***Data available online at http://www.astronautix.com/craft/esahicle.htm.t.

activities of the other nations. In short everything was done on the basis of "barter," namely, I will do this part if you will do another part. Thus, no provision had previously been made within the NASA budget planning process for any financial support for the Russians to continue these transport functions. The absence of explicit mutual commitments between the international community and especially the United States, which has already borne the major ISS cost burden, means that the Russians were in a very strong bargaining position with regard to the new Soyuz/Progress purchases. The fact that neither NASA nor Roskosmos released the prices of the Russian vehicles suggest that the prices were likely high [16].

In the recently disclosed purchase of the Soyuz vehicles, there was no indication as to whether there had been discussions about the possible future procurement of an expanded Soyuz/Progress design to accommodate a full crew. The alternative is the reactivation of the X-38 program, but this does not seem to be a viable option given the major cost overruns associated with bringing the space shuttle back to flight status. The bottom line is that because the Soyuz return capsule can accommodate only two, or possibly at most three, astronauts, the ability of the ISS to sustain a crew of four or more and have a CRV available would return there being two Soyuz/Progress units available at the ISS at all times.

Backup, Redundancy, and Fail-Safe Measures

There is no risk-free activity. The International Space Station is clearly a safer orbital craft than its predecessors in terms of life-support systems, margins of error, and redundancy in key systems and subsystems, etc. Nevertheless there are still subsystems that could fail and disable the ISS, all of the way from limited operations up to catastrophic failures. Scientists and engineers have argued that several systems should wisely be given greater redundancy, such as the oxygen generator and carbon-dioxide reduction system. There has also been concern about improved escape capabilities, improved capabilities to withstand intense solar radiation storms, improved airlock systems, improved onboard health care and remote medical systems, air and water-monitoring systems, upgraded broadband communications and IT systems, and more effective ways to provide thrust to keep the ISS in its proper orbit. All of these issues are addressed next and in Appendix D.

Potential Terrorist Threats

The possibility of a terrorist threat to either the space shuttle or the ISS seems remote to most people involved in the U.S. space program because the space shuttle facilities are reasonably well protected and that once in space the vehicles are physically remote from any would-be attackers. The nature of possible attacks on the ISS must be broken down into various elements.

As far as physical attack on the ISS is concerned, there are, in fact, several possibilities. It might be possible for an explosive or more likely a poisonous gas canister to somehow be smuggled onto a resupply mission coming either from the United States or Russia with a timer or remote triggering of such a device. Although this seems unlikely, protection measures should be undertaken against such possibilities originating from either a U.S. or Russian launch site (or in the future a European or even Japanese launch site).

It would seem desirable for systematic tracking and screening of all elements that are launched on ISS missions or resupply craft to be undertaken. This would be at all launch sites around the world with cargo or crew going to the ISS and would be carried out from the perspective of screening for terrorist implements and devices rather than simple inventory control.

Secondly, docking of the ISS with another vehicle is a delicate operation and if there were spurious signals generated to override the controls associated with the mating of the space station with another launch system, then the potential for harm to both the ISS and the other vehicle is great. Thus a thorough review should be made with regard to the possibility of enhancing redundancy and encryption, improved subroutine software, upgraded laser guidance hardware, and/or additional manual override capabilities related to docking systems. These design and operational changes would allow aborting the mating process on an instantaneous basis whether because of a software problem, an operator or mechanical error, incorrect laser instrument readings, or even a terrorist attempt to jam communications and IT transmissions at a critical time. Likewise, similar precautions should be taken against spurious commands that might be sent when the ISS is operating by remote control by ground operators (i.e., fly-by-wire) while astronauts are engaged in a spacewalk. All such possibilities should be carefully reviewed and design adjustments made if these are feasible and programmatically viable.

Thirdly, and seemingly most unlikely, it is possible that there could be some form of in-orbit attack. It has been suggested that a modified SCUD missile with an additional stage added or some other launcher in terrorist hands could possibly take a small payload of ball bearings, nails, etc. all of the way to loop around the moon. It would then return to Earth orbit in a transverse direction to release a deadly rain of debris that would have sufficient relative velocity to destroy or greatly damage the ISS and many communications or remote-sensing satellites as well. Such a deadly intent, if not detected before launch, would be extremely hard to stop once the payload was on it way to the moon. Such a type of mission, if it constituted an attack on the geosynchronous orbit, rather than low Earth orbit, could potentially destroy the tracking and data relay satellite (TDRS) system on which NASA operations and control of the space station greatly depends. Although this type of attack has been discounted by NASA engineers, it is included as a reminder that terrorist attacks can often take unconventional approaches that are difficult to anticipate.

Fourthly, the most likely terrorist threat of all would be an attack on ground-based control centers for the ISS, especially at a critical period such as during a rocket or thruster firing. Clearly perimeter security is needed at all control facilities around the world.

The most likely of all types of terrorist attacks on the ISS is one in which the tracking, telemetry and command functions are subject to either a virus in the control software, a jamming of tracking, telemetry, and command (TT&C) signals, or the overload of IT transmissions so that key communications could not get through on one or more of the channels reserved for this purpose. There could even be an attempt to send spurious commands to the ISS for it to vent oxygen, turn on or off heating or cooling systems, or misfire the gyro control systems. This would be difficult to accomplish because of encryption and other reverification controls that exist, but improved security is nevertheless advisable.

The extent to which IT and telecommunications channels are protected against such cyberattacks needs to be reexamined, security codes for such systems frequently updated, and overrides possible in near real time if alert alarms should sound. Commercial satellite systems have protected their spacecraft by requiring not only coded commands, but also by requiring ground instructions for the firing of stabilization jets to be authenticated at other TTC&M facilities. A review of protective best practices among U.S. civil and defense agencies, to ensure not only the security of the ISS but of other U.S. space assets, would seem advisable.

Safety Issues Resulting from the International Aspects of the Program

Russia and the United States currently represent the two major partners who participate in the launch and assembly of the ISS and thus play a key role in the management and control of its operations. The European Space Agency (ESA), the Japanese Aerospace Exploration Agency (JAXA), the Canadian Space Agency (CSA) are also key partners, and they have assumed specific roles for the construction of specific subsystems or tasks. All partners have invested billions of dollars into the project.

Further, from the outset, all partners have been vitally involved in the overall design, payload delivery, assembly, and operation of the ISS. Nevertheless, at times some partners have felt relegated to a secondary role. With the operation of the new European ATV in early 2006, the role of ESA, both in a substantive and literal sense, will be "elevated" [17].

When so many partners share critical joint responsibilities over a long period of time with investments totaling many billions of dollars, it is not surprising that disputes have arisen. In particular, this has occurred between NASA and the Russian Space Agency (RSA) (now known as Roskosmos) over what are considered to be safe ISS operations. Since the *Columbia* disaster, NASA has given new attention to ensuring the safety of operations onboard the ISS. Roskosmos, with many more years of onboard experience with space-station operations, considers itself "more flexible."

Sergei Gorbunov, a spokesman for Roskosmos, said the following on this topic: "Here in Russia, we are more flexible in our approach to technical problems .... The Americans are more conservative in dealing with technical problems, but this isn't a fault."[ttt]

An incident occurred in 2002, which highlights the differences in the approach to ISS operations between the two agencies. This incident was related to a set of batteries that the Russian Space Agency had installed on the ISS. It was revealed that the batteries had not been properly tested against approved test procedures. NASA believed there was a small possibility they could explode. The batteries never did cause an open dispute, but the batteries were installed despite NASA's objections [18].

Two additional incidents also suggest a problem of miscommunications or difference in approach to safety as seen from the NASA and the Russian perspective. In fact, members of NASA's ASAP safety oversight group resigned in September of 2003. In their resignation, they cited two incidents of miscommunications between Russia and the United States and how this resulted in the improper positioning of the station in orbit [19].

There is evidence that both NASA and Russia have learned from these incidents and are making changes to improve communications, to ensure proper system and subsystem testing, and to better manage the effects of these differences in philosophy with regard to ISS operations by the two agencies. Arthur Zygielbaum, a former NASA safety advisory board member said, "Since the batteries incident, complaints or concerns can be taken up the command chain more quickly." Even so, there does seem to be a different type of approach to safety issues. Shirley McCarty, former head of NASA's safety advisory board has stated the issue as follows: "It's a different philosophy. In the U.S. program you must prove it safe. The Russian approach is 'prove it's not safe'" [19]. The indication that comes from interviews conducted by the author is that this difference of approach continues, and this represents yet another reason in favor of the creation of an international entity with integrated authority to deal with critical safety issues. This is discussed in greater detail in Chapter 7, which addresses international space programs.

International Modules and Components of the ISS

The International Space Station is one of the largest international collaborative projects in recorded history. As described earlier, in addition to the United States, major forms of participation come from the Europe, Japan, Canada, and Russia. This international participation is reflected not only in the design and construction of the ISS in terms of its various components but also in terms of a high level of international experimentation. The major components of the ISS are as outlined here:

[ttt]Data available online at http://www.space.com/missionlaunches/ ap_iss_031110.html [cited 10 Nov. 2003].

1) **Europe:** Columbus European laboratory, automated transfer vehicle
2) **Japan:** Japan experiments module (known as Kibo), H2 transfer vehicle, and centrifuge accommodation module (CAM)
3) **Canada:** Canadarm2 and manipulator
4) **Russia:** Progress IM/Soyuz flights to the ISS, space suits, environmental systems, batteries and other components plus ground control and command centers
5) **United States:** rest of the ISS system (including shuttle launches for assembly and operations).

The international participation in this multibillion-dollar project is certainly beneficial in terms of spreading costs for this huge undertaking. The scope and scale of the undertaking would certainly have been far less without international participation, which is detailed further in Chapter 7.

Without the United States and Russia, there would not have been the capability to launch and integrate such a large structure in space. Further, Russian capacity to launch and resupply the crew and maintain the ISS in a proper orbit during the periods the shuttle has been grounded has been critical. The total shuttle grounding period as a result of *Challenger* and *Columbia* is now greater than six years. In the case of the loss of the *Challenger* in 1986, the hiatus was 2.5 years. In the case of the loss of the *Columbia* in 2003, the downtime has been more than three years, and the clock is still running. The shuttle was grounded from February 2003 through August 2005. Then after STS-114 in August 2005, it was again grounded and is likely to remain so at least through midyear 2006.

Uncertain Future for the ISS?

The ISS is currently 15 years behind schedule, its technology and subsystems are in many ways obsolete, the nature of space research and exploration objectives have changed greatly since the space station was conceived, and it will be hugely expensive to finish and maintain. The ISS and the space shuttle thus are in many ways precious "white elephants" that are too costly to abandon and too costly to operate. When the U.S. government is faced with a million-dollar problem, it can simply bury it and chart a new course. But the International Space Station at a projected total cost of $100 billion and an aging fleet of three space shuttle orbiters cannot be quietly discarded or swept under a "miscellaneous write off" at the end of the year audit.

Neither NASA, nor Congress, nor the White House took the good advice of the Rogers and the Payne commission in 1986 to develop a new space vehicle as soon as possible and to finish up the International Space Station as quickly as possible.

As Professor Logsdon has said, it took the *Columbia* accident to move NASA's space program back on a correction course, after 35 years of pursuing a space policy that had serious flaws. A new set of space vehicles, a new set of space goals, and an attempt to put a brave face on finishing the ISS and grounding the Space Shuttle reflects today's new reality. In moving forward, it is crucial to make sure that no more space accidents nor international misunderstandings further erode attempts to chart a new way forward for U.S. and international space exploration. In this respect the concerns that are set forth in Tables 5.1 and 5.2 and Appendix D are worth serious consideration.

References

[1] "NASA to Use Russian Spaceships for Flights to ISS," *Astro News*, 28 Dec. 2005, URL: http://www.astroexpo.com/news/newsdetail.asp?ID=23444& ListType=TopNews&StartDate=12/26/2005&EndDate=12/30/2005.

[2] Berger, B., "NASA: Finishing Station with ELVs Would Cost More, Take Longer," *Space News*, 10 May 2004, p. 8.

[3] Gugliotta, G., "Foam Cracks May Delay Shuttle Launch," *Washington Post*, 2 Dec. 2005, p. A3.

[4] Schwartz, J., "Minority Report Faults NASA as Compromising Safety," *New York Times*, 18 Aug. 2005, p. A15.

[5] "NASA Report on ISS Safety," NASA Headquarters, NASA-SP 2018 Washington, DC, 3 March 2004.

[6] Recer, P., "New Station Crew Was Launched Despite Safety Warnings," *Associated Press*, 23 Oct. 2003, URL: http://www.space.com/ missionlaunches/exp8_ap_031023.html.

[7] Sgobba, T., and Chiesa, S., "Toward an International Space Station Safety Authority?" International Astronautical Federation, Bremen, Germany, Oct. 2002.

[8] "Space Station's Safety Defended," *Reuters*, 1 Oct. 2003, URL: http://www. smh.com.au/articles/2003/99/30/1064819931106.html.

[9] Mendell, W., "Mediations on the New Space Vision: The Moon as Stepping Stone to Mars," International Astronautical Academy, Paper IAA 3.7.1.01, Oct. 2004.

[10] "NASA Revises Plans for the International Space Station," *The Washington Post*, 1 Feb. 2004, p. A3.

[11] John Glenn presentation, Remarks at the Smithsonian National Air and Space Exhibit Facility, Dulles, VA, 10 June 2004.

[12] "Reduction in Space Station Research Projects," *Space News*, 9 Feb. 2004, p. 7.

[13] de Selding, P., "Partners Agree to ISS Crews of 'More than Three: Details Sketchy,'" *Space News*, 23 July 2004, p. 6, URL: www.space.com/mission launches/isscrew_040723.html.

[14] Dunn, M., "NASA Criticized on Space Station Safety," *Associated Press*, 27 Feb. 2004, URL: http://cnews.canoe.ca/CNEWS/sapce/2004/01/23/ pf-323158.html.

[15] Sawyer, K., "Crew to Exit Space Station in Exercise," *Washington Post*, 23 Feb. 2004, pp. A1, A9.

16 "NASA to Use Russian Spaceships for Flights to ISS," *Astro News*, 28 Dec. 2005, URL: http://www.astroexpo.com/news/newsdetail.asp?ID=23444& ListType= TopNews&StartDate=12/26/2005&EndDate=12/30/2005.

17 de Selding, P., "European Officials Skeptical of U.S. Space Motivation," *Space News*, 17 May 2004, p. 6.

18 Statement of Allen Li, Associate Director, National Security and International Affairs Div., "Space Station—Russian Compliance with Safety Requirements," U.S. GAO Testimony Before the Subcommittee on Space and Aeronautics Committee on Science, House of Representatives, GAO/T-NSIAD-00-128, Washington, DC, Aug. 2003.

19 Astronaut Safety Advisory Panel (ASAP), "White Paper on Operation of ISS with Two Crew Members 11 April 2003," Aeroscience and Flight Mechanics Div., Boeing Space and Defense Systems Flight Mechanics and Analysis, STS-81 LN-100G Report STS-86 LN-100G Addendum, Houston, TX, April 2003.

CHAPTER 6
NASA's Unsuccessful X-Projects and the Prospects for New Private Space Vehicle Development

"NASA has encountered difficult lessons and delays in key technology projects. We've learned that more development along multiple competing paths is needed. We've learned that commercial markets are not growing as previously projected. But there are still possibilities to make access to space more robust."

—Dr. Row Rogacki, Director of the Space Transportation Directorate at NASA's Marshall Space Flight Center in the year 2000 when announcing NASA's program to develop new reusable launch vehicle by 2010

Radical Change in Developing Launch Systems

This chapter examines NASA's series of attempts to develop new personal reusable space vehicles and escape vehicles for the post space shuttle era. For a variety of reasons, these various development programs, which were initiated one after the other over the past 15 years, all ended prematurely and unsuccessfully.

There were at least two projects to develop escape capabilities for astronauts, as represented by the HL-20 and X-38 programs, as well as four projects to develop a personal reusable launch vehicle including the so-called space plane or scramjet developments. In a way, all of these projects are parallel in that they inevitably ended at the prototype design or the early the testing phases before the programs could be successfully completed.

NASA's world and its attitude toward developing launch systems has changed radically in the past few years. Many factors have led to this change. First, none of the X-programs were successful, and the need to make something actually work this time is enormous. Second, NASA is now clearly concentrating on Project Constellation in response to a presidential mandate. Thus there is less worry that NASA might yet again take its eye off the need to develop a replacement for the shuttle, but at the same time concern that its three-fold mission of getting the shuttle to fly, completing the ISS, and going to the moon and Mars might stretch its resources too thin and create conflicting priorities. Third, NASA now intends to contract with industry to provide crew access to the International Space Station (ISS) and low-Earth-orbit missions. All of these factors lead to growing interest, new commercial support, and substantial capitalization efforts behind entrepreneurial aerospace companies willing and able to undertake at least a part of the NASA mission. Many of these entities are seeking to provide new commercial access to low Earth orbit, space tourism, ... and more. All

> We are seeing new, different, and outside-the-box thinking. Both the nature of space travel and the players in the space business are being redefined and rapidly so.

of these elements of change suggest that tomorrow's launchers within the world of space transportation are not like their father's Oldsmobile. We are seeing new, different, and outside-the-box thinking. Both the nature of space travel and the players in the space business are being redefined and rapidly so.

In the next decade, one can expect to see a number of new manned space vehicles flying into space not only in support of NASA missions, but to support other commercial ventures including space tourism and possibly private space stations. A decade ago the idea of space tourism seemed exotic, but now several wealthy individuals have done it. Indeed thousands have actually signed up with Sir Richard Branson's Virgin Galactic and Rocketplane Ltd. with the prospect of their flights occurring as early as sometime in 2008. These will be initially be suborbital flights but high enough to pass the 50-mile barrier to qualify as astronauts.

The history of the various NASA crew return vehicles and personal launch systems over the last 15 years or so plus the efforts of such innovative companies as Scaled Composites, SpaceDev, and SpaceX go a long way to explain where we have been, in trying to develop new space-vehicle capabilities, and perhaps some useful insights into where we are going.

Escape Vehicle for Astronauts: HL-20 Program

The HL-20 was developed as a low-Earth-orbit transportation system to complement the space shuttle and to provide an escape capability from the ISS. The key objectives of the program were to provide safe, reliable, and low-cost manned access to space. Designed to be part of a personal launch system (PLS), the HL-20 was to utilize an expendable booster to reach orbit and could accommodate eight passengers and two crew members.

Investigations into the design of the HL-20 began at Langley Research Center during the mid-1980s, but it was not until after the Space Shuttle *Challenger* accident in 1986 that the program began to mature rapidly. The planners of the HL-20 believed that an alternate vehicle would be needed to support the proposed Space Station Freedom (now the International Space Station) in the event that the shuttle was unavailable. The design evolved from the earlier lifting-body reusable launch vehicle (RLV) or the space planes from the 1960s and 1970s, namely, the M2-F2, HL-10, and X24.

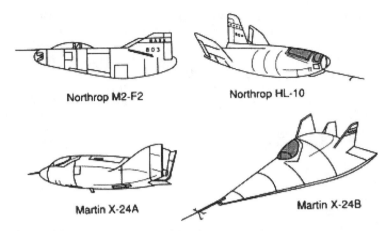

Figure 6-1   Lifting-body designs of the 1960s–1970 s.

Particular attention was also given to several aerodynamic features of the Russian BOR-4 that flew in the early 1980s to test thermal protection system (TPS) materials for the Soviet shuttle, the Boran (or alternatively the Buran). Figure 6.1 shows drawings of the previous lifting-body designs.

A significant amount of research and design went into the HL-20 in the late 1980s. A comprehensive aerodynamic and thermodynamic data-base was compiled, spanning the entire speed range the HL-20 would fly through. Several models were built, which showed that the lifting-body shape possessed good flying qualities in all flight regimes. Computational fluid dynamics (CFD) were used to study patterns of flow field phenom-ena, shock waves, and stability and control in regimes where wind tunnels could not duplicate the reentry environment. Extensive research was also conducted in flight and control to investigate the handling characteristics of the HL-20.

A full-size, nonflying engineering research model of the HL-20 was constructed by North Carolina State and North Carolina A&T Universities during 1990 for studying crew seating arrangements, ingress and egress, and equipment layout. The model provided the full-scale external and internal dimensions of the HL-20 for human factors research for the program.

During the early 1990s, the program was cancelled as the projected life-cycle cost of the HL-20 was estimated at approximately $2 billion. Instead, the now two-person configuration of the Russian Soyuz vehicle (with the possibility of three members in a true emergency) was chosen as the primary crew emergency vehicle or crew escape vehicle (CEV) that would service the space station in the event of the shuttle being unavailable. This CEV should not be confused with the current crew exploration vehicle that NASA is developing to go to the ISS, the moon, and eventually Mars.

The lack of crew capacity of the Soyuz severely limits its utility as a rescue vehicle, and indeed the shuttle remains the only effective escape system for a full crew of the ISS. (*Note*: There are proposals for an expanded Soyuz design that would allow for it to carry a full crew as well, but this has not been agreed or funded and the recent procurement of Soyuz/Progess vehicles by NASA as of December 2005 are of the conventional design with the 2.3-m capsule that accommodates two to three astronauts for return flights to the Earth. Likewise there have been thoughts of upgrading the European ATV so that it could return crew to the Earth's surface, but this major upgrade has not been funded either.)

Design Features

The HL-20 would have been much smaller than the space shuttle with an overall length of 29 ft (8.7 m) and wing span of 23.5 ft (6.9 m). It would have weighed 22,000 lb (10,000 kg) without crew compared to the shuttle empty weight of 185,000 lb (84,100 kg). With its wings folded, the HL-20 would actually fit inside the shuttle's payload bay, allowing transportation of the spacecraft to the space station. Figure 6.2 shows the size comparison between the HL-20 and the Space Shuttle.

To fully and effectively complement the space shuttle, the design of the HL-20 had to meet the following design characteristics: enhanced crew safety, low-cost operation, and ensured man access to space.

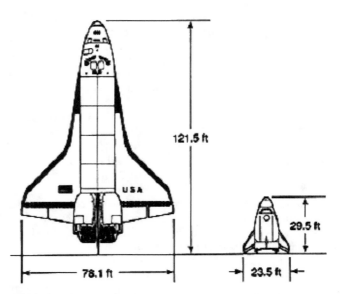

Figure 6-2   STS shuttle vs HL-20 (graphics courtesy Rockwell International Corporation).

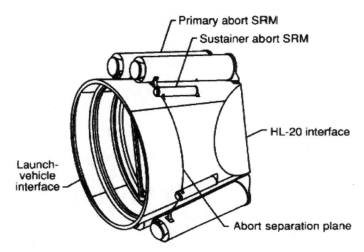

Figure 6-3 HL-20 launch escape system adaptor with abort motors (graphics courtesy of NASA).

Enhanced Crew Safety

Crew safety and survivability for various abort modes was of utmost importance during the design of the HL-20. The design did not have main propulsion engines or a large payload bay like the shuttle; thus, it was designed as a much smaller and more compact vehicle. This reduction in size made it more feasible to design an abort capability to safely recover the crew during critical phases of the launch and return from orbit. In short, it could carry crew to and from the ISS, but it was not a cargo-carrying vehicle.

On-the-pad emergencies (with the HL-20 mated to an expendable launch vehicle) were to have been accommodated in two ways, depending on the urgency of the situation. The interior layout had a ladder and hatch arrangement designed to allow rapid egress of the crew. This, of course, assumed that sufficient warning of an emergency would be available. In times of emergency such as a launch fire or explosion within the launch vehicle, the HL-20 was to be equipped with emergency solid rockets motors (SRMs) that could rapidly thrust the vehicle away from the launcher. Figure 6.3 shows the HL-20 launch escape system adaptor.

The ascent abort capability was studied for a launch from Titan Pad 40 at the Kennedy Space Center using a Titan III launch vehicle. Depending on the time of abort during ascent, the HL-20 was designed to have four abort-mode capabilities including the following:

1) **Return-to-launch site (RTLS)** is the first abort-mode capability. Prior to 20 s in the nominal ascent trajectory, the HL-20 must abort to the shuttle landing facility. From 20 to 64 s the HL-20 can abort to the Air

Force skid strip. After 64 s the HL-20 does not have sufficient energy for RTLS.

2) **The second is ocean landing by parachute.** For aborts initiated between 64 and 403 s, the HL-20 must land in the ocean by parachute. Similar to the Apollo program, a cluster of three parachutes would open to lower the vehicle to a safe landing.

3) **Transatlantic abort landing (TAL)** is the third abort-mode capability. After 403 s during nominal ascent, the first TAL site becomes available. The three space shuttle abort landing sites were chosen, namely, Amilcar Cabral, Banjul, and Roberts Field.

4) **The last capability is abort to orbit (ATO).** At 477 s after launch, the HL-20 can reach the nominal injection orbit of 50 n miles by 100 n miles. Nominal shutdown of the launch vehicle occurs at 495 s after launch [1–3].

The design of the HL-20 demonstrated complete ascent abort capabilities. The crew is saved throughout the ascent with the vehicle recovered intact in all abort modes with the exception of the ocean-landing mode. This is greatly superior to the space shuttle, where the crew basically has to "hang on" until the solid rocket boosters are spent. In the event that the shuttle cannot perform an RTLS or TAL, the crew would have to bail out of the shuttle's side hatch at approximately 20,000 ft. (i.e., about 6500 m)

During reentry, the large lift-to-drag ratio (L/D) of the lifting-body design would give the HL-20 great maneuverability, providing a cross-range capability of over 1000 n miles. This, combined with the capability to land on a 10,000-ft runway, would dramatically increase the number of landing opportunities. This would be important when returning sick, injured, or deconditioned space station crew to Earth as wheeled runway landings would be possible, permitting simple, precision recovery at many sites around the world [2].

Low-Cost Operation

Low-cost operation was imperative for the success of the HL-20 or any proposed PLS. The HL-20 was forecasted to have a low operating cost as it was designed for maintainability with the use of simplified subsystems and available technologies. The selection and design of subsystems would reduce the maintenance requirements, such as the elimination of main engines and payload bay, and the use of electric controls instead of hydraulic systems. One of the key elements of discussion and concern with regard to the HL-20 was that its TPS would be of a similar composition to the shuttle, but its much smaller size would significantly reduce inspection and maintenance times. The shuttle uses in excess of 24,000 ceramic tiles in its TPS with only 13% being similar in shape, whereas the HL-20 would have required only 1000 of which 70% are identical. Nevertheless, many believed that a ceramic-tile approach to thermal protection was not the best technology to use in terms of safety, reliability, and operational and maintenance cost. If this system were to be designed today, for instance, a metallic thermal protection system would likely be considered.

The vehicle could have been processed in a horizontal position with large exterior access panels permitting easy access for technicians working on the subsystems. These design changes and subsystem simplifications, along with the adoption of aircraft maintenance philosophies, were predicted to reduce the HL-20 processing man-hours to less than 10% of those used on the space shuttle [1].

Ensured Man Access to Space

At the time the HL-20 was being designed, it was viewed as essential that the United States have alternate means of getting people and valuable small cargo to low-Earth orbit and back should the space shuttle be unavailable. (*Note*: Currently this alternative access to space by a U.S. vehicle is not available, and apparently this will be the case for some years to come unless the X-38 program, as described next, were to be reinstated.) The primary mission of the HL-20 was thus envisioned to be to transport crew to and from the ISS. Other potential missions defined for a PLS include the orbital rescue of stranded astronauts, priority delivery and observation missions, and missions to perform satellite servicing. The HL-20 was modular in design. This would have allowed simple reconfiguration of the spacecraft to complete different missions. The basic design would remain unchanged, but interior subsystems and arrangements could be changed according to crew accommodations, duration, and equipment required for the particular mission. The HL-20 could also be attached to different launch vehicles depending on the specifications of the mission. The enhanced crew safety and high utilization potential of the HL-20 would have been ideal for many missions where it might have substituted for the shuttle and rendered substantial savings [3].

The HL-20 was designed in the mid-1980s and into the early 1990s to fill a perceived gap in the national space program and to provide safe, ensured human access to space. The design focused on minimizing life-cycle costs of the system by insuring simple operations, low-cost manufacturing, and high utilization potential. Lance Bush, lead engineer during the design of the HL-20, when interviewed on the subject stated that he believed the strengths of the HL-20 were in its high maneuverability, modular design, and its ability to land on a 10,000-ft (3000-meter) runway. These factors, combined with complete ascent abort capabilities, would have enhanced the safety for the crew and increased their survivability during an emergency [4].

The very high cost to actually build and deploy the HL-20 at an estimated $2 billion, at a time when the space shuttle and the ISS were making large claims on NASA's budget, was apparently the prime reason for the cancellation of this program. Yet today, in comparison to the projected cost of developing the crew exploration vehicle, the HL-20 program would seem to be very cost effective.

X-38 Lifting Body and Renewed Efforts to Develop a Crew Return Vehicle

It is unclear as to the extent to which the X-38 evolved as a follow on to the HL-20 program (developed out of the Ames Research Center) or as result of work that the Johnson Space Center had been conducting on lifting bodies since the 1960s. In any event, the X-38 program was initiated after the closeout of the HL-20 program, even though the HL-20 program had been fully prototyped. The ostensible purpose of the X-38 was to develop further the technologies required for a prototype emergency CRV for the ISS. The objective was to take advantage of commercial-off-the-shelf (COTS) technology for 80% of the vehicle. It was thus optimistically estimated that the cost of the X-38 program would be less than 25% of the cost of the previous CRV program. Although initially intended as only a CRV, the project designers envisioned that the vehicle could be modified later for use as a crew transport vehicle, to be launched on the Ariane 5 booster or another launcher. Figure 6.4 shows an artist's impression of the X-38 returning from orbit.

The X-38 concept began in 1995 at the Johnson Space Center (JSC) using data from past lifting-body programs and with flight tests conducted on the basis of a steerable parafoil concept that could be used by the CRV during landing. In early 1996, a contract for the construction of two full-scale atmospheric test frames was awarded to Scaled Composites, Inc., with the first being delivered to JSC in September and the second in December 1996. Scaled Composites, Inc., the company of noted aerospace designer Burt Rutan, received an additional contract in

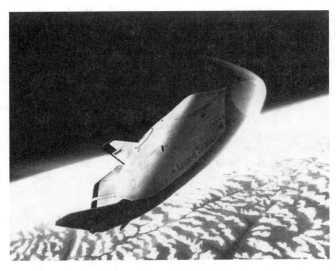

Figure 6-4   Artist's impression of an X-38 reentering the atmosphere (graphics courtesy of NASA).

October 1998 to modify the first X-38 demonstrator to incorporate the exact size and shape of the future CRV. All three prototypes were fitted with navigation, guidance, flight-control, and parachute deployment systems at JSC. From 1997 to 2001, the first three prototypes performed a series of captive-carry and free flights to test the vehicle's aerodynamics and stability characteristics during landing and the parachute's deployment and steering capabilities. A fourth X-38 was to be constructed at JSC and used for deorbit testing after being released from an orbiting shuttle. Two years short of completing the test-flight phase, NASA announced the cancellation of the X-38 program on 29 April 2002 as a result of budget pressures that were apparently largely associated with the ISS.

The X-38 design relied heavily upon the proven lifting-body shape of the X-23 and X-24A that were successfully tested in the 1960s. Extensive aerodynamic and heating characteristics were already measured from earlier wind-tunnel and flight tests. The use of parachute techniques developed by the Army for the landing phase simplified the internal systems and eliminated the need for pilot control. By combining the data from each of the programs and adding expertise gained from the space shuttle, the X-38 was able to merge many of the technologies needed for its planned missions.* Figure 6.5 shows a representation of the X-38 during landing with the aid of the steerable parafoil.

The X-38 design was to be used strictly as a CRV. It could have been modified later for use as a crew transport vehicle. It was to be equipped with only enough life-support supplies for nine hours free flying from the ISS in orbit. The X-38 was designed to be totally automated during landing, although the crew had the capability to switch to backup systems, control the orientation in orbit, pick a deorbit site, and steer the parafoil. The use of the steerable parafoil would have increased the safety of the crew over a conventional landing, as it would make the craft more maneuverable and drastically lower the speed upon landing. The X-38 had a nitrogen gas-fueled attitude control system and also included a bank of batteries for power. The CRV would have been able to transport a crew of seven. It was to have been 30 ft (or 9 m) long, 14.5 ft (or 4.4 m) wide, and represented a weight of a little over 20,000 lb (or 9100 kg). Many of these size characteristics were very similar to the HL-20.†

Previous programs to build a CRV, that is, the HL-20, estimated the total development cost to be over $2 billion. The use of available technology and off-the-shelf equipment significantly reduced the X-38's projected costs to an estimated $500 to $700 million for development and flight testing. This is a remarkably low cost for such a versatile vehicle and again quite significantly less than the projected costs of the crew exploration vehicle.

---

*Data available online at http://www.nasa.gov/missions/research/x38-main.html.
†Data available online at http://www.nasa.gov/missions/research/HL-20-main.html.

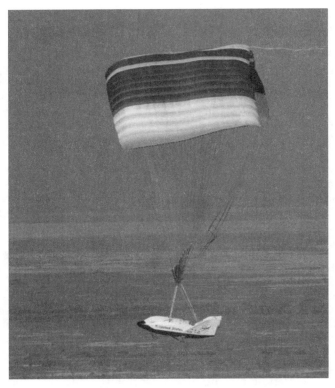

Figure 6-5   X-38 landing with the aid of a steerable parafoil (graphics courtesy of NASA).

The X-38 was an innovative project to develop the technologies for a crew return vehicle for the ISS. Although prematurely cancelled, the program showed that by using existing materials and technologies the cost of developing a functional CRV could be significantly reduced. With the current absence of the shuttle, the ISS is limited to a crew of two that can be only be evacuated with the use of the Soyuz in an extremely tight crew configuration. If operations on the ISS are to continue for the 2010–2020 time period, a vehicle such as the X-38, or a modified version of the Soyuz with expanded crew capability, should be available upon retirement of the space shuttle. NASA has recently issued, in January 2006, an RFP seeking bids from contractors to provide crew transport services. Time will tell the extent to which the responses from the aerospace industry will build on the experiences from the HL-20 and the X-38 vehicles in preparing their responses.

NASA has indicated to its international partners its plans to operate the ISS with a minimum crew of four, once the shuttle returns to flight on an ongoing basis. This commitment immediately highlights a problem of crew escape capability given the limited capacity of the Soyuz as an escape vehicle as currently configured. The dramatically different costs between the X-38 and the current CEV development program suggests that the use of more entrepreneurial approaches with off-the-shelf equipment, wherever possible, could lead to cost efficiencies in program developments.

RLVs and Space-Plane Development

NASA efforts to develop a second-generation RLV system that would be safer, more cost efficient, and better from virtually all program respects has been marked by a series of difficulties over the past decade.

Time after time there have been demonstration projects and systems studies of issues such as propulsion systems, escape vehicles, or safety requirements, but never has an actual RLV been fully developed. This is surprising in that it is now essentially 20 years after the Paine and Rogers commissions identified such a capability as a top priority for NASA.

The net result of resource claims by the shuttle and the ISS programs on NASA's budgets over the years has been to push all of the RLV programs further and further forward in time. This has undermined NASA's credibility about ever being able to deliver on any of its varying commitments to develop a safe RLV or to create a comprehensive space policy. The challenge of totally new technology and the need for safety clearly explains a good deal of these difficulties. Nevertheless, after the expenditure of billions of dollars during a period that now spans well over a decade, little tangible progress has been achieved. Lack of progress on these programs has not only undercut NASA's credibility but arguably has undercut support for future astronaut and exploration programs as well.

The programs to develop a new RLV have included the X-33, the X-34, the X-37, and X-43A.

In reviewing this complex history, it is hard to pick the most useful starting point, but because our focus is on safety one likely choice is March 2000, some six years ago. At that time, NASA's Marshall Space Flight Center published an official research announcement entitled "Second Generation RLV Risk Reduction Definition Program." It called for industry proposals as a first step in defining detailed requirements that would identify and even commence initial risk-reduction options, to enable a second-generation reusable-launch-vehicle competition in 2005. This was to lead *"to an operational system around 2010"* (emphasis added). This is worthy of note in that the under the presidential vision for space exploration announced in January 2004 the original objective for a proven flight-worthy version of the CEV was initially set for 2014. Only after major overhaul of the development schedule for this new vehicle, the NASA administrator has now said, in response to congressional pressure, that the vehicle "might" be ready by 2012. If the original plan unveiled in 2000 had been maintained, the "crisis" of the four-year gap between the grounding of the shuttle and a new replacement vehicle would never have emerged in the first place.

In 2000, however, the plan was to undertake a five-year, $4.5-billion effort. This effort was to start by identifying a technical approach to reduce the risk associated with building and operating next-generation launch systems and then enter into the full-scale development phase of the second-generation RLV in 2005. Row Rogacki, director of the Space Transportation Directorate at NASA's Marshall Space Flight Center in Huntsville, Alabama, stated in a NASA press release on the NASA web site: www.NASA.gov: "In the last several years, NASA has initiated several technology demonstration programs...and invested in specific concepts." At the time Rogacki was very optimistic about achieving an operational system by 2010 and stated: "We've made great progress and gained much insight into promising emerging technologies. We better understand the balance between commercial and government interests." He went on to put the nature of the challenge in perspective by saying: "...NASA has encountered difficult lessons and delays in key technology projects. We've learned that more development along multiple competing paths is needed. We've learned that commercial markets are not growing as previously projected. But there are still possibilities [as listed in the following] to make access to space more robust," he said. "This effort is part of the Administration's Space Launch Initiative intended to target these challenges."

1) Oversee 100-fold increase in safety over existing systems and a 10-fold reduction in the cost to launch payloads, from $10,000 per pound today to $1000 per pound in a decade.

2) Minimize technical and business risk for the full-scale development program, ensure NASA's requirements are met, coordinate with requirements of the commercial space industry, and support private ownership and operation of reusable launch vehicles and other potential systems.

3) Enable more than one commercial option for getting to the International Space Station and affordably meet NASA's near-term space transportation requirements while providing growth paths to meet future requirements.

This last objective, as just noted, is currently being actively pursued in terms of NASA's January 2006 request for proposal from the aerospace industry to provide commercial access to the ISS under contract with the U.S. government. This RFP seems to underscore NASA's current perspective that its mission lies primarily with moon, Mars, and solar-system exploration and sciences, while commercial entities (and the military) will increasingly address near-Earth space activities.

The NASA studies launched in 2000 were to cover Earth-to-orbit launch vehicles as well as in-space orbit-transfer vehicles, ground and flight operations, and the technology and organization required to support both. Clearly that perspective has changed.

NASA and its industry partners were thus supposed to take advantage of the various space transportation research programs, such as the

X-33, X-34, X-37, X-43A, and X-43C and the overall integrated advanced space transportation program, to reduce technical risk and create increased competition during the five-year risk-reduction phase. Further work on risk reduction would be not only a NASA-wide effort but would also involve cooperation with the U.S. Department of Defense.

The risk-reduction program announced in March 2000 was acknowledged at the time to be a result of NASA's industry-led space transportation architecture studies in 1998 and 1999 and the agency's integrated space transportation plan (ISTP) developed in the fall of 1999. In addition to a second-generation reusable launch vehicle, that plan addressed safety upgrades for the space shuttle, a crew return vehicle for the space station (i.e., X-38 program), and basic technology research. Essentially NASA failed against all of these objectives.

The following sections describe each of these essentially unsuccessful programs and note that none of them resulted in a reliable operational vehicle. The integrated space transportation plan that had presumably guided NASA programs at least from 1999 through 2003 was essentially scrapped by the new space vision of January 2004. This message that NASA intends to head in new directions and the ISTP is now history was clear not only in the announced plans by President George W. Bush, but reiterated by the clarifications of NASA's plans as indicated by Administrator O'Keefe in early 2005, by the Aldridge commission report in midyear 2005, and by the new NASA Administrator Michael Griffin when he assumed office in the spring of 2005.

The development plans of NASA for new space vehicles are now entirely shaped by Project Constellation. The development efforts related to X-33, X-34, X-37, and X-43A, and X-43C, to the extent they are relevant to NASA's future plans, must aid the development of the crew exploration vehicle, the crew escape capability, the crew launch vehicle, or the shuttle solid-fuel motor-based heavy-lift cargo vehicle.

Each of the various reusable launch vehicles discussed next has thus suffered not only from a variety of technical, management, and budgetary problems, but their relevancy to NASA's future development agenda has essentially evaporated.

The budgetary demands to sustain the space shuttle and to implement the International Space Station clearly claimed financial and human resources that adversely impacted all of the X-series programs.

X-33 Reusable-Launch-Vehicle Program

The X-33 Advanced Technology Demonstrator was designed to be a single-stage-to-Orbit (SSTO) RLV. The goal of the X-33 program was to demonstrate advanced technologies to increase launch vehicle safety and reliability and to lower the cost of putting a pound of payload into space from $10,000 to $1000. The X-33 was a half-scale prototype of Lockheed Martin's "VentureStar," a proposed fully reusable, commercial SSTO craft. Figure 6.6 shows an artist's concept of the X-33 RLV.

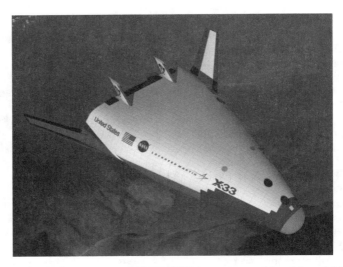

Figure 6-6   Artist's concept of X-33 RLV (courtesy of Lockheed Martin).

In July 1996, after a complex competitive process, NASA awarded Lockheed Martin's Skunk Works a contract to design, build, and test the X-33 technology demonstrator for their ambitious reusable-launch-vehicle program. Lockheed Martin's design was chosen over two other designs from Rockwell and McDonnell-Douglas Aerospace. The X-33 was scheduled to complete 15 test flights of varying speeds, altitudes, and distances beginning in July 1999.

The failure of a composite liquid-hydrogen tank in November 1999, along with constant weight growth and engine and stability problems, forced NASA to undertake a major reevaluation of the X-33 program. A new launch date of 2003 was targeted, but because of funding cuts the program was cancelled in March 2001 even though the first X-33 was over 85% complete. During the program, NASA committed $912 million to the building of the X-33 with Lockheed Martin and other contractors investing $356 million of their own funds [5].

The X-33 was a lifting-body design that incorporated two revolutionary linear aerospike rocket engines, lightweight composite materials, and a new metallic TPS. It was to be launched vertically, fly autonomously to altitudes of 60 miles and speeds in excess of Mach 13, before gliding to a conventional runway landing. The objectives of the X-33 were to demonstrate the use of linear aerospike rocket engines; a reusable cryogenic tank system including composite tanks for liquid hydrogen and liquid oxygen (*note*: tanks were later changed to aluminum because of design problems); thermal-protection-system durability with low maintenance and high performance over a large range of temperatures; complete autonomous guidance and navigation throughout flight; hypersonic flight with speeds over Mach 13; composite structures integrated with the thermal protection system; ability of a two-day turnaround between two consecutive flights;

ability of a seven-day turnaround between three consecutive flights; and the ability that a maximum of 50 personnel performing hands-on vehicle operations, maintenance, and refueling could successfully carry out flight readiness for two flights.

These were important and significant goals that implicitly contained major safety goals because the propulsion system, the TPS, and the maintenance and turnaround objectives, if met, would imply an extremely safe vehicle.

The X-33 was designed to utilize linear aerospike rocket engines that have lower operating costs and are more efficient than conventional engines. Instead of an exhaust plume of hot gas that shoots out through a bell-shaped nozzle, as in a conventional rocket engine, the hot gas is forced out along the outside walls of a tapered, rectangular ramp. This ramp serves as the inner wall of the nozzle while atmospheric pressure serves as the outside "invisible" wall. With increasing altitude and consequently decreasing atmospheric pressure, the aerospikes plume can widen, thus maximizing the engine's efficiency at all altitudes. Thrust direction and force levels can be achieved by varying the rate at which fuel flows to different parts of the engine. Figure 6.7 shows the difference between the nozzles on a conventional and aerospike engine.

Although the X-33 was only a half-scale prototype, its aim was to demonstrate technology applicable to future commercial RLV programs and specifically the proposed Lockheed Martin concept for "VentureStar."

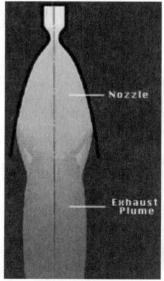
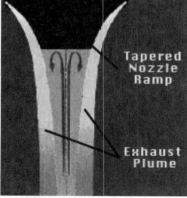

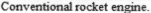
Conventional rocket engine. Aerospike engine.

Figure 6-7 Conventional vs aerospike engine nozzle (graphic courtesy of Boeing).

The safety of future flight crew or passengers was a major consideration in the design. The X-33 was designed to be a SSTO vehicle, negating the need for an expendable launch system. The smaller size and lighter weight would hopefully allow the spacecraft to be significantly easier to inspect and also allow easier repair of any damage.

The use of lightweight composite materials on the internal structure and fuel tanks and the integration of the structure to the TPS significantly reduced the weight of the vehicle. Manufacturing the liquid oxygen and hydrogen fuel tanks with composite materials was also believed to be safer as these materials are less susceptible to the extreme temperatures of the supercold rocket fuel. However after the November 1999 failure of the composite fuel tank, Lockheed Martin engineers realized there are were still a number of technical challenges to be overcome and thus resorted to a design that employed aluminum fuel tanks. It was still believed that the use of the aerospike engines would increase the safety of anyone onboard, as there would be no solid rocket boosters (SRBs) or external tanks like the ones currently used during shuttle launches. The use of SRBs and the external tanks is seen as having contributed to both the *Challenger* and *Columbia* accidents, as documented in the Rogers commission and the Gehman commission (CAIB) reports.

The thermal protection system of the X-33 was to have been composed of rugged metallic panels that were expected to reduce maintenance time and costs compared to that of the ceramic tiles on the shuttle. The new TPS design would undoubtedly have led to increased safety protection, as it was more resilient than the ceramic materials and the components were fewer in number and much less specialized in nature. This design was intended to aid prelaunch checkout and test and speeded postlaunch review and repair, and obviously such a design would have led to reduced costs.

Although the X-33 never flew and was cancelled in 2001 at a point where the program was projected to have been 85% complete, it did achieve some of its goals in the development of technology that could be used in future RLV programs. But now, the goal of developing such an RLV has been overtaken by the design objectives for the CEV. Valuable knowledge was gained from the development of the aerospike engines and in new metallic TPS materials and composite structures, but little of this can or will be applied to Project Constellation.‡

X-34 Program

The pilotless X-34 technology demonstrator was designed as a test bed for operations applicable to future low-cost, RLVs. The X-34 project (just as in the case of the X-33 program) sought to lower launch costs from the

---

‡Data available online at http://www.nasa.gov/missions/research/x33-main.html.

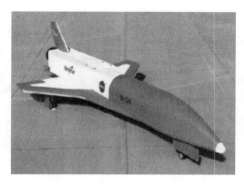

Figure 6-8   X-34 Technology Demonstrator (courtesy of NASA).

$10,000 per pound down to $1000 per pound and to demonstrate new technologies that would be pertinent to the viable operation of future RLVs. Figure 6.8 shows a completed X-34.

On 28 August 1996, NASA awarded Orbital Sciences Corporation a 50-month contract to design, develop, and flight test three X-34 vehicles. Orbital Sciences was the main contractor, with NASA also allocating additional funding to other companies for wind-tunnel testing, thermal protection systems, vehicle health monitoring, ground support, engine testing, and flight support. Between program launch in 1996 and its end in 2001, three airframes were manufactured, and a total of three test flights were completed out of an expected 27 flights. The three test flights were nonpowered, captive-carry flights attached to a modified Lockheed L-1011. A joint NASA/Orbital Sciences review of the project in 2000 concluded the "need to redefine the project's approach, scope, budget and schedule." To ensure safety and mission success of the X-34, it was judged necessary to increase government technical insight, hardware testing, and integrated systems assessments. As a result, the projected cost of completing the X-34 program at an acceptable level of risk rose significantly above the planned budget. NASA determined the benefits to be derived from the X-34 did not justify the costs, and the project was cancelled in March 2001.

The X-34 had a 27.7-ft (8.4-m) wing span and stood 11.5 ft tall (3.5 m) and was 58.3 ft (17.6 m) long. It was designed to be air launched from a modified Lockheed L-1011 and fly a preprogrammed suborbital flight profile before making an automated approach and landing on a conventional runway. The X-34 was expected to reach an altitude of up to 250,000 ft and speeds of Mach 8 with a cost goal of $500,000 per flight. A typical flight profile of the X-34 is shown in Fig. 6.9.

The X-34 was designed to be powered by the Fastrac, a single-stage engine that burns a mixture of liquid oxygen and kerosene. Designed and developed by NASA's Marshall Space Flight Center, the Fastrac provides 60,000 lb of thrust and would cost approximately $1.2 million per engine.

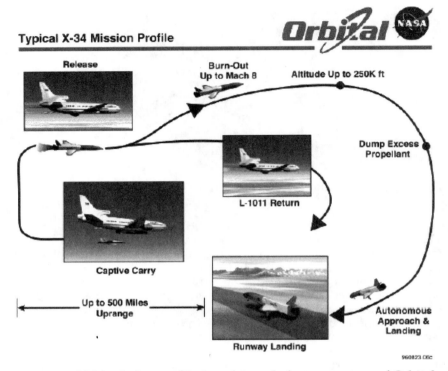

Figure 6-9   X-34 mission profile (graphic and photos courtesy of Orbital Sciences Corporation).

This is about one-fifth the cost of similar engines as it is designed for simplicity and low cost with significantly fewer parts and reduced design time.

To reach the goals of dramatically increasing reliability and lowering the cost of putting payloads into space, the X-34 was designed to demonstrate the following technical objectives: capability of 25 flights over a period of one year; capability of autonomous flight operations; capability of demonstrating safe abort; subsonic and hypersonic flight; integrated automated vehicle health monitoring and checkout; lightweight composite airframe structures that require minimal inspection; reusable composite propellant tanks with insulation; advanced Thermal Protection Systems capable of surviving subsonic flights even through an atmospheric condition of heavy rain and fog; integrated, low-cost avionics, including GPS and automatic landing techniques and landing in 20-kn crosswind.

The X-34 was designed as a test-bed demonstrator to study how new materials and design philosophies could lower the cost of putting payloads into space. Thus the three-fold objective of the X-34 development was to 1) reduce the cost of a commercial reusable launch vehicle; 2) create new opportunities for scientific, commercial, and educational space endeavors; and 3) significantly improve U.S. economic competitiveness in the world launch market.§

Although the X-34 program was cancelled and potentially prematurely so, it is reasonable to believe that, as in the case of the X-33, the lessons learned during the design phase of the X-34 will help engineers develop future low-cost RLVs. If this is not something that NASA undertakes, then perhaps commercial organizations might feel these represent viable business goals to pursue, particularly if such systems can be launched and controlled autonomously without crew aboard.

X-37 Program

The X-37 program objective was to design a reusable advanced technology flight demonstrator that would serve as a test bed for new airframe, propulsion, and operations technologies. Its prime objective was to help design a new space vehicle that would be safe and reliable yet reduce significantly the cost of putting payloads into space. The X-37 was a key part of NASA's space launch initiative that began in the 1990s. Figure 6.10 shows an artist's impression of the X-37 during flight.¶

In August 1998, NASA issued a research announcement for proposals for a flight demonstrator vehicle to "test and validate emerging technologies that could dramatically reduce the cost of space transportation."** In July 1999, The Boeing Company was awarded a four-year cooperative agreement to develop the X-37 valued at $173 million. The cooperative agreement was negotiated on the basis of a sharing arrangement, with Boeing contributing approximately $67 million in shared development expenses. Another $16-million contribution for the X-37 program came from the U.S. Air Force to support additional technology experiments. Boeing was awarded an additional contract worth $301 million in November 2002 to continue the development of the X-37 flight demonstrator. This $300-million contract called for the "development of an X-37 Approach and Landing Test Vehicle (ALTV) with a progressive series of approach and landing tests and the development of an X-37 Orbital Vehicle with an orbital flight test".**

Tests on the ALTV to validate the integrity of the airframe were successfully completed in July 2003 with atmospheric flight tests scheduled for mid-2004. The X-40A, an 85%-scaled version of the X-37, was

---

§Data available online at http://www.nasa.gov/missions/research/ x34-main.html.
¶Data available online at http://www.nasa.gov/missions/research/ x37-main.html.
**Data available online at http://www.nasa.gov/missions/research/ x37-main.html.

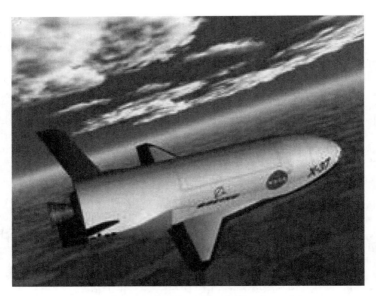

Figure 6-10   Artist's impression of X-37 in flight (graphic courtesy of NASA).

developed to reduce the costs and risk factors associated with the program. The X-40A proved the capability of the autonomous flight-control and landing system in a series of seven glide flights after being dropped from 15,000 ft by a heavy-lift Chinook helicopter. These tests were to have set the stage for a low-earth-orbital test flight of the X-37 in July 2006.[tt] These plans were, however, altered by the new space vision announced by President George W. Bush in January 2004.

The X-37 was the third advanced technology demonstrator, following on from the X-33 and X-34 programs. Unlike those programs that were intended to test technologies at lower speeds and altitudes, the X-37 was designed to operate in both the orbital and reentry phases of flight after being ferried into orbit by the shuttle or an expendable launch vehicle. The X-37, building on the X-33 and X-34 programs, demonstrated some 40 advanced airframe, propulsion, avionics, and operations technologies that are applicable to future reusable space vehicles. A major focus of this program was to develop a highly durable, high-temperature thermal protection system that would be easier to maintain than current systems.[tt]

The X-37 at 27.5 ft long (8.3 m) and with a 15-ft (4.5-m) wing span just fits into the shuttle cargo bay. The X-37's payload bay is 7 ft long (2.15 m) and 4 ft (1.2 m) in diameter and is able to carry up to 500 lb (227 kg). The X-37 was designed to be capable of conducting continuous in-orbit

---

[tt]Data available online at http://www.spacetoday.net.

operations for up to 21 days and was also envisioned to deploy various payloads or satellites and perform a variety of maneuvering operations before reentering the atmosphere and landing on a conventional runway. During reentry, the X-37 would fly at speeds of up to Mach 25.

The Astronaut Safety Assessment Program (ASAP) [6] has expressed concerns over crew escape from the International Space Station and has advocated an escape mechanism that would protect the onboard crew under three design reference missions: return of a sick or injured crew member; total evacuation of the ISS in the event it becomes uninhabitable, for example, after a total decompression; and unavailability of resupply for a prolonged period, for example, because of grounding of the space shuttle.

In their 1993 *Annual Report*, the ASAP presented a detailed assessment of the requirements for a generic CRV and drew the conclusion that the lowest risk configuration for a space station is one with two return vehicles, each of which can accommodate the entire crew.

Based on these recommendations, NASA decided to use a Soyuz as a return vehicle until a full-crew CRV was available, even though there is a severe limitation on the crew return capability of the Soyuz. The ASAP concurred with that approach as an interim expedient. The X-38 program (see Fig. 6.11) was developed to be a full-crew return vehicle, but this program has been abandoned. In its place, NASA continues to rely on the Soyuz as the only lifeboat for the International Space Station beyond the shuttle.

The X-37 was designed to be powered by a "clean" single AR-2/3 hydrogen peroxide and JP-8 (jet fuel) engine. These rocket propellants are considered to be more environmentally friendly and compact than commonly used propellants such as kerosene. The initial investment of $16 million from the U.S. Air Force was used to add specific orbital capabilities to the system's mission including solar arrays and a vernier engine system for orbital operations. The engine system would enable ultrafine

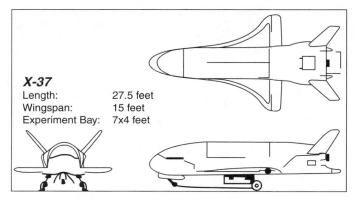

X-37
Length: 27.5 feet
Wingspan: 15 feet
Experiment Bay: 7x4 feet

Figure 6-11   Layout of the X-37 (graphics courtesy of Boeing).

and precision flight control allowing close in-orbit operations, while the solar arrays would increase the time the X-37 could stay in orbit.‡‡

The X-37 program was intended to demonstrate new advanced technologies that would increase the safety, reliability, and cost of space travel. Overall, the X-37 was to test a composite of some 40 new technologies in flight. The intention now is to combine relevant technologies developed in the X-37 program into Project Constellation.

X-43A and X-43C Space Plane (Hypersonic Craft) Development

The X-43A was the test vehicle of an experimental hypersonic ground and flight-test program, initially called Hyper X. The aim of the X-43A was to demonstrate airframe-integrated, airbreathing engine technologies that promise to increase payload capacity for future hypersonic aircraft and/or reusable space launch vehicles. Hyper X, until its cancellation in early 2004, was a $250-million joint program between NASA's Dryden and Langley Research Centers. Figure 6.12 shows an artist's impression of the X-43A in flight.

Hyper-X research began with conceptual design and wind-tunnel work in early 1996. Alliant Techsystems (known by its New York Stock Exchange symbol, ATK) has built three unpiloted X-43A research aircraft with extensive contributions from Boeing's Phantom Works. Each X-43A was designed to ride on an Orbital Sciences Corporation booster rocket, released from a NASA B-52 aircraft. During the first flight in June 2001, the combined booster and X-43A vehicle deviated from the flight path and thus were deliberately destroyed. Investigation into the mishap showed that there was no single contributing factor, but the root cause of the

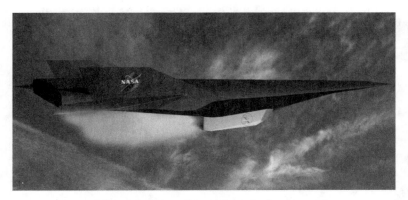

Figure 6-12   Artist's impression of X-43A in flight (graphic courtesy of NASA).

---

‡‡Data available online at http://www.space.com.

problem was identified as the control system of the booster. On 27 March 2004, the second X-43A flew successfully making it the first time an airbreathing scramjet powered aircraft has flown freely.§§

In this test, the modified Pegasus booster rocket carried the X-43A up to its test altitude of 95,000 ft, where it was released and the scramjet ignited. The scramjet engine operated for approximately 10 s, propelling the X-43A to its test speed of Mach 6.83. The third X-43A had a successful flight test in the fall of 2004 at the Edwards Air Force Base and performed to specifications by attaining speeds of Mach 10. The X-43A program, however, was terminated after this third test flight. Plans for a follow-on X-43C program, which would have been a joint NASA–U.S. Air Force project with flight models scheduled for 2007, have also been cancelled as a result of national budgetary pressures and the newly defined moon–Mars exploration program [7]. Instead, the Department of Defense has embarked on its independent X-43B program with a new billion-dollar contract awarded to Northrop Grumman.

The three X-43A vehicles were all identical in appearance. They were only 12 ft (3.5 m) long and 5 ft (1.7 m) wide. They were engineered, how-ever, with slight differences in simulating engine inlet variable geometry, so as to achieve higher hypersonic speeds.¶¶

The main innovation tested on the X-43A was, of course, the scramjet engine. This innovative engine has a simple design and, quite impres-sively, no moving parts. Rather than using a rotating compressor, like a turbojet engine, the forward velocity and aerodynamics of the vehicle compress the air into the engine. Hydrogen fuel is then injected into the airstream, and the expanding hot gases from combustion accelerate the exhaust air to create thrust. The X-43A craft itself is thus designed to be a part of the engine system; the front of the vehicle acts as the intake for the airflow, and the aft serves as the nozzle that accelerates the exhausted air. Figure 6.13 shows a diagram of the scramjet system.

The advantage of the scramjet engine is that the craft does not need to carry large amounts of liquid oxygen like a conventional rocket engine. Eliminating the need to carry oxygen will enable future hypersonic vehi-cles to be smaller and/or carry heavier payloads.*** The X-43A was an air-launched system utilizing a modified Pegasus rocket and a NASA B-52 aircraft. Figure 6.14 shows the flight plan of the X-43A vehicle.

X-43A Program Manager Joel Sitz, at NASA Dryden Flight Research Center, calls hypersonics the holy grail of aeronautics because it has taken about 40 years to execute a flight research project that validates concepts

---

§§Data available online at http://www.nasa.gov/missions/research/x43-main.html.

¶¶Data available online at http://www.orbital.com/Advanced Space/Hyper-X/index.html.

***Data available online at http://www.dfrc.nasa.gov/Newsroom/FactSheets/FS-040-DFRC.html.

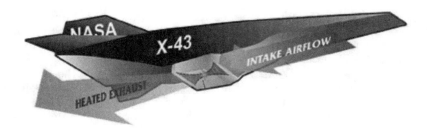

Figure 6-13   Scramjet engine system (graphic courtesy of NASA).

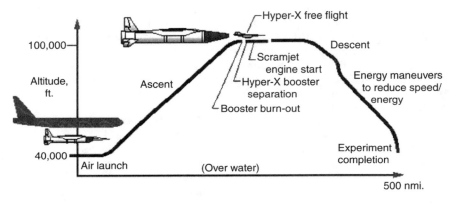

Figure 6-14   X-43A flight plan (graphic courtesy of NASA).

developed on the ground and researched in wind tunnels, but never proven in flight. The X-43A has supplied invaluable flight data to support the principles behind the scramjet engine. This project has successfully demonstrated the enabling technology to sustain an advanced propulsion system to support both future exploration and commercial applications.[†††]

Many advocates of hypersonic spaceflight systems feel that cancellation of the program at the time of first successful test flights represents a major misjudgment with regard to new space technology development. These critics, especially from the U.S. defense sector, point to the successive cancellations of the HL-20, X-38, X-33, X-34, and the X-43A/ X-43C programs and suggest that they reflect substantial management issues and strategic planning "confusion" in NASA programs that transcend budgetary constraints represented by the space shuttle and the ISS.

[†††]Data available online at http://www.boeing.com/phantom/hyperx.html.

Robotic Freighters and New Launch Concepts

The future of truly viable space exploration seems closely linked to finding new ways to doing things both more safely and more cost effectively in space. This might very well boil down to the idea of husbanding the use of astronauts to where it is absolutely necessary and using robotic systems wherever and whenever possible. This also suggests the need to simplify the design of vehicles when possible as well.

> The future of truly viable space exploration seems closely linked to finding new ways to doing things both more safely and more cost effectively in space.

This simplification might begin by using the space shuttle as a robotically controlled vehicle with no or very limited crew. The prime way to ensure astronaut safety in completing work on the ISS might very well be to use the remaining shuttle launchers as fully automated systems wherever possible—a concept that is reiterated in the final chapter of this book. With the Canadaarm2 fully in place, a good deal of the final construction of the space station should be possible without extended EVAs by astronauts, and cargo should be able to unloaded robotically as well.

A further extension of this concept for the longer term is to be able to create new lunar safe havens and industrial colonies. These lunar facilities would be equipped with automated material processing and self-sustaining technologies to generate food, water, energy, communications, housing, and basic materials support for astronauts.

California, Alaska, the Northwest Territorities, the Lousiana Purchase, and so on have turned out to be good investments in America's future. This was not only because they brought new territory to the United States, but because these new territories could support explorers and settlers to be self-sustaining for the essentials of life. Until one can think in terms of settlements on the moon or elsewhere as being regenerative and self-sustaining, space exploration will represent a drain on Earth's resources rather than potentially economically viable and successful systems.

The key to space enterprise becoming a viable longer-term high frontier might very well hinge on developing technology that allows science and exploration activities to be self-sustaining. The first essential step is to develop highly cost-efficient robotic freighters that can deliver machines and processors to the high frontier that allow the building of cities, the generation of power, and the growing of food.

L. M. E. Morin, a former NASA astronaut, at the sixth Space Resources Utilization Roundtable in Golden, Colorado, in 2004, set forth a so-called "biological growth" approach to rapid lunar industrialization. Morin's idea is that rather than developing heavy-lift vehicles that would launch massive lunar exploration apparatus from the Earth we should concentrate instead on "organic growth" model. In particular, this would involve the launch of a series of 1000-kilogram payloads known as in situ resource utilization (ISRU) packages. These payloads could almost immediately actually start to mine and start producing materials and creating new production units on the lunar surface. This would be done solely by robotic production that could double their mass in a year by production, on average, of 0.1 to 0.2 kg of new lunar-produced apparatus per hour. Under Morin's approach, the key would not be in new extremely heavy launch systems but rather in producing robotically capable production units that could be launched within the 1000-kg (2200-lb) payload capabilities of conventional rockets [8].

In the longer term, ideas such as electronic propulsion, nuclear heated plasma or ions, nuclear engines, solar sails, gravity accelerators, rail guns, advanced tethers, the so-called space elevator, or very sophisticated mass driver launching systems might be able to deliver much higher reliability and space launch systems at a reasonable cost in coming decades. The idea of using controlled chemical explosions and rocket propulsion as the logical and safest way into space will, over the long term, seem like a very quaint and ultimately silly idea.

The lessons of the shuttle have seemingly taught us not to try to combine all launch capabilities into a single system and, even more so, not to try to rely on a particular vehicle or technology too long.

What can be seen from the cursory review of new technology in Chapter 10 of this book is that many new technologies over the longer term might become safer, more reliable, more cost effective, and more versatile than current chemically based rocket-blasting processes. This might not be obvious today, but over the next 10 to 20 years concepts such as space elevators, ion engines, or solar sails might seem much more reasonable.

Finally, it can well be said that current plans to place the entire future of manned space flight into the single mold framed by Project Constellation has certain counterindicators as reflected in the shuttle experience. The idea of putting all of one's resources into a complex single system that is expected to represent the future of space exploration and space access for the next 20 years could very well serve to limit innovation and thwart new and outside-the-box solutions. The idea of spiral development within the CEV design process, which allows the gradual introduction of new technology, might, in time, ultimately prove to be of limited value. Thus, if in five to 10 years we should develop major breakthroughs in scramjet technology, ion engines, nuclear engines, rail guns, or even space elevators or solar-sail technology, the $104-billion investment in Project Constellation might prove an expensive investment in largely passé technology. This is not to suggest that we should not continue to develop CEV and CRV systems, but to keep an open mind to technological options and not close down R&D on other systems. Perhaps it is most important to keep private entrepreneurial approaches to space exploration alive and well.

Private Human Spaceflight Initiatives, the X-Prize, and the Future

During the 1980s and the Reagan administration, there was a shift in space policy to foster the development of private launch development programs. In the wake of the *Challenger* disaster, private commercial missions were removed from the launch manifest for the shuttle and thus transferred to commercial companies offering launch services.

A new unit was created in U.S. Department of Transportation to foster the development of private launch capabilities. This policy did not produce the desired response in the U.S. commercial launch-vehicle industry. In fact, it was the Ariane vehicles of the European commercial launcher program, developed by Arianespace and the European Space Agency (ESA) and the French space agency Centre National d'Etudes Spatiales (CNES), that quickly moved to become the dominant provider of launch services.

Since that time, U.S. companies have developed new and improved versions of Atlas, Agena, Atlas-Centaur, Delta, Titan, Titan-Centaur, Pegasus, and Taurus launch systems, etc. And now other U.S. systems are under development, such as Space X's launcher program and SpaceDev's DreamChaser. In the United Kingdom the Rocketplane Ltd. enterprise has also made significant progress. These systems might, in just a few years time, lead to a new resurgence in space commercialization and privately developed launch systems. Nevertheless the rest of the world still leads in the commercial launch business.

The inability of the U.S. conventional launch service providers, such as Lockheed Martin, Boeing, General Dynamics, Orbital Sciences, etc., to provide rocket systems that are price competitive with the world market for commercial flights has led some to believe that only new and truly entrepreneurial companies, able to "think outside the box," could produce highly reliable and cost-effective new launch capabilities.

Peter Diamandis, one of the three founders of the International Space University (ISU), and many others combined to create the Ansari X-Prize on the premise that creativity and entrepreneurial talent might provide the best ways forward. The $10-million Ansari X-prize was established to create incentives for an entrepreneurial group to develop an orbital space plane that could, within an eight-day turnaround window, launch two crews successfully into low Earth orbit (i.e., 62 miles or 100 km). Remarkably, a number of small space development organizations (a total of 27 of which six were considered serious contenders) embarked on trying to win the prize. Scaled Composites, headed by aerospace designer Burt Rutan and major financial backer Paul Allen, after a successful launch of SpaceShipOne in June 2004, were then able to go on to successfully claim the X-Prize [9,10].

Although the X-Prize and the exploits of Burt Rutan and Paul Allen captured the biggest headlines, other new private space initiatives are emerging. These include the new launch system being developed by Space X, the plans of Bigelow Aerospace to launch an inflatable "TransHab" facility into orbit to create a private space station, and other similar initiatives. In short, serious attempts to create private access to space are emerging from fantasy into serious possibility. Even Brad Edwards' ideas of building a space elevator are beginning to be taken seriously by entrepreneurial investors.

Perhaps most interesting of all are the plans of SpaceDev to develop a highly cost-effective and reliable DreamChaser launch system using a hybrid and "throttleable" solid fuel to provide access to low Earth orbit for manned or unmanned systems. This development, if successful, will allow Sir Richard Branson to proceed with his plans to take space tourists into near space via his Virgin Galactic venture.

The question that naturally arises is the extent to which the U.S. government (or international entities such as the International Telecommunication Union [ITU]) should, or need to, regulate such ventures.

The fact that Burt Rutan, with some $20 million in financing provided by Microsoft executive Paul Allen, has been able to achieve so much towards reusable spaceflight, while NASA's billions of dollars in expenditures have produced modest results, suggest that private space initiatives must be considered a critical pathway to the future.

Certainly the safety features of the Scaled Composite SpaceShipOne are in some ways superior to the shuttle in terms of offering an escape capability for virtually all of the flight and a lightweight structure and aerodynamic design that restricts descent flight speeds to about Mach 3. In short, the various innovative designs for the X-Prize competition not only show great ingenuity, but also suggest in many ways the high level of risk associated with the shuttle design—particularly in terms of limited escape capability and the need for a thermal protection system to withstands tremendously high temperatures [9,10].

Some of those interviewed in the GW University study process suggested that if NASA privatized more of its human space research programs and let entrepreneurial talent develop new human-rated space vehicles many problems would be potentially solved. The programs could be overseen and regulated by the Federal Aviation Administration, and private "astronauts" could sign waivers and accept higher risk assignments for higher compensation to enable accelerated development programs. Regardless of U.S. federal policy, the programs of Scaled Composites, Bigelow Aerospace, SpaceDev, SpaceX, and others are clearly headed in such a direction in any event. Certainly NASA's new program to offer prizes for innovation creates new opportunities to see how entrepreneurial talent can help develop interesting new technology that might indeed provide useful support for Project Constellation.

References

1 Stone, H. W., and Piland, W. M., "21st Century Space Transportation System Design Approach: HL-20 Personnel Launch System," *Journal of Spacecraft and Rockets*, No. 5, 1993.
2 Ware, G. M., and Cruz, C. I., "Aerodynamic Characteristics of the HL-20," *Journal of Spacecraft and Rockets*, No. 5, 1993.

3 Ehrlich, C. F., Jr., "HL-20 Concept: Design Rationale and Approach," *Journal of Spacecraft and Rockets*, No. 5, 1993.

4 Telephone Interview, Dr. Lance Bush of NASA, In person interview on the HL-20 Program, 29 April 2004

5 "Cancellation of the X-33 Program," *Space.com*, March 2001.

6 Status Report, Astronaut Safety Assessment Program (ASAP) NASA-ASAP 2002, Washington, DC, 18 April 2002.

7 Cambi, E., "Speeding into Oblivion," *Aerospace America*, Vol. 42, Issue 6, June 2004, p. 3.

8 Morin, L. M. E., "Biological Growth Approach to Rapid Lunar Industrialization Proposed," *Lunar Enterprise Daily*, No. 220, 12 Nov. 2004, URL: http://www.spaceagepub.com.

9 Booth, W., "Starship Private Enterprise," *Washington Post*, 22 June 2004, pp. A1, A8.

10 Schwartz, J., "Manned Private Craft," *New York Times*, 22 June 2004, pp. A1, A12.

CHAPTER 7
International Space Programs and Launch Systems

> "There are concerns around the world about the lack of
> clear, specific and tangible opportunities for international
> collaboration within Project Constellation. This concern is
> undoubtedly exacerbated by a reluctance among the
> world space community to commit to any new US space
> programs until existing commitments involving the ISS are
> successfully concluded."
>
> —*Joseph N. Pelton, Director, Space and Advanced Communications*
> *Research Institute, George Washington University*

International Cooperation at a Critical Stage

The U.S. manned space program is today heavily international. Indeed
the International Space Station is one of the largest joint international projects in human history. President Bush, in his new space vision, emphasized that it would have an international dimension, and the Aldridge
commission emphasized international participation as a key aspect of
Project Constellation—although just what this international role might be
remains more than a little unclear and elusive. Despite the important past
and present of international cooperation in space and the promised future
of joint space exploration, the details of where, when, and how remain
very sketchy. The $104-billion plan that the NASA administrator pre-
sented to Congress for Project Constellation was lacking in key details
about the international dimensions of this program.

As described in Chapter 5, the key partners in the International Space
Station program include Russia, Canada, Japan, and Europe. There are a
total of 16 national partners, and each of them has played a key role in the
design and construction of various parts of the ISS or in lifting critical
cargo into orbit. For the period of the shuttle grounding, Russian launch
vehicles and service modules remained the only way to ferry supplies to
the ISS, to position the station in orbit, and, in the event of an emergency,
to allow astronauts to escape from the ISS. Without Russian participation
the International Space Station would be in very deep trouble indeed.

The past, present, and future of NASA's space exploration program
depends, at least to some degree, on international cooperation. Clearly the
U.S. ability to ensure astronaut access to the ISS while the shuttle remains
grounded clearly depends on the Russian Progress and Soyuz vehicles.
Russian booster systems are key to keeping the ISS in its required orbit,

and the very earliest that the United States will have a replacement for the shuttle is year-end 2012. The Japanese H2 transfer vehicle (HTV) and the European automated transfer vehicle (ATV) represent additional systems to ferry supplies to the ISS and remove waste materials. The Jules Verne ATV is only just set for its maiden flight, and the HTV remains in development, and so the extent to which these supply systems can be relied on remains in question.

Thus the future of NASA's international cooperation in space seems to be at a critical phase. In November 2004, NASA hosted a widely attended international conference at the Kennedy Space Center to explore international participation in Project Constellation. Even China attended. But as of early 2006, major international issues remain open. Until the construction schedule for the ISS and the launch manifest for the remaining shuttle flights are resolved, this is likely to remain the case. The rest of the world is not about to leap into new space exploration commitments before pending ones are made good by the United States. The old saying seems to apply very aptly here: "Fool me once, shame on you. Fool me twice, shame on me."

The open issues concerning U.S. space cooperation and collaboration with its international partners include the following:

1) Concerns and questions about the full deployment of the ISS and all of its international components is an open issue (including major elements that have involved investments of billions of dollars by European and Japanese partners).

2) Another issue involves questions about the longer-term operation of the ISS with a "full" crew, the extent of the space station's ongoing experimental program and activities, and the nature of agreed and truly integrated safety standards and procedures. In this context, NASA, under new legislative authority, has now purchased a number of Soyuz launches and guaranteed U.S. astronaut access to the ISS to supplement the capability of the space shuttle. This bridges the gap until the initial CEV and CLV systems are being tested and until they are available for operational service as of end 2012. (*Note*: The NASA RFP seeking to contract for commercial contractors to ferry astronauts and cargo to the ISS should help to resolve some of these issues once the selection is made and longer-term access to the space station is further ensured.)

3) Finally there are concerns around the world about the lack of clear, specific, and tangible opportunities for international collaboration within the context of Project Constellation. This concern is undoubtedly exacerbated by a reluctance among the world space community to commit to any new programs until existing commitments involving the ISS are successfully concluded.

International Space Programs and Safety

Beyond the preceding specific concerns about how NASA and other space agencies might cooperate in the future, there is a philosophical question concerning the best approach to an integrated and systems-level safety program for the ISS. This preference for an integrated approach is directly opposed to the currently operational idea that one can simply divide up certain tasks and hardware objectives and then glue them together within the context of national franchises. The ISS approach of divided responsibility within the various national franchises runs counter to the idea that safety must be addressed at a systems engineering and almost organic level to succeed.

In short, there appears to be growing concern among some space safety officials that the memorandum of understanding between NASA and its international partners does not include specific provisions related to an overall approach to ISS safety. In particular there is concern that current ISS safety procedures and standards do not recognize the need for integrated operation of all of the modules in the overall station and that there is not one unified international safety and emergency control entity able to establish priorities in times of operational crises. There is no "ISS Safety Authority," and this has been critiqued by several of the program participants, especially from Europe [1].

There is provision for what are called partner safety review panels (PSRPs) that are responsible for the international partner franchises covering the various international components of the ISS such as the Japanese experimental module (JEM)—also known as Kibo—the Japanese centrifuge accommodation module (CAM), the European Space Lab Columbus, etc., but this does not constitute an integrated ISS safety authority. In fact, if one were to look at the ISS in political terms it would not be likened to a nation or even a city state, but rather to something more like a loose federation.

The concerns of safety experts such as T. Sgobba and S. Chiesa is that a federation of control centers and launch operations around the world, in the United States, Russia, Europe, Canada, and Japan, does not add up to the maximum degree of safety for the whole. There are those who question whether the PSRP franchise process is sufficient to deal with emergency situations wherein the safety of the entire ISS and its modules were threatened on an instantaneous basis. In such a case, there is significant question as to whether the "parts" would be able to respond on an integrated, safety-maximizing basis. In cases of survival priorities, the key question is whether each national unit might simply opt to save its own astronauts or module first?

There are concerns about a fully integrated approach to safety that go well back into the history of European and U.S. cooperation in astronaut-related space exploration and experimentation programs from 15 years ago. These concerns continue. Or at least press reports persist in recounting areas of dispute between the U.S. and ISS partners about safety procedures. The point of these concerns is that unless these issues are resolved in the near term international cooperation in the context of the even more complex (and dangerous) Project Constellation will undoubtedly be even more difficult. In this respect the ISS represents in microcosm the next steps of exploring and colonizing the moon and going on to Mars [2].*,†

Changing Nature of International Space Initiatives

The world of international space is changing in form, objectives, and participants. China recently joined the ranks of nations able to deploy astronauts to orbit. Europe has announced a new space action plan that clearly indicates a desire to obtain greater independence of action in space programs, both in terms of space applications (such as the newly evolving Galileo space navigation project) as well as manned space programs. Countries that have relied on the United States to achieve access to space for their astronauts via the shuttle are examining new options. Specifically, European and Russian collaboration is actively being discussed in the context of the Russian plans to deploy by 2012 a reusable spacecraft similar in context to the space shuttle.

It thus seems appropriate to review international manned space programs and their relation to the United States, both in general terms and more specifically in the context of the future manned space programs implicit in Project Constellation as well as ISS operations. In this review, the safety implications of these international programs are particularly emphasized.

Russian Programs and the Soyuz

The Russian space program dates back well into the 1950s, and over a dozen types of vehicles have been developed for military and civil programs over the years. The principal program for cosmonaut or human-rated space launches is the Soyuz/Progress launch system that overall has one of the best records of any program in the world.

The Soyuz launch system comprises the manned Soyuz spacecraft and an expendable Soyuz launch vehicle known as the Progress 1M. Both of these systems have evolved over time after originally being conceived in the 1960s during the race to the moon. The Soyuz launch system has been the backbone of the Soviet/Russian space program, and, with the shuttle fleet grounded, it is now the primary craft for the transportation of astronauts into and out of space. It has also been used to launch commercial payloads [3].

The Soyuz spacecraft is certainly the longest-serving man-rated spacecraft in the world. The original version was conceived during the early 1960s to gain essential experience in lunar flight in areas such as

---

*Data available online at http://www.charlest.n.net/stories/092403/wor_24nasa.shtml.
†Data available online at http://www.pbs.org/newshour/bb/science/jan=june 97/mir_6=25.html.

active maneuvering, orbital rendezvous, and docking. At the end of the 1960s and with the Soviet space program behind the United States in the race to the moon, the Soviet space industry focused on the Salyut space station as their new direction in manned spacecraft. In 1971 a new, modified version of Soyuz, the Soyuz Salyut 1-type, was created to allow docking with the Salyut space stations. However, disaster struck after Soyuz 11 experienced difficulties un-docking from Salyut 1 causing rapid depressurization of the reentry capsule and killing the three crew members onboard [4].

Since the Soyuz 11 accident, the Soyuz has been modified and improved many times to increase safety of the crew and enhance the versatility of the spacecraft. Variants have included the Soyuz Ferry, Soyuz T, Soyuz TM, and the latest version, the Soyuz TMA. These spacecraft have acted as crew transfer for the Soviet Salyut, Almaz, and Mir space stations. Since November 2000, first the Soyuz TM and then the Soyuz TMA have been the essential space vehicles that have ferried international crews between the ISS and Earth. With the grounding of the shuttle fleet after the *Columbia* accident, the Soyuz TMA became the primary crew transfer vehicle for the ISS [5]. After the reflight of the *Discovery* shuttle from 26 July to 9 August 2005, it became clear that the foam-shedding problem had not been successfully resolved. Thus the U.S. Congress proceeded to pass legislation that allowed an exception to the Iran trade restrictions that up to that point had prohibited the United States from purchasing additional Soyuz vehicles. As noted earlier, these additional Soyuz vehicles will thus allow the relay of crews to and from the ISS as well as help with resupply missions.

The efficiency and reliability of the Soyuz has increased with each upgrade, culminating in the current version, the Soyuz TMA. Like previous variants, the Soyuz TMA consists of an orbital module, a descent module, and an instrumentation/propulsion module, as can be seen in Fig. 7.1.

1) Orbital module is used by the crew while in orbit during free flight. Upon reentry the module separates from the descent module and is destroyed.

2) Descent module is used by crew during launch, reentry, and landing. The module contains the landing rockets, parachutes, and life-support systems used during descent.

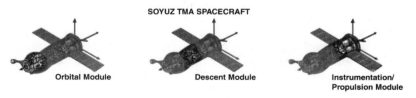

SOYUZ TMA SPACECRAFT

Orbital Module   Descent Module   Instrumentation/
Propulsion Module

Figure 7-1   Three modules of the Soyuz TMA spacecraft are highlighted in the figure (graphic courtesy of NASA).

3) The instrumentation/propulsion module provides the systems used for orbital maneuvering, instrumentation for guidance and control, and solar arrays that are attached to batteries to provide power. This module also separates from the descent module and is destroyed during reentry.

The Soyuz spacecraft is launched on a Soyuz launch vehicle with a trip to the ISS taking two days from launch to docking. The spacecraft can then spend up to one year docked before returning to earth in less than 3.5 hours [6].

Since the Soyuz was first flown in the 1960s, there have been a few accidents and malfunctions that have killed or endangered the flight crew onboard, as well as other less serious incidents. Cosmonaut Vladimir Komarov was killed during the Soyuz 1 flight in 1967 when the onboard parachutes entangled and failed to operate correctly. This accident led to the redesign of the parachute and landing system [7].

As noted earlier, three crew members died during the Soyuz 11 accident, and Soyuz 5, Soyuz 33, and TM-8 all experienced difficulties that resulted in either the abort of the mission or a "heavy" but not fatal landing. Because of the secretive nature of the Russian space program, it is also possible there have been other accidents that have not become public knowledge. Generally, however, the Soyuz spacecraft has shown a good level of reliability, and the safety of the crew has been improved with each new version [7]. Its overall performance record at 97.5% is quite similar to the shuttle's record of 98.2%. Further, the Soyuz has now had over 800 flights, compared to 114 for the shuttle. Most important of all, the Soyuz's safety record has steadily improved over time with design and system upgrades.

The Soyuz TMA increases safety, especially in descent and landing, over the previous Soyuz TM. The incorporation of smaller and more efficient computers and improved displays has allowed the Soyuz TMA to accommodate individuals of between 4 ft 11 in. and 6 ft 3 in. and 110 to 209 lb. Two new engines that fire 1 s before touchdown reduce the landing speed and the forces felt by crew members by up to 30% over the Soyuz TM. Also, a new entry control system and three-axis accelerometer increase the landing accuracy. The new components and entire TMA were tested more rigorously than any previous Soyuz, with ground, hangar drops, and airdrop tests completed before the spacecraft was declared flight ready. Each individual crew member has a specialized molded seat that fits tightly to reduce the forces felt upon landing.

During launch, the Soyuz is attached to an escape tower and launch jettison system that uses small rocket motors to propel the spacecraft away from the pad in case of an emergency. During a Soyuz-T flight in September 1983, the Soyuz launch vehicle caught fire, and the two-person crew completed the first off-the-pad abort. The crew survived the 20-g acceleration and landed close to the launch site [4].

Figure 7.2 shows a picture of the launch jettison system for the Soyuz in its most recent configuration.

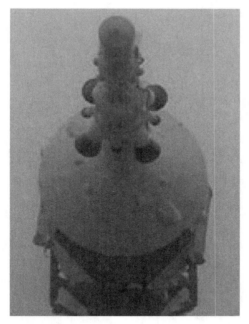

Figure 7-2   Launch jettison system of Soyuz.

Soyuz Launch Vehicle

The Soyuz launch vehicle is an expendable launch system that provides efficient and reliable launch services for manned and unmanned flights. This workhorse of the Soviet/Russian space program and the variants of the Soyuz, as already noted, have completed in excess of 800 launches. The 97.5% success record thus translates to a total of 20 major failures—with most of those occurring in the earliest years of the Soyuz's development. Figure 7.3 shows the launch of a Progress 1M/Soyuz mission to the ISS.

The Progress 1M/Soyuz evolved from the R-7A intercontinental ballistic missile used to launch Sputnik in 1957 and the Vostok that carried Yuri Gagarin into space in 1961 and also launched the first unmanned spacecraft to the moon. The Progress 1M/Soyuz launcher was introduced in 1966 as a three-stage rocket, and later models were produced with a variety of fourth stages. The Soyuz U/Fregat, which utilizes a highly adaptable, restartable Fregat upper stage, was developed in order to supply more power than previous versions. The Soyuz U was replaced by the Soyuz/ST launcher in 2005 to increase the performance and payload capacity of the launch system even further [3,8].

The Progress 1M/Soyuz consists of three or four stages topped with the payload accommodation. For missions to low Earth orbit or manned launches of the Soyuz spacecraft, the Progress 1M/Soyuz launcher uses three stages to reach orbit. For higher geostationary, elliptical and escape missions,

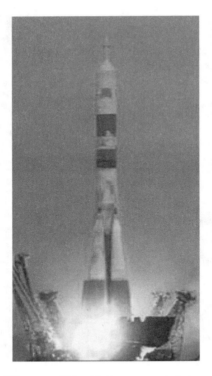

Figure 7-3 Launch of Progress 1M with Soyuz module bound for ISS (graphic courtesy of NASA).

a Fregat upper stage is added to supply greater thrust power. Table 7.1 outlines the payload capacity for a particular mission [9,10].

A mixture of liquid oxygen and kerosene powers the first three stages of a Soyuz launch with each engine having four combustion chambers and nozzles. The fourth stage uses storable hypergolic propellants (UDMH/N2O4) that provide for an easy restart capability. This flexible fourth stage can thus enable the Soyuz to carry out complex mission profiles. Because of their toxic nature, the use of hypergolic fuels always represents a safety concern for those aboard manned spacecraft. Currently, however, there are no plans to replace the UDMH/N2O4 with another fuel [8].

Table 7-1 Payload Capacity for Soyuz to Different Orbits (Information Courtesy of Starsem)

Orbit	Payload Capacity, tons
Low Earth orbit	5.0
Sun-synchronous orbit	4.4
Medium Earth orbit	2.1
Geostationary orbit	1.8
Escape	1.2

Further Improvement in the Safety of the Soyuz

The Progress 1M/Soyuz launch-vehicle system and payload are integrated horizontally in a hanger. The rocket is moved by rail and erected on the pad only two days before launch. Currently the Soyuz has a production rate of 9 to 12 launch vehicles per year in response to Russian Space Agency, commercial and ISS activity. Increasing the production rate to a higher level to support an accelerated finish of the ISS could very well represent a safety hazard in that production of these vehicles must be carefully monitored and subsystems must remain under stringent quality control.

The new Soyuz TMA design that adds two new engines to soften landing impact represents a useful safety measure. Likewise the new entry control system and three-axis accelerometer that increase landing accuracy represent clear safety enhancements. Also, the recent move to provide crew members with satellite telephones and enhanced GPS locational capability are additional safety precautions.

The Soyuz launch system has sustained a success rate of over 97.5% over a nearly 30-year period. Most significantly it has had only one major accident in the past 15 years. The long string of successful launches was broken in October 2002, when a suspected engine failure on the Soyuz U launcher caused an explosion 29 s after liftoff killing one person and injuring eight on the ground. Despite this accident, the Soyuz has proven reliability and robustness, and it is the only human-rated launch system within Russia [4].

The Soyuz launch system's reliability and adaptability are its greatest traits. It can be utilized in a variety of ways, from transporting crew or supplies to the ISS to launching satellites and exploratory missions with a modified Soyuz launcher. It is difficult to directly compare the Soyuz and the shuttle because the designs are quite different. The Soyuz uses an expendable Progress 1M rocket to obtain Earth orbit and a capsule return to come back to the Earth's surface. Each Soyuz is a "new creation," whereas the shuttle, as a reusable craft, carries with it the history of stress and atmospheric heating that accumulates with each mission. Thus one can anticipate that Soyuz vehicles will likely continue to improve their safety record as engineering upgrades are made, but in the case of the shuttle the wear of age and stress of launch and deorbit can erode safety margins. Certainly, the Soyuz history of 800-plus flights greatly outweighs the 100-plus flights of the shuttle, but nevertheless safety concerns remain [5].

Recent history with the Soyuz TMA includes mishaps or near mishaps that have not been publicly disclosed in full, and, as a consequence, details of these problems are limited. According to a NASA source, who has requested anonymity, "We are only one mistake away with a Russian Soyuz space capsule accident and then we would have no capability to support human spaceflight. For example, during the Soyuz incident in 2003, the Soyuz spacecraft experienced life endangering accelerations in excess of 9 g's and landed 250 nautical miles off target."

An open source report describes the following event:

> In May 2003 the crew of Soyuz TMA-1 landed some 440 km (275 miles) short of their planned landing target in Kazakhstan. A malfunction had caused their descent vehicle to perform a ballistic rather than a controlled re-entry. After two hours of searching, rescue aircraft picked up the signal from its radio beacon and located the descent module. All involved expressed frustration that the crew was not able to communicate with mission control or, even if they did, that they would not have been able to give their location to the recovery team.‡

As noted earlier, this problem has been solved by adding a GPS receiver and a satellite phone to the Soyuz craft for future missions, but the malfunction in the capsule return process has not yet been adequately addressed. Although the use of commercially available satellite-based navigation and communications service equipment might seem prosaic, it makes perfectly good sense to utilize these capabilities, but only as backup. For example, the high accelerations experienced by the Soyuz TMA-1 capsule could have damaged the vehicle and/or injured the persons onboard to the extent that the crew might not have been able to open the capsule hatch or extricate themselves out of the capsule enough to make these commercial communications and GPS systems operate [6 and 7].

It is fortunate that the Soyuz TMA-1 vehicle had the conventional aircraft emergency locator transmitter (ELT) system that allowed the search aircraft to find the capsule that was 440 km off the intended landing zone. The typical ELT system transmissions at 121.5 MHz suffer from reflections off the local terrain that greatly complicate the ability to find the location of the ELT device in a timely manner. This early ELT system is reported to have a 97% false-alarm rate and typically functions in only 12% of crashes. There is also a much superior system using 406-MHz transmissions of the COSPAS–SARSAT international program. However, use of the 406-MHz system could require from tens of minutes up to an hour to produce a clear-cut location before search and rescue teams could begin their operations [8].

A newer innovation is the personal locator beacon (PLB) that allows rescue forces to home in on a beacon once the 406-MHz satellite system has got them "in the ballpark" (about two to three miles). Some newer PLBs also allow GPS-derived location information to be integrated into the distress signal. This GPS-encoded position dramatically improves the location accuracy down to the 100-m level or better, depending upon the availability of correction signals from the WAAS (wide-area augmentation system) operated by the U.S. Federal Aviation Administration (FAA) and other international partners in Europe and Asia [9].

---

‡Data available online at http://www.Spaceref.com [cited 27 Oct. 2003].

International Modules and Components of the International Space Station

The International Space Station is one of the largest and most expensive international collaborative projects in recorded history. Major forms of participation come from the United States, the European Space Agency, Japan, Canada, and Russia. This international participation is reflected not only in the design and construction of the ISS in terms of its safety, its various modules and operating components, but also in terms of a high level of international experimentation. As also summarized in Chapter 5, the major non-U.S. components of the ISS are as outlined here: for Europe the automated transfer vehicle and the Columbia laboratory; for Japan the Japan experimental module (known as Kibo), the HII transfer vehicle, and the centrifuge accommodation module (CAM) (Note NASA has now canceled the CAM); for Canada the Canadarm 2 and the mobile service system (or Manipulator or Canada Hand); and for Russia the various launch systems and modules as well as key life-support systems (i.e., space suits, oxygen generators, and other components such as batteries, etc.).

International participation in the ISS project is beneficial in terms of spreading the costs for this huge undertaking, plus it allows a much wider range of research competencies to work on this megaproject. The scope and scale of the undertaking would certainly have been greatly reduced without the resources and technology added to the project through international participation. Without the United States and Russia, there would not have been the capability to launch and integrate such a large structure in space.

Despite the program and cost benefits of international participation, the international nature of the ISS program has given rise to a number of difficulties as well and in some cases concern for increased risk factors and reduced safety [10].

Japanese Participation in the ISS

Japan participated in the ISS from the outset and has been one of the most enthusiastic partners. Their participation includes the Japanese engineering module known as Kibo, the HII transfer vehicle, and the centrifuge accommodation module (CAM). In total these modules and the HII launch system represent several billions of dollars of investment and a substantial portion of the NASDA (now JAXA) annual budgets over the past few decades.

Japanese Experimental Module (known as Kibo)

The Japanese experimental module (JEM), or Kibo, was designed to be a major contribution to the International Space Station (ISS) and Japan's first human space facility. The JEM was designed to focus on space medicine, biology, Earth observations, material production, biotechnology, and communications research.§ Figure 7.4 shows an illustration of the completed JEM.

---

§Data available online at http://www.nasa.gov.

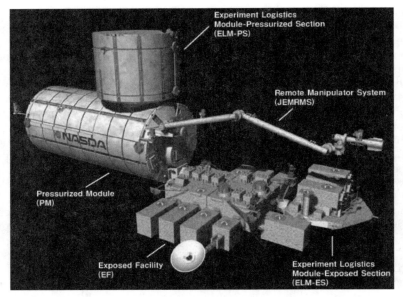

Figure 7-4   Kibo—Japanese experiment module (graphic courtesy of Spaceandtech.com)

Kibo consists of two main components: the pressurized module (PM) for microgravity experiments and the exposed facility for experiments in the space environment. The PM provides an environment where up to four astronauts can complete bio and material experiments in a microgravity environment. The exposed facility is a unique platform on the ISS that is continuously exposed to the space environment. Experiments on the exposed platform can range from Earth observation and communication systems to scientific, engineering, and materials science experiments. There is an airlock separating the components, and both have experiment logistics modules (ELM) that allow in-orbit storage for the experiments.[1]

In addition to the research facilities, the Kibo will have a remote manipulator system (RMS) and an interorbit communication system unit (ICS). The RMS consists of two robotic arms that are operated from a computer console inside the pressurized module. These robotic arms support operations outside of Kibo with the main arm capable of lifting up to 6.4 metric tons and the small fine arm handling more delicate operations. The ICS allows direct communication between Kibo and Mission Control at the Tsukuba Space Center to facilitate transfer of system, payload, and video data for scientific operations.

---

[1]Data available online at http://www.nasa.gov.

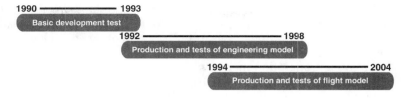

Figure 7-5 Original Kibo development schedule (graphic courtesy of JAXA).

The development of Kibo was divided into three stages: 1) basic development test stage; 2) engineering model production and test stage; and 3) proto flight model production and test stage. The original development schedule of the Kibo can be seen in Fig. 7.5. Just as is the case with every phase of the ISS, the grounding of the shuttle system has substantially delayed the JEM–Kibo system and in this instance on the order of four to five years. This is because the deployment of JEM will likely require three Shuttle launches.

The second stage of development was completed in October 1998 with the production of two engineering models for testing. Tests on these two models allowed the final module to be developed and produced. The completed JEM was unveiled in Japan in October 2001 with final testing conducted in following months.[**]

The pressurized module of the Kibo was transported to the Space Station Processing Facility at Kennedy Space Center (KSC), arriving on 30 May 2003. The additional components were expected to be transported in 2003 with the entire module scheduled to undergo preflight testing at KSC before its scheduled 2004 launch. However, the *Columbia* accident in February 2003 severely disrupted the assembly timetable of the ISS. Consequently, the assembly of the Kibo is not likely to be completed until 2009 or so. Indeed the reduced launch schedule for the shuttle could lead to questions about the United States completing the deployment of the JEM. An unwillingness by the United States to deploy the JEM would seriously jeopardize U.S.–Japanese space cooperation and even overall international relationships given the huge investment made in this module by the Japanese government.

There are several safety implications related to the JEM (Kibo). These include the following:

1) The first is environmental and aging issues related to a highly complex mechanism waiting in storage for five years or more even if stored in special pressurized storage units. (Although retesting and certification can certainly take place prior to launch, the possibility of wiring connections becoming loosened, the effects of oxidation, or other environmental effects are certainly highly undesirable.)

[**]Data available online at http://www.space.com.

2) The separate airlock system on the JEM for conducting experiments outside the ISS raises several issues related to the atmospheric seals against leakage, the operation of the air pumps, and other controls related to the proper control of this mechanism.

3) Kibo system operation inside this module is to be controlled from the Mission Control Room from the Tsukuba Space Center in the Ibaraki region of Japan. The issue of normal operational and emergency distribution of resources of the ISS such as power, crew resources (food, water, and oxygen), and communications is now governed by a negotiated agreement. In an emergency situation, however, there is a question as to whether "distributed" control of individual modules (particularly for the Columbus, JEM/Kibo/U.S. facilities, etc.) will be the most effective mode of operation [11].

4) The fundamental safety issue, of course, is the need for three shuttle missions to lift the various parts of the JEM (Kibo) up to the ISS and the installation of this very large and complex system after being in storage for four to five years. On the plus side, however, the communications system that is a part of the JEM (Kibo) is an alternative or backup way to provide a fail-safe communications link to the ISS. Further, if the JEM is indeed inhabited by as many as four research crew, this should provide increased life-science testing with regard to the problem of living in the space environment for long periods of time. These additional data will be key in preparing for future lunar missions.

Centrifuge Accommodation Module

The centrifuge accommodation module (CAM) is a laboratory module dedicated to gravitational biology research that was also designed to be installed on the ISS. Unfortunately this key component of the ISS has now been canceled. The main purpose of the CAM is to study the long-term effects of varying gravity levels on the structure and function of living organisms and to test methods for countering any negative results caused by those variations. The results obtained could be important for future manned missions as it could supply information on the health, safety, and productivity of humans during long-term space travel. Figure 7.6 shows an illustration of the centrifuge accommodation module.[††]

The CAM consists of a centrifuge rotor, a life-sciences glovebox (LSG), and the module itself. Originally scheduled to be developed and constructed in the United States, a 1998 agreement was reached with NASDA [now the Japan Aerospace Exploration Agency (JAXA)], whereby Japan would build the CAM and centrifuge rotor to offset the cost of launching the Japanese experimental module (JEM) aboard the space shuttle.[‡‡]

[††]Data available online at http://iss.sfo.jaxa.jp/iss/contribution/ issjpdoc 3_2_e.html.
[‡‡]Data available online at http://www.boeing.com/defense-space/space/ spacestation/components/centrifuge_module.html.

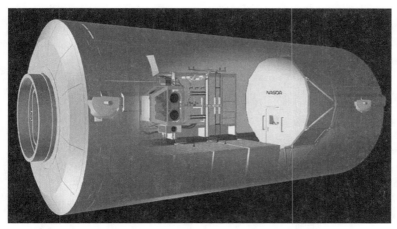

Figure 7-6   Centrifuge accommodation module (graphic courtesy of JAXA).

The United States is to provide the LSG, CAM racks, and other hardware, and once in orbit the CAM is to be operated as a U.S. facility. The CAM was originally scheduled to be launched aboard STS-134 in 2006; however, this date has been pushed back and is still to be determined depending on the return-to-flight activities.§§

The CAM is 29 ft (8.9 m) long, 14.4 ft (4.4 m) in diameter, and has a launch weight of 10 tons. It is designed to house the centrifuge rotor and LSG and has 14 rack locations, four for experimental hardware and 10 for storage. The centrifuge facility contains an 8.2-ft (2.5-m)-diam centrifuge rotor (CR) mounted in the end cone of the CAM. At 1825 kg the rotor will be the largest to have ever flown in space and is capable of providing artificial gravity levels ranging from 0.001 to 2 g. The centrifuge is designed to house microorganisms, plants, and small animals and can accommodate up to eight habitats at any time. It will allow research to be done on these specimens to test the effects of varying g levels. Figure 7.7 shows a diagram of the centrifuge rotor.§§

The life-science glovebox or LSG is an enclosed work environment that would enable astronauts to complete experiments with biological specimens and chemicals while remaining safely out of contact with the rest of the ISS. Within the LSG, ISS crew members are to use gloves that are incorporated into the glovebox to manipulate specimens. The LSG was designed to be used for scientific procedures such as dissection and microsurgery on small research animals, tending to bacterial and microorganism cultures, and the seeding and harvesting of plant specimens. It has a working volume large enough for two crew members to work in

---

§§Data available online at http://www.spaceref.com/iss/elements/cam.html.

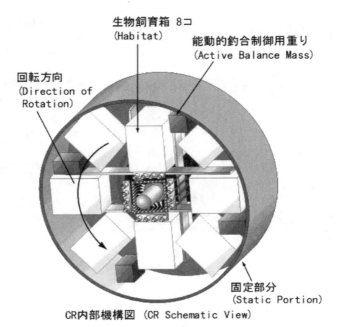

生物飼育箱 8コ
(Habitat)

能動的釣合制御用重り
(Active Balance Mass)

回転方向
(Direction of
Rotation)

固定部分
(Static Portion)

CR内部機構図 (CR Schematic View)

Figure 7-7   Centrifuge rotor (graphic courtesy of JAXA).

and will be maintained at temperatures between 18–27°C. Although the CAM was initially due for launch in September 2004, the deployment of this unit, which is to be operated as a U.S. facility, is currently in question as ways to reduce the number of shuttle launches continues to be explored.¶¶

Figure 7.8 shows a diagram of the life-sciences glovebox.

The development and integration of the CAM to the ISS, along with the Columbus and JEM, would bring number of the station's laboratories to three. The safety implications of the CAM are essentially the same as those noted with regard to the JEM and thus will not be repeated.¶¶ Even though the CAM was built for the United States and is intended to be staffed by U.S. scientists, a decision not to deploy this very sophisticated lab facility would be seen by the Japanese government as a strong negative both in terms of current ISS and future international space cooperation. The fact that this project was in effect carried out as a "trade-off compensation" between the United States and Japan, however, could make it easier for the United States to not deploy the CAM, in the event limited shuttle launch capability should make this necessary.

¶¶Data available online at http://www.spaceref.cam/iss/elements/com.html.

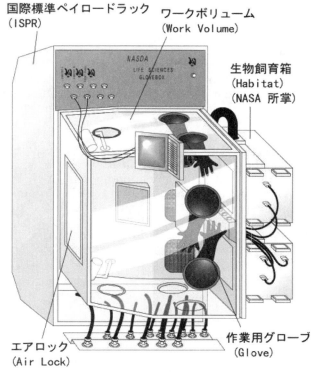

国際標準ペイロードラック
（ISPR）

ワークボリューム
（Work Volume）

生物飼育箱
（Habitat）
（NASA 所掌）

エアロック
（Air Lock）

作業用グローブ
（Glove）

Figure 7-8   Life-sciences glove box (graphic courtesy of JAXA).

The Japanese HII Transfer Vehicle (HTV)

The HII transfer vehicle is designed as a four-module unit that is about 4 m in diameter (13 ft) and 10 m (33 ft) in length and is composed of four components that include the logistic carrier pressurized section, the logistic carrier unpressurized section, the power module, and the propulsion unit.

The HTV is designed to carry out independent flights from the ISS with the rendezvous between the HTV and the ISS being accomplished by use of the ISS remote manipulator systems (SSRMS) that will capture the HTV and secure it for crew transfer from the pressurized section of the HTV to the space station. The experience with the Japanese experimental test satellite ETS-VII to carry out robotically controlled docking in space served as a precursor to this more ambitious space project.

The navigation and guidance system (SIGI for Space Integrated GPSR/IMU) that uses a combination of accelerometers and ring laser gyros has been designed by Honeywell of Tampa, Florida, and has been fully tested to control the capture and docking of the HTV with the ISS.

The HTV program has been postponed as a result of the *Columbia* accident and difficulties with the HII program. The safety concerns with regard to the HTV system are several. The close manuevers to the ISS for capture by the SSRMS is a safety concern as well as the performance of the SIGI in that the GPS system was designed for exact location on the Earth's surface and not well out into space in low Earth orbit. In short some degree of accuracy is not achievable several hundred kilometers off the Earth's surface.***

In light of the sizable delay in the deployment of the HTV system, its deployment might usefully be reexamined both from a safety and fiscal savings standpoint. Such reexamination by both JAXA and NASA of the HTV program would thus consider whether redeployment of resources might be advisable at this time, particularly if the European ATV system performs to specifications. One alternative would be to see if the Progress IM/Soyuz, and especially the Ariane 5/ATV, might be substituted for the HTV (assuming the ATV proves successful in initial flights). In this case Japan/JAXA would be able to reinvest resources in other programs.

Canadian Participation–Canadarm2

The Canadarm2 is a robotic RMS that is an essential component of the ISS and one that plays a key role in the station's assembly and maintenance. A major part of the remote manipulator system known as the mobile servicing system (MSS) is yet to be installed. The MSS is capable of moving equipment and supplies around the station, servicing instruments and other payloads, and supporting astronauts in space. Figure 7.9 shows Canadarm2 after installation on the ISS.

The MSS has been considered key to the construction, maintenance, and servicing of the ISS, and it consists of three separate but integrated parts. An artist's impression of the completed three components of the MMS can be seen in Fig. 7.10.

The basic elements of Canadarm2 were launched aboard the space Shuttle *Endeavor* in April 2001. The design incorporates seven motorized joints, and, when fully extended, it extends to 17.6 m (57.7 ft). The Canadarm2, because of the "relative weightlessness of outer space," is capable of handling large payloads. It was initially designed to be able to help the shuttle dock with the ISS, but this remains only an option in an emergency.

One of the key benefits of the Canardarm2 is that unlike the shuttle's Canadarm it can be relocated and is not fixed to one spot. Up to 10

***Data available online at http://www.jaxa.jp/missions/projects/rockets/ htv/booknumber_e.html.

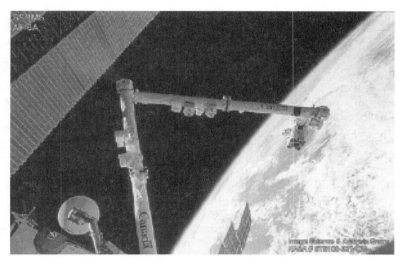

Figure 7-9   Canadarm2 on the ISS (graphic courtesy of NASA).

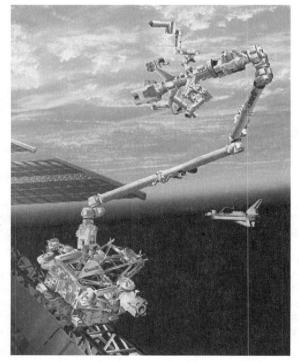

Figure 7-10   Artist's impression of mobile servicing system of the ISS (graphic courtesy of NASA).

construction sites would ultimately be possible using this relocatable feature. The RMS has two identical hands on each end that allow it to inchworm its way around the station, grabbing hold of conveniently positioned power data grapple fixtures (PDGF). PDGFs are round antenna-like devices that provide Canadarm2 with power and computer links as well as physical attachment to the ISS. These fixtures are to be added strategically in order to allow the arm to maneuver itself completely around the station.[†††]

The mobile base system (MBS) is the second major component of the MSS. This system was installed during the STS-111 flight in June 2002 and is a movable aluminum platform that provides lateral mobility for the Canadarm2 and other equipment. The MBS fits on the American-built mobile transporter and runs on tracks around the station. Combined with the Canadarm2, these two components have the capability to transport and lift construction equipment to different work sites on the ISS that expand as the station's construction is completed. This capability potentially increases the speed at which construction and maintenance can be completed on the station.[‡‡‡]

The final component of the MSS is the special purpose dexterous manipulator (SPDM) or Canada Hand, which is an attachment for the end of the Canadarm2. The Canada Hand is a highly advanced two-armed robot that is capable of handling delicate assembly tasks currently performed by astronauts during EVAs. Utilizing sophisticated feedback mechanisms that allow it to touch and feel much like a human hand, the Canada Hand will perform subtle operations such as installing batteries, power supplies, and computers in addition to simple structural elements. The Canada Hand will substantially reduce the amount of time astronauts spend outside the station on dangerous EVAs. Currently, the Canada Hand is to be launched soon after the space shuttle transportation system is able to return to flight during 2006.

There are relatively few safety implications for the Canadarm2 once the various elements are in place, except on the positive side. The completed facility will be able to reduce astronaut EVAs associated with construction, and, as noted earlier, EVAs are one of the greater risk elements because of the hazards of orbital debris, possible suit decompression, etc. Further, the fully deployed Canadarm2 facility, complete with video-camera capabilities, will allow improved reconnaissance for examining the shuttle's thermal protection system or investigating the impact and possible damage to the ISS caused by orbital debris. Thus, although there are clearly hazards associated with completing the full installation of the Canadarm2 and the Canada Hand, there are clear safety advantages that result from this highly flexible capability being onboard the ISS. These Canadarm2 technologies can, of course, be reapplied on the surface of the moon or Mars. Undoubtedly these additional applications will

---

[†††]Data available online at http://www.nasa.gov.
[‡‡‡]Data available online at http://www.canadaonline.com.

occur as the advantages of robotic systems operations are increasingly recognized within space exploration programs.

There will continue to be intense pressure within NASA and the U.S. government to limit shuttle missions and reduce ISS costs. In essence there will be a search to identify elements that might be "subtracted" from the ISS full build-out program. In this respect a clear set of criteria needs to be developed against which launch priorities might be set. Criteria that might be considered appropriate and relevant include the following:

1) Does it involve a significant and previously agreed international commitment?

2) Does the launch of a particular module or component raise or lower astronaut safety?

3) Does the mission either speed or slow ISS construction?

4) Would ISS operation and scientific mission over the longer term be more difficult and more dangerous without it?

The Canadian Canadarm2 and MMS capability seemingly score very high with regard to all four criteria. The prime safety concern, however, is whether the flexible PDGF will operate as designed. This is a new and unproven capability (at least in space) that should be tested thoroughly on the ground and in space before committing the use of these systems to astronaut operations in a life-dependent mode.

European Space Programs in Support of the ISS

The European Space Agency (ESA) has been a crucial partner in the International Space Agency and has assisted the project in many different ways. The two prime contributions are the ATV and the Columbus laboratory.

The ATV is an automatic, unmanned transport vehicle that will be used for the periodic supply of the ISS and is capable of carrying about three times more cargo than the Russian Progress/Soyuz. Thus the ATV can supply the ISS with food, water, oxygen, nitrogen, and propellant in order to keep the station operational, and it can also be used to raise the orbit of the ISS or to perform collision avoidance with debris. In these respects the ATV adds major new safety capabilities to the ISS after it is successfully docked. The ATV is launched aboard the Ariane 5 as a final stage. The entire ATV apparatus is destroyed in the Earth's atmosphere during the return flight after spending up to six months docked to the ISS. Figure 7.11 shows an artist's representation of the ATV.

The ATV was first proposed in the mid-1980s as a way to transport unmanned cargo to space stations. Early studies focused on using a modified Ariane 5 upper stage, but in 1992 the ESA decided a propulsion module combined with a cargo module would be more efficient and would

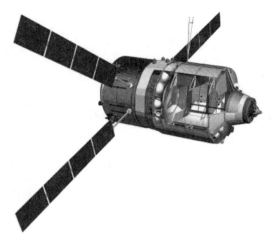

Figure 7-11   Automated transfer vehicle (graphic courtesy of ESA).

also add more capability once docked with the ISS. ESA signed a $470-million contract with Aerospatiale, a division of European Aeronautics Defense and Space Company (EADS), in 1998 for the development of the ATV.§§§ In July 2004, ESA signed a $1-billion contract with EADS for the production of six additional ATVs in addition to the first ATV, named the Jules Verne. The first flight of the ATV was initially scheduled to take place in September 2004; however, software integration and propulsion bay issues delayed the test flight.

The two prime objectives of the latest space walk (i.e., EVAs) by the two remaining space-station crew were to carry out critical repairs and also to prepare the ISS for docking with the Jules Verne ATV.

The ATV is designed to play the role of a cargo and logistics vehicle for the ISS and in this regard will complement the smaller and less capable Russian supply vehicles if the European system proves successful. After its launch aboard an Ariane 5 launch vehicle, the ATV will take two days to reach the ISS. One of its key safety features is that it can be docked either automatically or manually. After unloading, it can stay attached to the ISS for up to six months to provide orbital maneuvering capability before being refilled with trash and deorbited. The vehicle and the trash will then be burned up in the atmosphere during reentry. There are conceptual studies of how the ATV could be extended to provide for a crew return capability, but such a program has yet to be formally approved or funded. Figure 7.12 shows an artist's impression of the ATV rendezvousing with the ISS.

The ATV consists of two modules known as the cargo module and the spacecraft module. The cargo module is composed of two sections, one

§§§Data available online at http://www.astronautix.com.

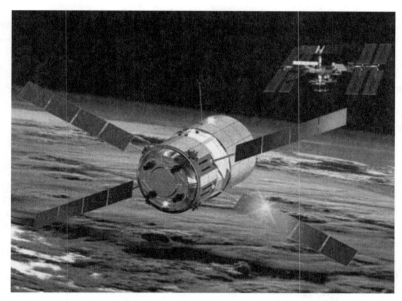

Figure 7-12   Impression of ATV and ISS (graphic courtesy of NASA).

pressurized and one unpressurized. The pressurized section has room for up to eight racks to stow standard ISS cargo transfer bags that carry items such as food, clothing, and equipment. The unpressurized section holds several titanium tanks containing the water, oxygen, nitrogen, and propellant that can be transferred to the ISS. The cargo module also contains the docking equipment and most of the spacecraft's avionics in the front section of the module.¶¶¶ Table 7.2 below lists the payload capabilities of the ATV.

The spacecraft module has four main and 28 smaller thrusters for maneuvering itself and the ISS in space. After docking, the ATV will be able to change the ISS's attitude with its smaller thrusters or use the four main thrusters for debris avoidance or to maneuver the station to a higher orbit. Reboosting the ISS is an important mission objective for the ATV because of its increased propellant capacity and the future limited supply of the Russian Progress/Soyuz vehicles.¶¶¶

The launch weight for the ATV, at 20,750 kg, is nearly three times that of the Progress M1's 7150 kg, and it is capable of carrying nearly three times the cargo and propellant for the ISS. The increased size will also make it easier for the ISS crew in loading and unloading the ATV. Figure 7.13 shows a comparison between the sizes of the two spacecraft.

¶¶¶Data available online at http://www.esa.int.

Table 7-2   Technical Characteristics of the ATV

Characteristic	Value
ATV dimensions	
Length	9.79 m
Largest diameter	4.48 m
Span with solar arrays deployed	22.28 m
ATV mass	13,084 kg
Maximum launch weight	20,750 kg
ATV cargo mass	
Dry cargo	1500–5500 kg
Water	0–840 kg
Gas (nitrogen, oxygen)	0–100 kg
ISS reboost and attitude control propellant	0–4500 kg
Total cargo upload capacity	7667 kg
Waste download capacity	6500 kg
ATV propulsion	
Main propulsion system	4×490 N thrusters
Attitude control system	28×220 N thrusters
Propellant	Monomethyl-hydrazine fuel and nitrogen-tetroxide oxidizer

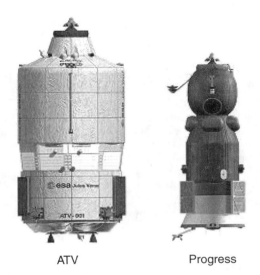

ATV   Progress

Figure 7-13   Comparison between ATV and Progress (graphics courtesy of ESA).

ATV Role in Resupply of ISS

The ATV is scheduled to play a vital role in resupplying the ISS over the coming years. An extra vehicle capable of reaching the ISS will alleviate the reliance on Soyuz/Progress missions and increase the safety of the crew onboard. The ATV also marks the first European contribution of hardware to the ISS operating system. The design, manufacture, test, and launch of the ATV spacecraft over the coming years represents the largest part of the European multibillion dollar investment in this program, although the Columbia Laboratory described next is also of great significance.

The safety implications of the ATV are essentially four-fold:

1) **The first is the risk of docking and separation from the ISS.** There is danger of misfiring of thrusters and of computer, communications, or ranging data error that would somehow result in a collision of the ATV and the ISS. There is also some danger that the docking and undocking mechanisms might not work properly, which could also create safety concerns. The fact that automated and manually controlled docking is possible is clearly an asset from a safety perspective. Also the fact that there are 28 smaller thrusters of 220 N thrust and four larger thrusters of 490 N thrust is also significant in that failure of a number of thrusters would still allow a high degree of maneuverability.

2) **The second safety implication is an unproven space vehicle.** The ATV is essentially the top stage of the now well-proven Ariane 5 vehicle, and the thrusters on the ATV did not require new technology. The four main thrusters, backed up by the lower power thrusters, mean that the risks associated with the ATV propulsion system for docking and undocking are very small in terms of achieving needed power. However there is the issue of a stuck valve that would prevent the shutdown of a thruster's firing, which could be a serious problem. Extra careful testing of the thruster valves and the capability to achieve emergency shutdown is therefore considered to be highly desirable. The guidance, avionics, and solar-array deployment systems are also areas of concern, and these will be tested during the two-day mission before the ATV actually attempts to dock with the ISS.

3) **Orbit-raising capability is the third safety implication.** Because of the grounding of the space shuttle, the orbit-raising capability for the ISS is currently limited to Russian vehicles. The ATV will not only add an important new capability to relay supplies to the ISS, but also help ensure against excessive decay of the ISS orbit caused by the Earth's gravity and such factors as unexpected solar storms.

4) **The final implication is orbital maneuver capability to avoid debris.** The ATV adds significant new maneuverability that could be key to avoiding a collision with a significant element of debris.

European Columbus Laboratory

The Columbus is a pressurized, habitable research module that is one of the main contributions to the ISS by the ESA. Once assembled at the station, the

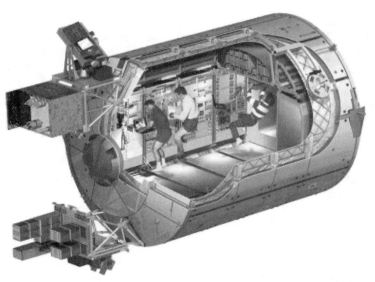

Figure 7-14   Columbus European laboratory (graphic courtesy of ESA).

Columbus is designed to provide internal payload accommodation for experiments in the fields of materials and fluid sciences, life sciences, and technology development. In addition, an external payload facility will host experiments and applications in the field of space sciences and Earth observation. Figure 7.14 shows an artist's cut-away impression of the Columbus Laboratory.****

The main contractor for the Columbus is Astrium GmbH, based in Bremen, Germany, plus there are several subcontractors. To achieve cost benefits, the basic design is based on the multipurpose logistics module (MPLM), which is a transport module provided to the ISS by the Italian Space Agency. The internal configuration of the Columbus laboratory provides 10 international standard payload racks (ISPR) for active research payloads with three extra for passive stowage. The exposed payload facility consists of two separate support structures attached to the end cone of the module that allows direct exposure to space for research.**** This direct exposure to space requires an additional airlock, just as the case for the JEM, and thus this feature provides another area of safety concern. Extensive pre-launch testing, however, will re-verify the airlock performance.

Table 7.3 outlines the dimensions and payload capacities of the Columbus laboratory.

****Data available online at http://www.esa.int.

Table 7-3 Columbus Laboratory Capabilities

Characteristic	Value
Columbus space laboratory dimensions	
Total module length	6.871 m
Largest diameter	4.477 m
Total internal volume	75 m³
Total volume of payload racks	25 m³
Mass	
Mass without payload	10,300 kg
Launch mass	12,800 kg
	(2500 kg payload)
Maximum payload mass	9000 kg
Maximum on orbit mass	19,300 kg
Environmental control	
Supported crew	3
Cabin temperature	16–30°C

The Columbus laboratory has undergone extensive testing to ensure that the module will be adaptable to the ISS and function correctly in orbit. The Columbus crew trainer has been developed to allow ISS astronauts to train in an exact replica of the interior of the module that simulates its functional characteristics. One trainer makes up part of the Space Station Training Facility at NASA's Johnson Space Center (JSC) while there is another at the European Astronaut Center in Cologne ("ISS Columbus"). Figure 7.15 shows a mock-up of Columbus undergoing verification of external operations in the JSC Neutral Buoyancy Laboratory.[††††]

Once in orbit, operation of the Columbus laboratory will take place at the Columbus control center (Col-CC) in Oberpfaffenhofen, Bavaria. The Col-CC is part of the German Space Operations Center (GSOC). Operations will be carried out under the leadership of the German center in close cooperation with the ESA and NASA. The responsibilities of the GSOC and Col-CC during Columbus flight operations include systems control and monitoring; coordination of the European payload operations activities; operations of the European communications network, including ATV communications support; and planning and coordination of all activities mentioned over the lifetime of the Columbus, which ESA anticipates will be 10 to 15 years.

Just as in the case of the JEM/Kibo, the issue of a separate communications network and operational control center offers redundant communications to the ISS, but it also raises the issue of overall ISS control and

---

[††††]Data available online at http://www.spaceref.com/redirect.ref? url-www. gsoc.dlr.de/columbus.htm&id-1163.

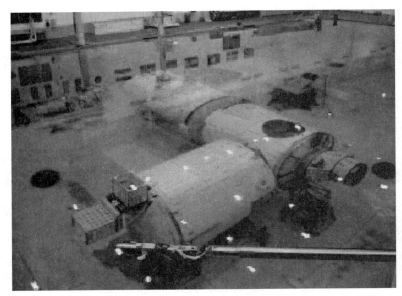

Figure 7-15   Columbus mockup in JSC Neutral Buoyancy laboratory (photo
courtesy of NASA).

operations in emergency situations where there might be a need to ration
power, exercise environmental controls, and marshal other scarce
resources. Unified controls for the ISS related to power rationing, emergency evacuation, etc. are therefore clearly needed. The International
Association for the Advancement of Space Safety (IAASS) has, in particular, flagged this issue and recommended possible solutions in terms of ISS
management safety standards and integrated safety processes.

There is also an issue of the planned operational timeline. If the
Columbus laboratory and the JEM are deployed in the 2007 to 2009 time
period and operated for 15 years, this would imply continuous in-orbit
support through 2022 or even to 2025. However, NASA with its priority
shifted to support Project Constellation might seek to end ISS operations
earlier than that date. Certainly continuous safe operation of the ISS,
with its many aging components (and dated technologies) for this
extended period, will represent a huge challenge for space safety and risk
reduction.

Columbus is currently awaiting launch at NASA's Kennedy Space
Center. Originally scheduled to fly in October 2004 onboard STS-124, the
grounding of the space shuttle has pushed that date back to an estimated
2007 time frame. Once in orbit, it will attach to Node-2 on the ISS and is
expected to have a 10–15-year usable life. The lab's cost was approximately $1.4 billion to design and develop. As a result of the delayed
deployment of several years, substantial cost overruns are being incurred

because the integration and launch preparation teams must be kept together until launch.

Once assembled at the ISS, the Columbus laboratory will be the main workplace for the scientific and technological activities of the European astronauts onboard the station. It will enable the ESA and its research partners, including the United States, to acquire valuable experience in long duration spaceflight and the operation and utilization of in-orbit infrastructure.

If the Columbus laboratory is launched and installed in the ISS in 2007, it would require operation of the ISS through 2022 to achieve its projected lifetime. The same issue also applies and, even more so, to the JEM/Kibo because it might not be deployed until 2009. This extended ISS operational lifetime, that is, perhaps through 2025, is substantially longer than is projected by current U.S. budgetary plans.

Finally there are some safety concerns with regard to the Columbus laboratory that in many ways mirror those with respect to the Japanese Kibo module (or JEM). These concerns include the following:

1) The need for retest of the module after several years of "mothballing" because of the grounding of the shuttle fleet is the first concern. (This module, of course, is also stored in a pressurized and environmental controlled facility, but wiring, seals, gaskets, and other components could be an issue after several years of storage.)

2) Second are the concerns about the performance of the airlock system that allows the Columbus to perform external experiments. (Again, as in the case with the JEM/Kibo, the airlock system was designed to high standards, and its performance is likely to be faultless. Nevertheless, particular test of the airlock performance is important.)

3) The independent control center for this research facility is not under a unified system or centralized ISS safety authority.

4) There is a need for thorough checkout of the complex Columbus laboratory after it is launched and installed on the ISS before it is officially activated and crew placed within this facility.

European Overall Space Policy Guidelines and Action Plan

The European space policies are complex. This is because of the number of countries involved and because the European Space Agency, headquartered in Paris, France, and the European Union, which acts through the European Commission and is headquartered in Brussels, Belgium, include different member countries. At this point both entities are involved in defining and funding European space programs, and there is not always agreement on space priorities and programs.‡‡‡‡

---

‡‡‡‡Data available online at http://www.space.com/news/spacestation/iss_ esacomp.html.

On 11 November 2003, the European Commission presented a policy paper on "Space: A New European Frontier for an Expanding Union." In this policy paper a detailed proposed action plan is set forth. Space technologies were identified as playing a key role in helping the European Union achieve its main objectives: faster economic growth, job creation, and industrial competitiveness, enlargement and cohesion, sustainable development, and security and defense. The paper was jointly developed with the European Space Agency, and it calls for substantial additional spending on space. It also recommends action to ensure Europe's independent access to space, enhance space technology, promote space exploration, attract more young people into careers in science, and strengthen European excellence in space science.

According to this new policy paper, European space policy is to be implemented through a new multi-annual European space program that would determine priorities, set objectives, allocate roles and responsibilities, and define annual budgets. Further this program is to be reviewed and updated every five years and is to include a new comprehensive plan that would incorporate research and development, infrastructure development, and services and technology.

In the action plan, space industries are seen as a key contributor to job creation and competitiveness in the European Union (EU) in many crucial high-tech sectors, especially telecommunications, information technologies, and robotics.

Today, the European space sector directly employs over 30,000 people in about 2000 large, medium, and small space companies. Thus, according to the action plan, the restructuring of the EU space industry is of critical importance for its future survival. To attract the necessary investment for the future, the EU space industry will need a steady flow of work, in particular from a strong public procurement market. Under the plan, an increase in space expenditures in the range of 2.3% (about 2.7 billion euros) to a high of 4.6% (or 5.4 billion euros) would support this new space program. What is significant about this plan is that it envisions a separate European access to space, greater independence from the United States with regard to space and defense-related issues, and less willingness to cooperate with the United States in future international space missions. As a part of this process, which officially started in 2003, the first test satellite in the European space navigation satellite system, Galileo, has now been launched and is in testing. Further, there are plans under discussion for a joint Russian and European project to develop a new launch system that might in many ways parallel the NASA crew exploration vehicle.§§§§

Several ministerial level officials in Europe have expressed skepticism about the new U.S. space vision in terms of European participation, but Europe's representatives were nevertheless key participants in the international coordination meeting organized by NASA in November 2004 [12].

---

§§§§Data available online at http://www.esa.int.

Conclusions and Recommendations

International space cooperation, for almost 40 years now, has had strong implications as to how space-faring countries of the world interact politically, economically, and even culturally. The International Space Station was seen as a way to link the developed nations of the world together to cooperate in the area of high technology and scientific discovery. The problems with the two shuttle accidents that have led directly to six, going on seven, years of delay in the deployment of the ISS, in addition to other delays, have now put the program almost 16 years behind schedule. This has led to significant inflation and cost overruns. There have been major systems redesign, problems with onboard noxious gases, oxygen generators, space suits, micrometeorite damage, and gyro stabilizer to name just some of the key ISS issues. Further there have been differences of approach between NASA and the Russian Space Agency on safety issues, which have undercut the anticipated success of this ambitious project, not to mention concerns expressed by other participating space agencies. Unfortunately, the cost of the project has now run to an estimated $100 billion when direct and indirect costs are considered. These cost escalations have led to proposals for possible ways to reduce the scope of the ISS and its experimental program. In short, the problems with the shuttle and the ISS, the new dimensions and plans of other space-faring countries, and the shifting priorities created by Project Constellation do not represent the optimum launchpad for U.S. space cooperation in the coming decade. Quite simply the ISS has fallen far, far short of its initial goals. It is not productive, however, to cry over spilled billions of dollars and lost opportunity. Much can still be gained by improved strategic planning.

Clearly it is important to restore the "success levels and measures" that are expected to be achieved by the ISS against a realistic time line for operation, experimentation, and project completion. Until all of the international partners see merit and value in working with the United States on this project through to its completion, further international collaboration will likely be impaired. Despite these issues involving the ISS, efforts to define meaningful new areas for international space collaboration between NASA and its space partners should be given priority now. Going to the moon, exploring the moon and going on to Mars are hugely challenging, expensive, and technologically difficult efforts. Effective cooperation can help. Not only can it help reduce costs and spur technological progress, but it can contribute to international cooperation and collaboration in many other sectors as well. In this respect, NASA might be well served not only by seeking cooperation with other space agencies around the world, but also by involving private entrepreneurial ventures from among the Organization for Economic Cooperation and Development (OECD) countries as well.

> Quite simply the ISS has fallen far, far short of its initial goals. It is not productive, however, to cry over spilled billions of dollars and lost opportunity. Much can still be gained by improved strategic planning.

In taking further steps to make the ISS more successful, it is highly desirable to set and to agree on realistic scientific, technological, and industrial development goals and objectives against a time-line. It is also essential to establish clearly integrated safety criteria, emergency rules, and operational procedures for times of emergency that can be invoked by a single point of authority that is mutually agreed by all ISS partners. These procedures should cover not only power, environmental control, and systems operations, but also allow for development of emergency procedures and operations that include in-flight repair, increased training for emergency actions, and accelerated departure from the ISS should it need to be abandoned under crisis conditions. Improved self-diagnostics, detection, and alert systems as well as video and reconnaissance capabilities should also continue to be upgraded to reflect new and emerging technologies. This integrated ISS safety authority would also be involved with the planning of in-orbit sparing and any needed in-orbit repair for reconstitution of the ISS and/or the shuttle for safe operation. If meaningful and coherent cooperation cannot be created among all of the ISS partners on this one specific, high-tech project, it is hard to envision how cooperation can be achieved on larger and more difficult issues. One might hope that the ISS could actually help to develop models for collaboration on issues of true global importance such as global warming and renewal energy—issues that are key to the survival of our great grandchildren and indeed the human race.

The various issues set forth in the entirety of this section should be considered and implemented wherever practical. The most fundamental of these recommendations would be the resupply and escape capability for the ISS. Fortunately, action has been taken by the U.S. Congress to acquire Soyuz capability for the resupply, orbital orientation, and escape from the ISS, and a pathway forward is now open for astronaut rescue and crew rotation.

Despite the various difficulties and problems, there are still many positive lessons that can be learned from the ISS experience that might be successfully applied to future international cooperation and collaboration in space. These lessons include the following:

1) The concept that international cooperation does not always need to involve specific collaborative participation in a physical sense with joint development of space equipment or launch of hardware on partner launch vehicles is the first lesson. International collaboration can also mean sharing of data and program information that is carried out on a parallel basis. Nevertheless collaboration is most rewarding when there is direct joint involvement at the hardware or software level.

2) The creation of an international space safety authority centered around specifically identified space projects could facilitate transnational cooperation for a variety of undertakings, including space agencies and most significantly new private entities involved in space projects. This international space safety authority might undertake such actions as a) setting of common standards of measurements; b) interface specifications for different modules and launch systems; c) common power, atmospheric

and environmental standards, etc.; d) mechanisms for a varying number of countries to share information or collaboration on a variable number of joint or parallel projects or even lunar test beds and sites; e) escape and hazard assessment procedures; f) liability provisions for equipment and astronaut operations; and g) provisions for the participation of private, entrepreneurial entities in space operations and transport that include safety standards, personal and corporate liability and other relevant understandings [13].

It is currently believed by most participants that the ISS should operate for at least another decade in orbit, that is, through 2016, even though some partners might wish to continue operation until 2025. Russia has indicated the value of the ISS having a longer-term role as an international spaceport. Agreement as to the lifetime of the ISS, together with a setting of goals and objectives against a timeline, is a critical missing step that needs urgent attention. This should be followed by a further refinement of safety procedures, updated self-monitoring safety equipment, escape and rescue operations, and unified safety operations control (under a single point of control) has considerable merit. In this regard the IAASS can likely play an essential role.

Study of these safety procedures, safety operations and detection, and recovery and repair equipment for their possible application to future international space cooperation in the areas of space applications, space sciences, and space exploration is also strongly urged. In this respect, the use of automated and robotic equipment over human operations should be reemphasized in these future space planning activities. In short, the use of robotics and automated systems should be the initial default choice for space missions and especially for lunar exploration.

> In short, the use of robotics and automated systems should be the initial default choice for space missions and especially for lunar exploration.

References

1 Sgobba, T., and Chiesa, S., "Toward an International Space Station Safety Authority?" International Astronautical Federation, Bremen, Germany, Oct. 2002, pp. 1–8.

2 ESA Internal Memo QS/90/213/60 to ESTEC Director and Report DNVID-51-000, European Space Agency, Noordwijk Netherlands, July 1989, pp. 1–10.

3 de Bakker, L. "Soyuz, a Trusted Spacecraft." RADIO Netherlands Transcript, Amsterdam, Netherlands, 13 April 2004, pp. 1–3, www.radionetherlands.Nl/features/science/0404!

4 "A Brief History of Space Accidents," Jane's, London, 3 Feb. 2003 pp. 23–44.

5 Sietzen, F. Jr., "Soyuz: The Space Workhorse," Aerospace America, Vol. 38, Issue 8, 27 Aug. 1999.

6 "Space Station Assembly: Russian Soyuz," NASA, Report NASA SP-1801, 18 June 2003.
7 Pike, J., "Soyuz Launch Vehicle." Annual Report of the Federation of American Scientists, Washington, DC.
8 Starsem, The Soyuz Co. www.starsem.com
9 Braeunig, R. A., "Rocket Propellants," 1996, http://users.commkey.net/braeunig/space
10 "Manned Space Flights Are Pointless," PRAVDA.Ru, 4 April 2003, p. 1, http://english.pravda.ru/science/tech04-04-2003/
11 "Outline of Kibo Operation System." www.iss.sso.jasa.jp/iss/kibo/develop-ahead-e.
12 de Selding, P., "European Officials Skeptical of U.S. Space Motivation," *Space News*, 17 May 2004, p. 6.
13 Finarelli, P., "International Cooperation in the Implementation of Space Exploration," 14th Japan-US Science Technology and Space Applications Program (JUSTSAP) Workshop, Nov. 2004, pp. 1–8.

Additional Reading

de Montlivault, J.-L., and Record, R. "The Certification of Manned Spaceflight," *Bulletin Technique du Bureau Veritas*, No. 1, 1991, pp. 8–17.
"International Spacecraft Rendezvous and Docking Conference-Working Group 4: Safety and Reliability," ESA Internal Memo QS/90/213/60 to ESTEC Director, Noordwijk, Netherlands, 9–12 July 1990, pp. 1–12.
Jones, R. I., "Application of Airworthiness Requirements to HERMES Space Vehicle," College of Aeronautics, Cranfield, England, UK, April 1987.
Shirai, T., "A Common Approach to Safety-JAXA PSRP Franchise," Cooperation in Space ISS International Partners Meeting, JAXA Safety and Product Assurance Office, April 2004, pp 1–18.

Web sites

"The Amazing Canadarm2, "http://science.nasa.gov/headlines/y2001/ast18apr_1.htm.
Klotz I., "Analysis: NASA, Russia at Odds Over ISS," http://washingtontimes.com/upi-breaking/20040421-121152-9548r.htm [cited 21 April 2004].
"Canadarm2", http://www.space.gc.ca/asc/eng/csa_sectors/human_pre/iss/canadarm2/canadarm2.asp [cited 17 Jan. 2002].
"A Canadian Base in Space," http://canadaonline.about.com/library/weekly/aa060902a.htm.
"Centrifuge," JAXAhttp://iss.sfo.jaxa.jp/iss/contribution/issjpdoc3_2_e.html [cited 1 Oct. 2003].
"Europe Sends NASA New Viewport for Space Station," http://www.space.com/missionlaunches/iss_cupola_040908.html [cited 8 Sept. 2004].
"ESA: Automated Transfer Vehicle," http://www.esa.int/export/SPECIALS/ATV/ESAE021VMOC_0.html.
"Europe Sends NASA New Viewport for Space Station," http://www.space.com/missionlaunches/iss_cupola_040908.html [cited 8 Sept. 2004].

"H-II Transfer Vehicle Project Topics," JAXA Launch Vehicles and Space Transportation, http://www.jaxa.jp/missions/projects/rockets/htv/back number_e.html [cited 28 May 2004].

"Japan's ISS Unit, Kibo, to Begin Final Testing Next Month," http://www.space.com/missionlaunches/japan_kibo_011020.html [cited 20 Oct. 2001].

"JAXA: Space Station," http://iss.sfo.jaxa.jp/index_e.html.

"International Space Station," http://en.wikipedia.org/wiki/International_Space_Station [cited 8 Sept. 2004].

"International Space Station Program Payload Flight Equipment Requirements and Guidelines for Safety," http://jsc-web-pub.jsc.nasa.gov/psrp/docs/SSP_52005B.pdf.

"International Space Station and Japanese Experiment Module—Kibo," http://iss.sfo.jaxa.jp/iss/index_e.html.

Thirkettle, A., Patti, B., Mitschdoerfer, P., Kledzik, R., Garigioli, E., and Brondolo, D., "ISS: Columbus," http://esapub.esrin.esa.it/bulletin/bullet109/thirkett.pdf.

"ISS Kibo (Japanese Experiment Module—JEM)—Summary," http://www.space andtech.com/spacedata/platforms/iss-kibo_sum.shtml [2001].

"ISS Astronaut Activity Report, JAXA ISS Astronauts," http://iss.sfo.jaxa.jp/astro/reprot/2002/0203_e.html [cited March 2002].

"ISS Elements: Centrifuge Accommodation Module (CAM)," Spaceref.com, http://www.spaceref.com/iss/elements/cam.html.

Kridler, C., "NASA Weighs Options for Station Escape Craft," http://www.space.com/missionlaunches/fl_crv_020811.html [cited 11 Aug. 2002].

"Outline of Kibo Operations System," JAXA Space Station, http://iss.sfo.jaxa.jp/iss/kibo/ctl_e.html [cited 19 Dec. 2001].

"Promoting Kibo Development," http://iss.sfo.jaxa.jp/iss/kibo/develop_ahead_e.html [cited 31 Oct. 2002].

"The Russians Are Coming," http://aerospacescholars.jsc.nasa.gov/HAS/cirr/ss/4/5.cfm [cited 21 June 2004].

"Space Station Assembly: Russian Soyuz," NASA, http://spaceflight.nasa.gov/station/assembly/elements/soyuz/index.html [cited 18 June 2003].

Schneider, M., "U.S. and Russia View Space Station Safety Differently," Associated Press, http://www.space.com/missionlaunches/ap_iss_031110.html [cited 10 Nov. 2003].

"Z1 Integrated Truss Segment," http://www.shuttlepresskit.com/STS-92/payload76.htm.

"Zverda," http://www.shuttlepresskit.com/ISS_OVR/assembly2_overview.htm [cited 6 July 2000].

CHAPTER 8
Project Constellation

"Project Constellation is sort of a retro Apollo program on steroids."

—*NASA Administrator, Michael Griffin at a September 2005*
news conference

"Just how the Moon will be 'used to go to Mars' and why it
will be 'used to go to Mars' has been the subject of a great deal of
misunderstanding and has been misrepresented to bolster the view
that the Vision for Space Exploration is unrealistic."

—*Wendell Mendell, NASA Johnson Space Center, Meditation on the*
New Space Vision, International Astronautics Congress, 2004

New Space Vision

The review of the space shuttle, the International Space Station, and other
NASA development programs for launch systems undertaken over the
last 15 years, as addressed in the previous chapters, focused primarily on
experience of the past and the near-term future. But what of the longer-
term future? Are NASA's plans for space exploration, as represented by
Project Constellation, going in the right direction? How safe will these
new programs be for future astronauts? Will mistakes of the past be
repeated? This chapter explores Project Constellation and the safety of
U.S. astronauts for the coming decade.

President George W. Bush, in many ways, stood NASA on its head
when he proclaimed at NASA Headquarters in January 2004 a new presidential vision for space exploration [1]. The President explained his
vision to a specially assembled group of astronauts that included Eugene
Cernan, the last astronaut to go to and return from the moon, and Pete
Aldridge, whom he asked to head a group to help flesh out the details.

Also present at the jam-packed NASA auditorium was a host of
NASA officials and assembled guests (including the author of this book).
The plan was visionary in its scope and broad in its implications for ongoing NASA programs. This vision set forth a plan to restore the space shuttle to flight in accord with the CAIB recommendations, to reorient the ISS
to a program to test astronauts for extended missions to the moon and
Mars, and to complete the ISS by 2010 and ground the shuttle fleet by that
time. This timetable for grounding the space shuttle depended on the
launch vehicles of other countries (largely Russia) until a new crew
launch vehicle and crew exploration vehicle would be ready in 2014.
The prime objective would be to develop this new class of launch and

exploration vehicles that would allow astronauts to go to the ISS, the moon (for long durations)... and ultimately to Mars!

This "Moon, Mars, and Beyond" vision was the first time in many years that a clear set of long-term goals had been given to NASA at the presidential level. In the months and now years that have followed, this new vision seems to have reinvigorated NASA's employees and given them clearer purpose. However, the implementation has proved difficult, and

This "Moon, Mars, and Beyond" vision was the first time in many years that a clear set of long-term goals had been given to NASA at the presidential level.

Congress and the new NASA administrator have intervened to change the program in many significant ways. A number of critics have asked whether the goal was to go to the moon or Mars? Senator John Glenn noted that once one developed a launch system that could go to the moon you were then 85% or more capable of going to Mars. Thus, he asked, was the objective to send astronauts back to the moon or go to Mars, and why were the two goals intertwined when they really did not need to be? Others such as Senator Kay Bailey Hutchison from Texas questioned the wisdom of the four-year gap between the proposed grounding of the shuttle and the planned availability of a CEV that could go to and return from the ISS. In response to the timing of the shuttle grounding, the NASA administrator has now "scrapped" the planned fly-off contest between the prime contractors and advanced the timetable to have the crew launch vehicle and the crew exploration vehicle available by possibly as early as year end 2012. NASA has also issued an RFP to U.S. aerospace industry to seek bids for a contract to build vehicles that can ferry astronauts and supplies to the ISS in the post-2010 time period and proposed to devote some $500 million of NASA's funds to this end.

It also became clear that the new vision was to be accomplished without a large new appropriation going to NASA for this purpose. The costs of this program, that is, Project Constellation, were to be paid out of savings that came out of grounding the shuttle by 2010; savings related to the ISS downsizing; reductions in shuttle launches (now down to about 10 fewer than before the new vision was announced); savings that came from reducing space science, educational or other programs; or savings achieved by stretching the "Constellation" exploration program so that the objective actually became that of just going to the moon by 2018. (Thus the manned-Mars mission, when viewed through the lens of a more or less constant budget for NASA, has almost "shrunk away" to obscurity—at least in terms of being achieved within a generation.)

Then there were other management and operational problems at NASA. These included continuing cost overruns associated with the return to flight program for the shuttle, the resignation of NASA Administrator Sean O'Keefe in the Spring of 2005 to become President of Southwest Louisiana State University, accounting problems with NASA's audited accounts for the 2001 to 2004 period, and the ongoing problems with the shuttle that became apparent with the reflight of the Space Shuttle

Discovery (STS 114) in midyear 2005. When a new NASA administrator arrived, in the form of Michael Griffin, formerly an executive of Orbital Sciences and a former astronaut, the number of future shuttle flights was cut by 10. Consequently, plans to "finish" the ISS and resupply the Hubble are now to be accomplished by "about 18" flights rather than the previously manifested 28 flights. In fact NASA Administrator Griffin has now said that he was no longer aiming at a specific number of shuttle flights but was working instead toward an expeditious but orderly retirement of the shuttle over the next five years—enough time, he thinks, to finish the space station. As a *New York Times* editorial puts it, he "wants to shuck off the Shuttle Program when feasible" [2].

This program was named Project Constellation, and despite efforts to accomplish its many objectives with a virtually steady-state budget (NASA's 2006 budget did increase slightly to $16 billion, and the proposed 2007 budget is about $17 billion) it has now become clear that NASA is currently projected to be something like $3-billion short of funds over the next few years to do all of the things that it plans to accomplish. Despite moves to cut costs and a $1-billion increase in budget, NASA does not have sufficient funds to accomplish its various science programs, to undertake the remaining shuttle missions, to complete the ISS, to refurbish the Hubble telescope, and to develop the new CEV-related capabilities and the solid rocket booster launcher needed to achieve Project Constellation. The new NASA administrator has found that pursuing the new space vision and finishing everything else on NASA's plate is a daunting task.

Nevertheless, NASA has tried very hard to move Project Constellation forward. Congressional overseers, as already noted, have asked that the new launch system and the new crew exploration vehicle be ready for use as near to the time that the shuttle is grounded as possible. This means bringing the new launcher systems and the CEV online years earlier, instead of having the new launch capability fully qualified for astronaut use by 2014 as first envisioned. This acceleration could of course entail some safety risks and cutting of corners in the design phase. Most particularly, it has meant the end of the proposed fly-off between Lockheed Martin on one hand and Boeing–Northrop Grumman on the other.

At the start of Project Constellation, NASA Administrator Sean O'Keefe brought Admiral Craig Steidle onboard to head a newly established Exploration System Mission Directorate (ESMD) to lead Project Constellation. Retired Admiral Steidle had headed the Joint Strike Force (JSF) fighter jet program at the Department of Defense, which developed the JSF jet by soliciting contractors through a broad area announcement (BAA) process. This ultimately ended in the two major prospective contractors engaging in a fly-off contest, which showed that all key performance objectives would be met. The "winner" was selected on the basis of actual hardware rather than a set of drawings and performance specs. This system undoubtedly produces reliable results, but it can also be expensive and time consuming.

During 2005, key members of Congress and the new NASA administrator both declared that they were committed to find a way to reduce costs and shrink the schedule for development of the crew launch vehicle and the crew exploration vehicle. The only way that could be envisioned to fly the CEV to the ISS at an earlier date was to abandon the Joint Strike Fighter fly-off model and to select the winning CEV contractor on the basis of their design proposals. The new NASA Administrator, Michael Griffin, and his new Associate Administrator for Program Analysis and Evaluation, Scott Pace, apparently concluded that the fly-off approach would consume too much at the early end of the Project Constellation budget and make the development schedule too long.

To accomplish the desired savings of time and money, Administrator Griffin initiated a process known as the Exploration Systems Architecture Study (ESAS) that suddenly threw some 400 NASA employees into a streamlining process. Admiral Steidle resigned, and the management of the program was returned to various NASA centers. The key elements of the ESAS study were essentially to use a design for the lunar exploration spacecraft that was closely patterned on the idea of simply creating a larger version of the command module used for Project Apollo and the Russian counterpart program that deployed a Zond capsule. The thought apparently was that because of the very exhaustive studies that had been carried out to support the design of the Apollo capsule and the success of the 17 Apollo missions this would allow a great deal of engineering work to be eliminated. This approach also had many pluses from a safety point of view—past experience, proven technical model, a minimum of new state-of-the-art technology, full-envelope escape capability, and the separation of crew and cargo.

This ESAS process has pushed NASA to choose the contractors that will design and manufacture these systems at a much earlier date and on the basis of "paper designs" rather than a hardware fly-off contest. Once again, NASA programs were clearly driven by schedules and budgeting and congressional intervention rather than science and engineering. There can be a reasonably good argument that the adoption of a design that is very much like "a retro Apollo program on steroids" has a very strong safety focus. The proven capsule design is clearly technologically easier and very likely safer than trying to design a reusable craft based on a new "super shuttle" concept. It is ironic, however, that Roskosmos has announced plans as of early 2006 to develop a new reusable launch system that seems to be a modernized version of the shuttle by 2012 [3].

Crew Exploration Vehicle

The prime objective of Project Constellation is to develop a new crew exploration vehicle (CEV) that can be launched via newly upgraded conventional expendable launch vehicle (i.e., a crew launch vehicle) that is to be based on adaptations of the shuttle liquid fuel engines.

This design for the CEV, which is based on economies of design as well as heightened concerns with safety, envisions the use of a capsule that will be able to use proven heat-shield technologies and shapes that are designed for return to Earth from the moon. This return from the moon requires the maximum amount of deceleration and therefore the highest heat gradients. The current design of the CEV thus envisions a shape and concept that is very much like an enlarged Apollo command module. Instead of a capsule that is 3.9 m in diameter with accommodation for three astronauts, the CEV is 5.5 m in diameter and plans to accommodate four astronauts. Figure 8.1 shows a cross-section view of the current design [4].

The development of this new human-rated launch system constituted the prime focus of NASA's manned space-vehicle development program during 2005. In September 2005, the complete architectural design of the new launch system and of the CEV (as it emerged from the ESAS process) was announced amid much fanfare. Perhaps the most surprising aspect of

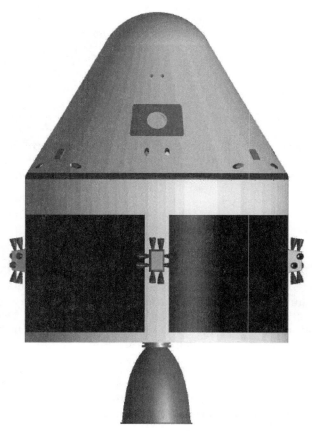

Figure 8-1   Reflects an artist conception of a cross section of a crew exploration vehicle (graphic courtesy of NASA).

the announcement was that this program would have a total price tag of $104 billion over the next 13 to 14 years—or just over $7 billion a year of NASA's $16 to 17 billion annual budget. Exactly how much backing Congress is willing to give to this program over the long term remains a bit sketchy [5].

The requested $438 million in new funding for this new program, sought for the FY 2005 budget, was reduced as a result of newly found fiscal austerity on Capitol Hill in the fall of 2004 [6]. Nevertheless NASA found sufficient funds to move ahead with the design that was announced in September 2005 and continues to award contracts critical to the overall program.

The advent of Hurricanes Katrina and Rita, the related costs of recovery, the domino impact of these disasters on the cost of gasoline, jet fuel and natural gas, plus the high cost of the war in Iraq clearly impacts the willingness of Congress to support what had now become largely a new lunar exploration program. Nevertheless, some modest increases in NASA funding were ultimately approved for FY 2006, with a significant boost in the funds for Project Constellation. The President's FY 2007 budget provides even more substantial support, but there are a dozen years remaining in Project Constellation until its culmination in 2018.

In short, mounting a sustained space exploration program that takes over a dozen years to implement will likely remain a struggle for NASA in years to come. Clearly the strategic guidance from the current White House is to accomplish this program within the limits of a $16 to 17 billion a year budget and on the basis of achieving new economies related to the phase out of the shuttle program and reduced expenditures on the ISS. These economies, however, can translate into safety concerns for both of these programs.

Current Status of the Development of a CEV

On 14 January 2004, President George W. Bush announced more than Project Constellation. He announced the specific goal to develop and test a new spacecraft, the Crew Exploration Vehicle, by 2008, and to conduct the first manned mission no later than 2014. Under the latest plan, the crew exploration vehicle, in one specific configuration, is to be capable of ferrying astronauts and scientists to the space station within the next six years. In short, the more conventional retro-like Apollo design and the elimination of the fly-off between the two prime candidates to build the system is expected to advance the first phase of the program by at least a couple of years.

The main purpose of the CEV, according to President Bush, was to design a spacecraft that "will be to carry astronauts beyond Earth orbit to other worlds. This will be the first spacecraft of its kind since the Apollo Command Module" [7]. Almost ironically, it turns out that this program, as defined in the fall of 2005, is very much an expanded and updated version of the Apollo program that uses new technology sparingly and employs a cautious design to achieve increased reliability and give primacy to astronaut safety.

As a first step in the design process, NASA funded 11 study proposals in August 2004 to examine design concepts. Three of these contracts examined lunar exploration objectives (i.e., Raytheon, Science Applications International Corporation, and SpaceHab). The other eight contractors [i.e., Andrews, Draper Labs, Lockheed Martin, Northrop Grumman, Orbital Sciences, Schafer, Boeing, and T/Space (Transformational Space)] defined concepts for the CEV. Further, there were two study teams from the NASA Exploration Directorate and the Launch Services Directorate that examined many alternatives for Project Constellation as well. The Launch Services Directorate investigators carried out a "bottom-up" exploration of existing capabilities in terms of rocket and launch systems (including the ability of existing U.S. rockets to be upgraded to human-rated capabilities), while the Exploration Directorate engaged in a "top-down" investigation of new modes of approach to developing the CEV [8].*

These design studies produced the concepts announced in September 2005 by NASA Administrator Michael Griffin to develop a module that can be launched on a conventional rocket based on the employment of the space shuttle rocket engines. The announced design was envisioned to produce a new level of human-flight reliability. The CEV, with a crew aboard, would be launched on a new rocket system, based on a cluster of five shuttle liquid rocket engines. This design separates the cargo rocket from a separate launch of the crew, its capsule, and an escape system. This approach greatly adds to the astronaut safety associated with this system's overall design.

The specific launcher configuration would allow a crew module to fly into orbit and then connect with the lunar-based propulsion system that would be launched by a heavier lift system based on two solid rockets (again directly derived from the shuttle design). On the return from the moon, the lander system would remain on the lunar surface, and the capsule with a proven heat-shield capability would make the descent through the Earth's atmosphere. The key to the concepts are modular systems that can fit together to accomplish different missions and the use of components from the shuttle propulsion system that have been generally very reliable (i.e., the liquid-fueled rocket engines). This design obviously abandons the shuttle thermal protection system that has proven to be complex, costly, and ultimately dangerous.

Initially there was some thought to producing a reusable flight vehicle as depicted in the Lockheed Martin concept shown in the following, but the lower cost capsule, such as was used in the Apollo program, plus the reliability factors associated with a capsule return (as proven by Apollo and Soyuz) led to the present design configuration.

---

*Data available online at http://www.astroexpo.com/news/newsdetail.asp? ID-15535 [cited 24 Aug. 2004].

Emphasis has been placed on the idea that the CEV will have a modular design to allow new capabilities to be added in later years and provide versatility for differing mission requirements. Ultimately, the capsule-shaped design was chosen because of its proven flightworthiness during the Mercury, Gemini, and Apollo programs.

Project Constellation envisions more than the production of a single vehicle because NASA is planning to use what is called a "spiral development model" as first set forth by Admiral Steidle. There will be variants of the CEV that will evolve over time to undertake more and more demanding missions and, for instance, to accommodate longer duration stays on the moon. The plans include the initial CEV that can support trips to and from the space station in low Earth orbit, CEVs that can travel to lunar orbit and land on the moon, and ultimately CEVs that also travel to the moon for long-duration stays as well as a CEV designed to go to destinations beyond the moon, such as Mars or other designations.

Today there are two large teams competing for the CRL and CEV contracts. One is headed by Lockheed Martin and the other by Boeing and Northrop Grumman. This competition is to provide a complete design for the CEV, the emergency escape capability, the human-rated crew launch vehicle based on the use of five shuttle engines, and a vehicle with the heavier lift system powered by the solid-fuel launchers for cargo that can lift materials to low Earth orbit.

In addition to the competition for the basic designs of these various spacecraft and launch vehicles, subcontractors will supply the CEV with life-support systems, rocket thrusters, and onboard navigation. In late December 2005, NASA announced the selection of five firms in response to a request for proposal for "Flight Critical Systems Research" that had been issued on 3 January 2006. Chosen for the multiple award were ARINC Engineering Services, LLC, Annapolis, Maryland; Boeing Company, Phantom Works, Seattle; Honeywell Corporation, Minneapolis; Lockheed Martin Aeronautics Company, Fort Worth, Texas; and Rannoch Corporation, Alexandria, Virginia. The work by these contractors will be on an as-needed basis, with task orders for specific work that will be completed among the five contractors with a value of up to $35 million. The work under these contracts is to be in four major areas: flight dynamics guidance and control; crew systems and aviation operations; reliable and robust avionics systems; and flight critical systems analysis and integration.

There is a fundamental policy issue concerning the award of these relatively minor contracts in the overall $104-billion program. This is the management of the program, the integration of design, and the possibility that critical safety elements are overlooked when there are to be so many contractors involved in designing the hundreds of elements that go into such a long-term and complex project [9].

NASA leadership does seem particularly attuned to the issue of safety, given not only the *Columbia* accident but also the discouraging nature of the shuttle reflight in the summer of 2005 and the latest problems discovered with the cracks in the PAL foam ramp. A safety review process has been established within NASA to be carried out in November 2006 with extensive interviews at the various NASA centers, where the CEV and and other launcher development programs are currently underway. Although this safety review process with regard to Project Constellation is commendable, there remain the following concerns:

> NASA leadership does seem particularly attuned to the issue of safety, given not only the *Columbia* accident but also the discouraging nature of the shuttle reflight in the summer of 2005 and the latest problems discovered with the cracks in the PAL foam ramp.

1) Will the review and interview process only involve NASA personnel, or will outside safety, design, and independent safety verification experts be consulted in this review process?

2) Will the newly established International Association for the Advancement of Space Safety (IAASS), which has now assembled a great deal of expertise in space safety, be allowed to participate in the safety review process?

3) What mechanisms will be established within NASA to better integrate its safety review and independent verification processes that is today a complex matrix of capabilities spread throughout its NASA Engineering and Safety Center, its various NASA centers, the independent technical authority, the inspector general's office, and so on?

4) Will the development program for the new launch systems, based on the clustering of five liquid-fueled shuttle motors for the CRV and the use of solid rocket motors for heavy lift capabilities, undertake a thorough review of these rocket motor systems based on past difficulties and launch problems to see if design concerns can be improved by means of a bottom-up engineering review. In particular, the detailed shuttle technical review as presented in Appendix C to this book should be used as one input to such a thorough design quality review.

Design of the CEV and Its Safety Engineering

NASA envisions that the CEV will be designed to carry four astronauts to the moon. It can be used in different configurations to lift crews (or operated robotically) to lift larger amounts of cargo.[†]

Overall, the design associated with the CEV seems to employ a lot of lessons learned. It uses the best of the rocket propulsion systems from the space shuttle, includes lessons learned from components used in the ISS program, and it adapts a good deal of the technology and systems design

---

[†]Data available online at http://www.astroexpo.com/news/newsdetail.asp? ID-15535 [cited 24 Aug. 2004].

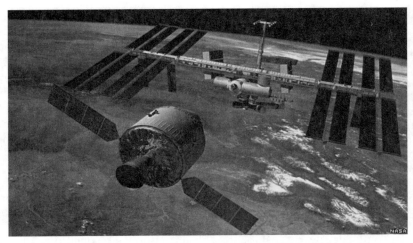

Figure 8-2 Artist's conception of crew exploration vehicle with solar panels deployed as it approaches the International Space Station (graphic courtesy of NASA).

that derive from both the Apollo Program and the Soyuz vehicle designed by the Russian Space Agency.

Spiral Development Concept for the CEV

The design for the CEVs is intended to be modular in nature so that various vehicles can be deployed in a series of spirals for different types of missions.‡ Spiral One represents the test flight and early deployment stage. The first rendition of the CEV is to be capable of carrying crews into orbit for test flights and able to provide a capability for astronauts to travel to and from the International Space Station. (This configuration is shown in Fig. 8.2.)

The Spiral Two stage is to represent what might be considered the early lunar expedition spacecraft. This vehicle design would be designed to be capable of staying on the moon for up to a week and then returning to Earth, whereas alternative configurations would be able to continue to support missions to the ISS. This configuration is shown in Fig. 8.3.

Spiral Three of the CEV would represent what might be called a mature lunar expedition spacecraft, capable of extending human presence on the moon for up to three months. This could be used to establish an initial lunar base.

The Spiral Four configuration is, of course, not yet clearly defined. This final iteration would presumably be able to support a Mars mission or other longer-term missions beyond the moon.

---

‡Data available online at http://www.astroexpo.com/news/newsdetail.asp? ID-15535 [cited 24 Aug. 2004].

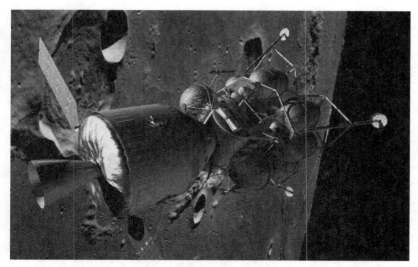

Figure 8-3   Artistic conception of CEV that could provide short-duration visits to the lunar surface (graphic courtesy of NASA).

At Boeing/Northrop Grumman and Lockheed Martin, the corporate heads of the two teams that are developing the CEV are currently competing to develop the best design, manufacturing, and deployment plans. As described earlier, because of schedule and budgetary constraints, the idea of a fly-off competition in 2008 has now been shelved, and a decision by NASA must be made solely on design concepts.

Figures 8.4 and 8.5 show preliminary concept designs that came from these companies several years ago. These advanced designs have now been overtaken by a more conservative design approach. Apparently Roskosmos intends to deploy a system that resembles this concept with regard to their own lunar exploration program.§

The current schedule that NASA hopes to follow (as shown next) in the development of the CEV has thus been considerably compressed. Instead of a fly-off in the 2008 time period, selection of prime contractor is foreseen in the relatively near future:

1) Near term—contractor and final design for the Spiral One CEV and initial crew launch-vehicle (CRL) system capable of going to the ISS is to be selected by NASA, based on the head-to-head competition between the teams headed by Lockheed Martin and Boeing–Northrop Grumman

2) 2008—finalization of the final design for the lunar spacecraft and future mission modes as represented by the Spiral Two development

---

§Data available online at http://www.astroexpo.com/news/newsdetail.asp?ID-15535 [cited 24 Aug. 2004].

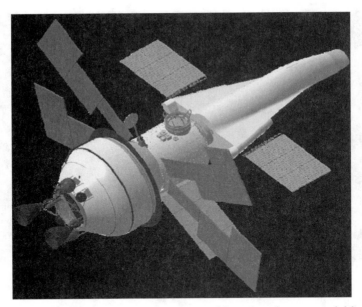

Figure 8-4   Enhanced CEV concept with reusable rather than expendable approach (graphic courtesy of Lockheed Martin).

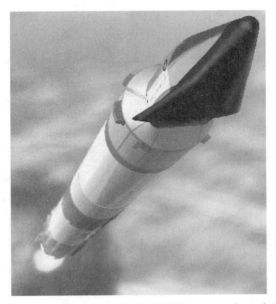

Figure 8-5   Lockheed Martin wing-shaped CEV concept aboard Atlas launch vehicle (graphic courtesy of Lockheed Martin).

3) 2012—flight model of the CEV capable of test flights and then going to the ISS

4) 2013–2014—first unmanned flight of lunar spacecraft

5) To be decided based on unmanned flights—first manned flight of lunar spacecraft

6) 2018—moon landings by astronauts in lunar spacecraft

The originally announced budget request associated with Project Constellation included $428 million for FY 2005 with an average of about $6.6 billion per year to be spent in the ensuing five years. However, this has now been overtaken by a more detailed and longer-term schedule and budget.¶

The final program concept involves the development of a number of new launch systems. These include a complete new launch system for astronauts (crew launch vehicle based on a cluster of liquid motors adapted from the shuttle), an unmanned robotically controlled launch system for the launch of cargo going to the moon (based on two solid fuel rockets adapted from the shuttle program), plus the crew exploration vehicle and the escape vehicle [10].

The wisdom of using separate vehicles for crew and cargo has been a long held tenet of space safety. The idea of using shuttle orbiter tested liquid-fueled motors to create a human-rated launch system that would be much like that shown to the right in Fig. 8.6, whereas the heavy cargo lifter that would use the reliable solid fuel motors as also recycled from the shuttle program would look like the launch system as shown to the left.

This entire development program of Project Constellation vehicles and systems, as announced in September 2005, entails a projected budget of $104 billion over a 12-year period that culminates in the operation of a new astronaut lander in 2018 that would be capable of long-duration stays—perhaps several months [11].

With the limited remaining lifetime of the shuttle and serious concerns about its reliability, the development of a new astronaut-capable launch and Earth-return capability, such as the CEV, is crucial for continuity in NASA's astronaut program. Despite the intensive design efforts represented by NASA's ESAS process and the now revamped plans for Project Constellation, there are a number of issues that remain open and unresolved.

These start with technical issues such as selection of the preferred contractor for the launch systems and the exploration vehicle, the safety reviews concerning the designs for the CRL, the CEV, the escape vehicle, etc. as scheduled for November 2006, and the need to carry out extensive qualification tests in coming years with the new systems and their "spiral development" [3].

Even larger questions arise with regard to the extent that Congress, the OMB/Executive Branch, and the ongoing political process will be

---

¶Data available online at http://www.projectconstellation.us.

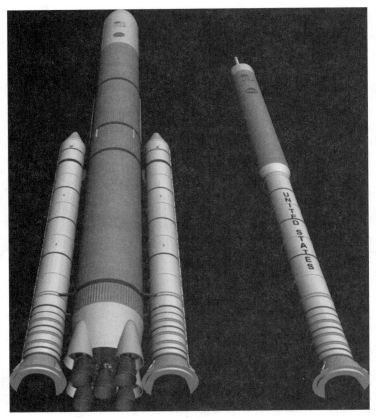

Figure 8-6   Smaller human CLV is shown to the right while the larger cargo launch system for Project Constellation is shown to the left.

willing and able to provide the very significant funding for Project Constellation to sustain NASA's implementation of this program and achieve the lunar landing in 2018. In short, it will take a persistent political will and perhaps some good fortune to sustain such a space program for essentially 13 years—not the most "lucky" number for a space program. Intervening variables such as terrorist attacks, wars, natural disasters, or other unanticipated events can undercut the needed funding. Further, Congress can also impact the schedule and funding by seeking to redeploy NASA funds for ISS research, for nuclear propulsion development, space sciences, education, or other space-related activities. Other presidential administrations in the future might simply redefine or revise national priorities. Finally, NASA has said that Project Constellation will ultimately be international in scope. At least two international coordination meetings have been held with potential international space partners concerning such collaboration, but nothing very specific has yet emerged.

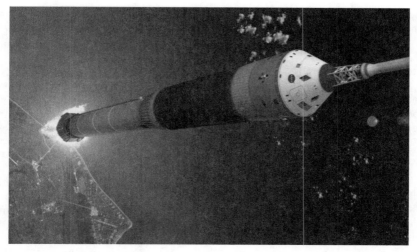

Figure 8-7   Crew launch vehicle mated to the crew exploration vehicle in space (graphic courtesy of NASA).

The overall design at this point, however, has all of the critical hardware being designed by NASA and built by U.S. contractors. The crew launch vehicle will carry the crew exploration vehicle and the splashdown capsule, as shown in Fig. 8.7, while the solid rocket booster will launch the lunar lander and the departure stage from the moon as shown in Fig. 8.8. Perhaps there can be equipment and facilities to be used on the lunar surface that might come from the international community, such as

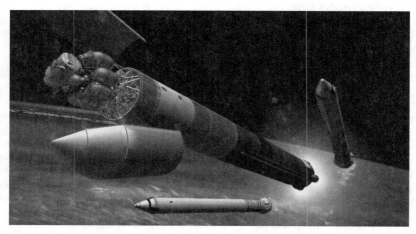

Figure 8-8   Solid-rocket-booster cargo system in space (graphic courtesy of NASA).

life-support systems, power generation, experimental labs, lunar rovers, or automated material processing capabilities.

International Collaboration and Cooperation

Because of past coordination problems, there is the potential for disputes about the stringency of safety practices and disagreements about the degree of autonomy that applies to various ISS national franchises. To a certain extent, NASA has assumed that if the United States leads the way in investing in new space vehicles to go to the ISS, the moon, and beyond, the rest of the world will simply follow suit and assume various subsidiary roles that the United States might request of them. This is not, however, the scenario that is playing out in the rapidly changing world of space activity, exploration, and even industrialization. In short, Russia, Europe, and China appear to be evolving their own plans separate from the United States, whereas other private space initiatives seem to be pursuing yet other options.

> In short, Russia, Europe, and China appear to be evolving their own plans separate from the United States, whereas other private space initiatives seem to be pursuing yet other options.

The following seeks to recap some of the current initiatives that seem to be pursuing parallel and not necessarily complementary programs with regard to space exploration and commercialization. The striking aspect of this review is the extent to which international space projects appear to be "diverging" rather than "converging."

Italian Lunar Telescope Project

The Italian News Agency ANSA announced in early January 2006 the plans of the Italian Space Agency to build a large telescope on the moon using robotic technology. The aim of the project is to expand knowledge of the moon, Earth, and the universe as well as develop new types of telerobotic technology. Rather than being a manned exploratory mission, the telescope will be built by robots and positioned in a lunar crater to give a new perspective on the Earth as well as the rest of the solar system and indeed the entire universe. This innovative project was announced by the head of the Italian Space Agency (ASI), Sergio Vetrella, on 4 January 2006 as part of the agency's plans for the future. The telescope, freed from interference from the Earth's atmosphere and the Van Allen belts, will be able to look deeper into space than Earth-based equivalents. The lunar telescope project, which will involve implanting the telescope parts within a lunar crater, will provide new information on the moon's resources. ASI has initially earmarked some 150 million euros for the project and will seek additional funding from the ESA and other international sources.

The current plans anticipate that the first robots will be sent up between 2010 and 2012 with the projected completion of the entire project by 2021. The head of ASI indicated that "the goal of the project is to gain more knowledge of the parts of the universe not visible from the Earth, as well as looking at our own planet with extreme precision." The so-called "modular robots," which will join together to form the lunar telescope, are currently planned to be launched to the moon aboard the Russian Vega launcher [12].

This innovative Italian lunar project is of special note for several reasons. First, it is envisioned as a thoroughly international project with the ESA, the Russian Space Agency, and NASA as likely key participants. Secondly, it is a very significant space science project that is likely to return important new information about the moon, the Earth, the solar system, and the universe yet be accomplished at relatively low cost, in comparison to Project Constellation. This is because of very innovative engineering, reliance on robotic technology rather than using astronauts, and because of international cost sharing.

Indirectly, this Italian-led project raises questions about the U.S. Project Constellation in terms of its scope, cost, schedule, and objectives. In short, if NASA were to design and send robots to the moon first, to develop key infrastructure to support an astronaut base, and then later develop manned launch systems that could go to the moon and Mars, could the project be designed at lower cost and perhaps with higher levels of safety margin? Might not new crew-based vehicles be able to benefit from more advanced launch systems such as electric ion or nuclear propulsion or even "space elevator" or tether-based systems? The basic question is to what extent does human exploration of the moon and Mars require humans? If robotic machinery plus video cameras can be used to send mechanized test beds, material processing units, and various sensors to celestial locations as the first stage of exploration, might this make more sense in terms of cost, results, and safety? Would this be particularly so if these robots could first build life-support systems, material processing, mining and radiation protection infrastructure, before sending astronauts at very high cost into harms way? If existing and lower cost launch systems of the United States, Europe, Japan, or Russia could support these robotic missions, without the super reliability required for astronaut-rated systems, do these questions become even more relevant?

Chinese Lunar Exploration Strategy

The U.S. plans to explore the moon and send humans into space are no longer the only game in town. The Chinese manned space program has advanced rapidly in the past few years with several human launches into space. The last launch was covered with live video coverage that signaled particular confidence in the Chinese vehicles. In October of 2003, the Chinese launched their astronaut Yang Li Wei into low Earth orbit for a 21-hour space trip to become the third country in the world, after the

United States and Russia, to accomplish this feat. In the latest launch aboard the Shenzhou VI spacecraft, two Chinese astronauts successfully completed a five-day mission that was televised around the world. China has announced its own plans to develop and launch its own low-Earth-orbit space station as well as to send its astronauts to the moon, perhaps before the United States completes its Project Constellation undertaking.**

In light of the high cost of space programs—particularly of manned space programs—that would go to the moon or Mars, the logic of trying to pool resources and capabilities to avoid duplication and overlap between and among China, Japan, Europe, Russia, the United States, and other space-faring nations would seem to make a great deal of sense. Clearly political agreement might be difficult to accommodate all players in a single program, but three or four parallel projects to send astronauts to the moon seems excessive. The idea that the United States, Japan, China, and perhaps Russia in partnership with Europe might all develop manned space launch systems that could go to the moon and beyond seems highly duplicative. The consequence might not only be money spent needlessly, but the likelihood that resources saved could have been invested in safer and more reliable space vehicles.

Russian Space Agency Initiatives in Cooperation with Europe

At this time, there are discussions ongoing between Russia and Europe to create an equivalent vehicle to the CEV that could be launched on Russian Progress vehicles or perhaps upgraded versions of the Ariane 5 launch systems. This new configuration, which would represent an upgrade of Soyuz or Vega crewed vehicles, would in many be ways parallel to the U.S. Project Constellation undertaking. In light of the fact that Russia and Europe (along with Japan and Canada) are key partners in the International Space Station, the emerging situation where the U.S. program would be essentially in direct competition with the Chinese efforts and the joint Russian/European efforts would appear to represent program duplications. The result might be that more money would be spent, less space science would be completed, and the risk to future astronauts might have increased. It is still early enough in these various programs, and especially the European and Russian efforts (including the next generation of the European ATV), that program planning might be changed. At the very least, it might be possible for the NASA CEV and the Russian/European program to be sufficiently aligned so that the various programs could be made to be compatible so that they could serve as backup rescue vehicles should the need arise.

One might very logically raise the question of U.S. strategic and national defense issues in such considerations. But the U.S. civil space and

---

**Data available online at http://www.astroexpo.com/news/newsdetails.asp? ID-23559&ListType-TopNews&StartDate-1/2/2006&EndDate-1/6/2006.

national defense space programs are now once again separated with the Department of Defense undertaking the development of a personal space vehicle that could provide reliable and quick assess to low Earth orbit (i.e., the X-43B programs *et al.*) while NASA is directed toward vehicles for moon and Mars exploration to meet civil space sciences goals. As will be noted next, the integrated space transportation plan, which had NASA and DOD jointly seeking to develop a personal space vehicle for rapid access to low Earth orbit, is no longer a part of the NASA mission.

Private Commercial Space Initiatives

Finally NASA planning with regard to Project Constellation must take into account private space initiatives as well. For many years Congress has questioned whether NASA R&D is sufficiently far in advance of regular commercial development programs and whether billion-dollar budgets related to R&D by both NASA and DOD were a "give-away" to aerospace corporations that might develop the technology for commercial purposes in any event. Even more recently there have been entrepreneurial companies that have shown that new technology could be developed more cost effectively by smaller and more innovative firms. The question thus becomes whether entrepreneurial business models might allow new breakthrough technologies to be developed more rapidly and at lower cost than the aerospace giants. In this stable of contenders—as noted in Chapter 1—are such individuals and organizations as Burt Rutan's Scaled Composites, the founders of Rocketplane, Ltd., Elon Musk's Space X, Jim Benson's Space Dev, Robert Bigelow's Bigelow Aerospace, Brad Edward's Space Elevator Corporation, Sir Robert Branson's Virgin Galactic, and Burt Rutan's SpaceOne venture as backed by Microsoft's Paul Allen. These innovative individuals, driven by new incentives such as the Ansari X-Prize, and perhaps just the "devil may care" challenge of creating new and innovative solutions, show us different approaches from the conventional models. These outside-the-box efforts to conquer space have shown the potential for new launch systems breakthroughs, better management techniques, cost savings, and even safety innovations.

New low-cost and reliable launcher systems, new approaches to space safety, and new plans for private space stations and even lunar projects have emerged at a rapid-fire pace in just the last few years. The FAA has sent to Congress serious proposals as to how private organizations might send individuals into space—not only in terms of space tourism, but also in the context of private space exploration and industry. A detailed exploration of each of these new initiatives is beyond the scope of this book, but clearly they are relevant and exciting aspects of 21st century space exploration that deserve close attention by policy makers, the general public, and healthy respect by the various space agencies around the world. Certainly the U.S. Air Force has taken Elon Musk's Space X program and the Falcon launcher so seriously that it has contracted for several low-cost launches. If Space X's Falcon vehicles that were developed on a shoestring in comparison to conventional methods should be successful, it might ultimately alter the entire space industry.

Status of NASA's Lunar Exploration Program

NASA's latest attempt to move forward with new human-rated space vehicles has focused on the exploration of the moon, on the basis that NASA and U.S. initiatives would continue to lead the way and that this effort needed to be successfully completed before a serious and safe manned Mars project could be contemplated. Thus, the idea of an astronaut mission to Mars appears to have been pushed even further forward in time and currently seems on the order of two decades away.

One of the clear innovations associated with the revised planning is that the human space exploration program will henceforth be strongly integrated with robotic vehicles and new transport systems that can ferry cargo to and from the ISS and perhaps even to the moon and beyond. There can be no doubt that robotic capability to replace some degree of astronaut activity could and would reduce costs and perhaps accelerate schedules. Certainly the safety review of Project Constellation now planned for November 2006 should carefully consider the possibility of increasing robotic missions and capabilities.

What is clear from the Project Constellation plans, as now presented by NASA, is a fundamental departure from the previously endorsed integrated space transportation plan. This plan was the road map endorsed by NASA and Congress as late as 2003. It included the development of a personal reusable launch vehicle (i.e., the pathway being developed via the X-33, X-34, X-37, and X-43A and X-43C programs) to provide quick and flexible access to low Earth orbit. This type of program has now been discontinued by NASA and turned over to the U.S. defense agencies.

There were many, including several individuals interviewed in the GW University study and those on the CAIB, who felt that the prior attempt by NASA to create an integrated space transportation plan had the problem of trying to do too many things with too many conflicting objectives. Many of the previous programs, such as X-33, X-34, X-37, and X-43A, to develop what might be called a personal reusable space plane were premised on a joint DOD and NASA effort. This attempt at a joint NASA and Air Force development program for a "personal space plane" was complicated by conflicting objectives and applications. The recent cancellation of the X-43A and X-43C by NASA, followed by the DOD award of a new contract totaling very nearly $1 billion to Northrop Grumman in order to develop an X-43B personal reusable launch vehicle, underscores this decision for the development of such a system under military funding [13].

NASA has obviously shifted other priorities as well. Project Constellation has meant a deemphasis on nuclear power development (i.e., the redlining of Project Prometheus), some reduction of space science and solar and planetary research (including possible sidelining of the highly innovative Project Sophia high-flying telescope initiative), as well as a clear reduction in the scope of the ISS and its scientific research program. These changes, together with an attempt to phase out the space shuttle as soon as possible and reduce the number of the shuttle missions to 18 (down from 28) have obvious implications for the safety of the shuttle and the ISS.

Issues, Concerns, and Opportunities Involving the CEV

As just noted, NASA's new emphasis will be on developing new human-rated spacecraft for longer range and extended missions.

In August 2004, NASA planners formally announced the process for developing the next generation of spacecraft that will be able to do a variety of things but not provide quick access to near Earth orbit for small crews. This objective will presumably be handed off to the U.S. DoD and the X-43B project. The prime focus of NASA is now on tasks that involve the ferrying of cargo to near Earth and beyond, robotic control missions and vehicles that can safely take astronauts to and from the moon, and eventually support Mars missions as well. NASA has thus made good on its claim that it was seeking fresh ideas and concepts as inspiration for the CEV. In this respect they clearly examined all of the predecessor programs, both in terms of taking from and using the best aspects of the space shuttle program and even going back to Project Apollo of the 1960s and applying principles of simplicity and seeking to achieve the safest possible design.

The greatest emphasis of NASA is to implement Project Constellation and realize the CEV as soon as possible. This clearly raises questions about the status and quality of attention devoted to the space shuttle and the ISS. It certainly appears to be the case that many people who were associated with either the space shuttle or ISS programs are now applying to work on Project Constellation and in many cases moving to this more exciting and future-looking program. This migration of staff can be seen as a somewhat worrisome safety issue for the successful completion of the reflight of the space shuttle and the completion of the ISS.

Certainly NASA personnel are also examining other design concepts that go beyond the first versions of the crew exploration vehicle. These include consideration of the possibility of a large cargo carrier that might be needed to support the moon landings and subsequent bases and that would presumably be a robotically controlled vehicle. But at this time, the focus is on developing the two competing CEV designs that have been underway since the second half of 2005.[††]

Two clear conclusions can be drawn from the current status of planning in terms of safety and risk minimization considerations. First,

---

[††]Data available online at http://www.astroexpo.com/news/newsdetail.asp? ID-15535.

the use of a robotically controlled heavy-lift system, as developed from one of the new launch options that use a configuration of shuttle liquid fuel motors, would likely provide cost efficiencies and improved astronaut safety simply by not having crew aboard such missions to the moon. If the planning proceeds on the basis of launching more robotic missions for scientific, exploration, and construction activities on the moon, NASA might well consider reducing the current number of astronauts by a significant degree. With some 240 active participants in the NASA astronaut training program at this time, the current level of staffing would seem much higher than required even with the accelerated development of the CEV. In short, there apparently will be at most 18 more launches of the shuttle as an outside number and having more robotic launches without crew in the future could add both economies and safety to the NASA exploration program.

Second, the nature of planning for the CEV and the upgrading of existing launch systems appears very heavily focused on achieving the lowest cost and simplest method to develop launch propulsion systems. The use of the shuttle engines for the new launch systems is but one of the indications that this is the case.

The new systems for long-duration missions, that is, for three months or so, are apparently being designed as a simple spiral and modular extension of the CEV. Criteria related to safety and risk reduction, such as systems that might include artificial gravity for a long-duration mission to Mars, do not appear to be aspects included in the longer-term planning. There seems to be lack of emphasis (or even inclusion) in the initial design concepts of such possible aspects as artificial gravity, enhanced radiation protection, and/or increased shielding for debris and micrometeorites. A modular design process would seem to include limited ability for such safety-related upgrades.

Clearly such considerations would add considerably to cost and could also add to the construction and deployment schedule. In light of existing budgetary constraints, these design elements will undoubtedly be left to later design processes.

The key observation related to astronaut safety—and this goes all the way back to the Mercury program—is the consistent finding that safety must be "designed in" rather than "added on" to launch systems and must be an ingrained part of the organizational culture. In terms of many elements of the CEV design, human safety and simplicity have had a major impact. Nevertheless, increased consideration of robotic missions, design of modules that offer better protection against space hazards, etc. should not be neglected as the launch system design matures.

CEV and Lessons Learned from the Shuttle Program

The longer-term future, extending beyond the CEV and any new heavy-lift vehicle, is wide open in terms of the many options that might be employed in the design. The thought that the CEV systems now being designed would form the basis of spacecraft that would remain operational and be the building blocks of launch systems for the 2015 to 2020 time period is in many senses worrisome. The idea of a spiral deployment in some ways suggests a possible "repeat" of the shuttle program. This is to say that the CEV, just like the shuttle, might somehow be extended to have a 30-year lifetime. In light of new technological development, new launch systems, and other safety innovations, it is difficult to see how the CEV can remain safe over such a long period of time. Interviews with NASA personnel indicate that spiral development is not meant in this sense at all. Instead spiral development is meant to emphasize modular design so that new technologies can be seamlessly introduced as they become mature. Thus useful subsystems can still be employed as new technologies are integrated into systems of the future. This concept might seem and indeed be sound, but its effective implementation (in terms of safety, technical innovation, and cost efficiency) will very likely prove extremely difficult. It also assumes that the way forward will be simple extensions of existing launch technology—an assumption that history has shown time and again to lack validity.

Space launch-vehicle systems that operate for 30 years, during a period of intense technology innovation, do not really make sense, either looking backward or forward in time. Thus there is reason to believe that major new technological innovations in launching systems, such as those discussed in Chapter 10 of this book, can bring increased performance and greater safety to future astronaut missions. Trying to design a system that "spirals" to cover a lifetime of 20–30 years, if mismanaged or misinterpreted in coming years, could lead to significant additional astronaut risk. We have concerns that this could lead to designing a system that becomes technologically obsolete if spiral development were misinterpreted to mean extended technology and components past their points of obsolescence. Care must therefore be taken to ensure that Congress and high-level government officials do not misinterpret spiral development and in future years push the CEV technology past a point of diminishing returns, both from the sense of economic efficiency and even more importantly of safety.

Therefore, before final decisions are made about a long-term multi-use launch system, a careful review should be undertaken of relevant problems that have been encountered with the shuttle program's design, implementation, operation, and plausible upgrade.

Safety-related problems from the shuttle era that deserve special consideration include such aspects as the following:

1) The first problem is the outmoded, expensive, and customized shuttle thermal protective system (TPS) that has been maintained well past its point of diminishing returns and where much improved technology now exists. (In this respect the capsule return approach might indeed make a great deal of sense.)

2) The next problem is the inability to upgrade various safety and astronaut escape systems caused by the limitations in the shuttle design

and particularly its use of a solid rocket motor. (Again this constraint is not present in the current designs for the new launch system or the CEV.)

3) The third problem is the inability to get replacement parts from many suppliers over the longer term. (This is a problem that has no easy answer and remains a significant problem in designing a space launch system that would have a protracted lifetime.)

4) Turnover of personnel dedicated to maintenance and refurbishment of highly specialized systems is the next problem. (Again this is a problem that has no easy solution for a long-lived space program.)

5) The false economies of trying to extend the lifetime of high-technology systems more than five to seven years when innovations in materials, ASIC chips, electronic systems, propulsion systems, and even life sciences are now moving so very rapidly ahead.

What is suggested in Chapter 10 is that there are truly many new types of technologies that on the 10- to 20-year time horizon might be much safer and more durable, reliable, and low cost than near-term technology, and that a spiral-deployment approach to the CEV, if misinterpreted at a later date, could well limit important new options for manned space programs of the future not only in terms of safety but in terms of performance. Future robotically controlled launch systems and even space exploration probes could have a particular impact on the wisdom of trying to design launch programs and the CEV for very long lifetimes.

These various options, such as ion propulsion, nuclear propulsion, tethers, space elevators, gravity-gradient systems, solar sails, lunar-based rail guns, or mag lev accelerators all merit careful consideration. A program that allows for the exploration of these types of new options could be highly productive. These programs could be conducted at low cost, representing only a small percentage of NASA's budget, through such avenues as the NASA Institute for Advanced Concepts (NIAC), the Small Business Initiatives Research (SBIR) program, plus innovations attained via private enterprise, university research, and prize money, which could potentially be highly productive.‡‡

In truth, the last 30 years in launch-vehicle development has produced modest gains, and the time is long overdue for one or more major breakthroughs to occur by sponsorship of research into truly new and innovative ideas that are discussed in detail in Chapter 10.

There remains not only the question of developing new technology but also new management, capital financing, and operational concepts that move forward astronaut exploration programs as well as their efficiency and safety. Wendell Mendell, who has been involved in the study of lunar colonies for almost 40 years, has recently set forth some ideas about institutional arrangements relating to missions to both the moon and Mars. In his article he suggests that NASA needs not only a strategy for exploring the moon and Mars, but an exit strategy that ensures a

---

‡‡Data available online at http://www.nasa.niac.gov.

transition to other entities that can take over the operational stage of this activity from a safety, financial, and international institutional perspective. If there is to be a transition to the private sector of responsibility for transportation of people to outer space and the establishment of settlements, then the question of human safety in space enters an entirely new domain for which careful thought and planning is essential [14].

Organizations such as the National Space Society, the Space Foundation, and the large aerospace corporations have embraced the new space vision and the plans for the crew exploration vehicle, the crew launch vehicle, and the cargo delivery vehicle as outlined by NASA as well as current plans to finish the ISS, but there are clearly critics. These critics include those that operate the site http://www.nasaproblems.com. These critics suggest that the near-term operation of the shuttle is more dangerous than NASA has claimed and that the planning concepts on which Project Constellation is based are needlessly expensive in scope and design—and more dangerous than advertised. Certainly GAO and U.S. Department of Defense reviews of the program have found a number of difficulties. If NASA is to succeed in the future, it needs clear-cut and viable plans forward. Certainly critical review of both Project Constellation and deployment plans by Congress, the Office of Management and Budget, and the scientific community (i.e., the National Academies of Science and Engineering) is warranted before the actual production of hardware begins.

References

1   *The Vision for Space Exploration*, NASA Publication, NP-2004-01-334, Washington, DC, 2004.
2   "Mismanaging the Shuttle Fixes," *New York Times*, 19 Aug. 2005, p. A20.
3   Sietzen, F., Jr., "Heir to Apollo: Shaping the CEV," *Aerospace America*, Vol. 44, Issue 1, Jan. 2006.
4   Leary, W., "NASA Planning Return to Moon Within 13 Years," *New York Times*, 20 Sept. 2005, p. A7.
5   Broad, W. J., "Space Vision: The Experts Split Again," *New York Times*, 20 Sept. 2005, p. A15.
6   "Panel Cuts Bush's Budget Request for NASA," *Washington Post*, 9 Sept. 2004, p. A 7.
7   Bush, President George W., "New Space Vision," speech at NASA Headquarters, Washington, DC, 14 Jan. 2004.
8   "NASA Selects 11 Contractors for Exploration Studies," *SatNews Daily*, 3 Sept. 2004, URL: http://www.satnews.com/stories11/472.htm.
9   "NASA Selects Flight Critical Systems Technology Providers," *Astro News*, 12–13 Dec. 2005, URL: http://www.astroexpo.com/gateway.asp.
10 Gugliotta, G., "NASA Unveils $104 Billion Plan to Return to the Moon by 2018," *Washington Post*, 20 Sept. 2005, pp. A-1, A-11.
11 Leary, W. E., "Nasa Planning Return to Moon Within 13 Years," *New York Times*, 20 Sept. 2005, pp. A-1, A-15.

[12] "Italians to Build Telescope on Moon," *Astro News*, Italian Space Agency Release via ANSA, 4 Jan. 2005, p. 4.

[13] "DOD Awards Nearly $1 Billion Contract to Northrop Grumman for X-43B Development," *Nasa News*, 13 Sept. 2003, p. 11, URL: http://www.spacenews.com.

[14] Mendell, W., "Meditations on the New Space Vision: The Moon as Stepping Stone to Mars," International Astronautical Academy, IAA Paper, 3.7.1.01, Oct. 2004.

Additional Reading

"Advanced Space Transportation research," NASA Inst. for Advanced Concepts, *http://www.nasa.niac.gov*.

Berger, B., "Discovery Opens Last Chapter for Space Shuttle Born of Compromise," *Space News*, Vol. 16, No. 32, 15 Aug. 2005, pp. 1, 4.

Gugliotta, G., "Foam Cracks May Delay Shuttle Launch," *Washington Post*, 2 Dec. 2005, p. A3.

"Mismanaging the Shuttle Fixes," *New York Times*, 19 Aug. 2005, p. A20.

"NASA Selects Flight Critical Systems Technology Providers," *Astro News*, 12–13 Dec. 2005, URL: http://www.astroexpo.com/gateway.asp.

Park, R. L., "The Dark Side of the Moon," *New York Times*, 22 Sept. 2005, p. A31.

"Project Constellation Update," http://www.projectconstellation.us.

Schwartz, J., "Minority Report Faults NASA as Compromising Safety," *New York Times*, 18 Aug. 2005, p. A15.

Schwartz, J., "A Wide-Eyed Astronaut Becomes a NASA Critic," *New York Times*, 24 Jan. 2006, pp. D1, D4.

Tierney, J., "Go West, Young Astronaut," *New York Times*, 5 Dec. 2005, p. A31.

CHAPTER 9
Lessons Learned in Space Safety and Ongoing Issues

"That's the beauty of offering prizes; a little money buys a lot
more R&D than you would ever get by giving the funds to
NASA. Prizes spurred Charles Lindbergh and others to quickly
turn aviation from a stunt into an industry."

—*John Tierney of the* New York Times

"NASA officials characterized the external tank as 'safer',
'the safest ever' or even 'fixed' when there was no objective
data to support the claims ... there were 'adjustments
of performance standards' when targets could not be met."

—*Minority Report of the Stafford–Covey Task Force charged
with certifying that the CAIB recommendations had been met
before the shuttle's return to orbit*

"An FBI-led watchdog agency has opened a investigation into
multiple complaints accusing NASA Inspector General
Robert W Cobb of failing to investigate safety violations
and retaliating against whistle-blowers."

—Washington Post, *front page report, 3 February 2006*

Two New "Disturbing" Developments

There is now broad agreement, both within and outside NASA, that the
shuttle program needs to be phased out of operation and replaced with
new vehicles—and just as soon as possible. This course of action, unfortunately, was outlined by the Rogers commission and the Payne commission in 1986 right after the *Challenger* disaster, but these recommendations
were not heeded. Had the recommendations made in 1986 been acted on
then, there is a good possibility that the *Columbia* accident might never
have occurred.

It is the finding of the 2005 George Washington University safety review
study, as well of many others, that the replacement of the shuttle should be
accomplished just as soon as possible, but this is apparently not imminent
and could easily to be another four to five years. The factors arguing for
early retirement include 1) many of the technologies used in this launch system are now out of date; 2) the thermal protection system has demonstrated
major weaknesses in safety, performance, and cost efficiency; 3) there are
wear-out and fatigue problems with many components; 4) the combination

of liquid-fueled and solid rocket boosters is problematic; 5) there is no full-envelope escape capability; 6) the foam-shedding problem has proved difficult to resolve; and 7) the shuttle design is overly complex and cannot be made significantly safer without, in effect, "starting over" with new concepts. It is clear for these reasons, and more, that new systems can be designed to be both safer and more cost efficient.

Despite the extensive efforts to improve the safety of the shuttle in the ongoing return-to-flight program (at an estimated total of direct and indirect costs of some $2 billion over a period of three years), very serious concerns still remain. The enormous complexity of the shuttle, with its 2.5 million parts and huge number of subsystems (including particularly the nearly 30,000 parts of the thermal protection system), simply does not allow significant improvement in safety. Curtailing the deployment of certain elements of the ISS to reduce the number of shuttle flights currently appears to be one way to both reduce costs and improve safety. Serious NASA commitments to ISS partners to launch the JEM, the Columbus Laboratory, etc., however, significantly limit such options to ground the shuttle sooner by virtue of reducing its remaining flights beyond the reductions now anticipated, that is, from 28 down to 18 launches.

The 25-member panel, chaired by astronauts Stafford and Covey, that was charged in 2003 with overseeing NASA's effort to implement the findings and recommendations of the *Columbia* Accident Investigation Board (CAIB) issued a report in August 2005 that generally signed off on the reflight efforts. However, seven of the voting members issued a minority report that was generally scathing in its critique of NASA's efforts and suggested that three of the most important recommendations had not been implemented. This minority report suggested that when three key efforts became too difficult to achieve NASA managers simply redefined the objectives. These were 1) to eliminate foam and ice debris during launching, 2) to toughen the orbiter's outer skin, and 3) to develop techniques to repair a damaged craft while in orbit. The report went on to say that NASA managers and officials "must break this cycle of smugness substituting for knowledge [1]."

NASA Administrator Michael Griffin had sufficient concerns about the safety of the shuttle that in April 2005 he ordered a review of specific risk issues, such as whether liftoff debris had been sufficiently addressed, and he delayed the STS-114 launch of the Discovery by two months so that such concerns could be addressed in some detail. In the wake of the recurrence of significant liftoff foam debris that just missed the orbiter, Administrator Griffin then ordered a grounding of the shuttle and proceeded with a management shakeup. Most notably, Admiral Readdy, who had overseen the reflight campaign, left NASA [2].

One of the most recent and disturbing developments, following the disappointing STS Mission 114 in August 2005, was the subsequent discovery of cracks in the so-called protuberance air load (PAL) ramp. This ramp was designed to divert foam debris at liftoff away from the orbiter. This feature had been added on the advice of the CAIB. Shuttle Program

Manager N. Wayne Hale explained in a public statement in December 2005 that inspections have now shown cracks in the PAL ramp that had apparently been caused by contraction and expansion as the supercooled liquid-hydrogen and -oxygen fuel is added to the orbiter's fuel tanks. Hale has indicated that if the decision is made to remove the PAL ramp this would add four months on to the time that the shuttle would remain grounded [3].

The other perhaps even more disturbing event was the February 2006 disclosure that the FBI had launched a formal probe into NASA's inspector general's office concerning allegations that serious safety violations had not been investigated properly and that whistle-blowers who made complaints concerning safety issues were punished rather than protected. Specific incidents that are apparently under investigation involve a 2002 shuttle launch in which the shuttle's backup command destruct system was not functioning and the range "red" condition was overridden by the range commander without NASA engineers being made aware of these conditions. Another complaint involves the cancellation of funding for upgrades to deteriorating gantries, launchpads, and other shuttle infrastructure that had not been carried out in a proper manner. Apparently the shuttle program wanted these upgrades made, but the funding was killed without the inspector general's investigators being able to find out who had made this decision. The essence of the allegations appears to center on the relationship between the NASA inspector general and the former NASA administrator when these and other incidents occurred [4,5].

There are many lessons to be learned from the U.S. manned space program over the last four decades. If these earlier "lessons learned" had been properly applied to the shuttle, results might have been different. The most important of these lessons learned included the following: 1) limiting the number of waivers to a minimum and fixing problems rather than finding ways to make allowances for them, 2) providing full-envelope escape capability, 3) separating crew and cargo wherever possible, and 4) avoiding combining different launch propulsion systems of liquid and solid fuels.

> Applying these four lessons learned to the shuttle design and operation might well have prevented both the *Challenger* and *Columbia* accidents or at least allowed for the successful escape of the astronauts.

Applying these four lessons learned to the shuttle design and operation might well have prevented both the *Challenger* and *Columbia* accidents or at least allowed for the successful escape of the astronauts.

There is a danger, however, in trying to plan the way forward by trying to fight the last war. The future of space exploration and space safety must therefore look to the future, while learning from the past.

This chapter seeks to review lessons learned from Mercury, Gemini, Apollo, Skylab, the shuttle, the International Space Station, the various X-projects whereby NASA undertook to develop either a personal space vehicle or an astronaut escape system, and even from Project Constellation efforts to date. Finally, this chapter explores the possibilities for new space development and enhanced space safety that might be found either within the private and entrepreneurial sectors of the aerospace industry as well as from international developments and experience.

Safety is more than good design, or quality control, or effective management or learning from historical experience, or technical innovation. In fact, space safety also involves more than just making better spacecraft for astronauts—it includes a myriad of things that range widely over such diverse areas as better safety processes for aerospace workers and NASA technical engineers on the ground; safety precautions for range safety; effective means to protect nuclear power supplies on space systems; protection of astronauts against radiation, micrometeorites, and the effects of low-*g* environments; and an overall safety culture in which all NASA employees and contractors are universally and passionately committed to space safety. In such an environment "corners are not cut" to meet budget or schedule demands by risking the lives of astronauts or space program workers.

Looking to the Future of Space Safety

In looking to the future, NASA must ensure the development of new and improved launch systems. These should allow for separation of crew and cargo, simplicity of design, launch-to-land full-envelope escape capabilities, and more creative exploitation of more and more capable robotic and avionic systems. Currently, NASA safety practices and programs are contained within many diverse units that cut across more than a dozen centers and scores of disciplinary competencies and program elements. Ultimately, there is an argument for NASA to take a comprehensive and fresh look at safety from an organic and a simplified viewpoint. Safety must be approached as a system rather than a collection of parts, and it must be engineered and designed in rather than trying to use reliability testing to "weed out" weak links. Ultimately safety must be a state of mind and an inbred culture.

> Safety must be approached as a system rather than a collection of parts, and it must be engineered and designed in rather than trying to use reliability testing to "weed out" weak links.

Application of many of the findings presented in this chapter can improve safety practices as well as promote the design of systems that are substantially safer and more cost efficient. Important improvements can come in many ways—through the use of the latest thermal protection materials, improved propulsion systems, and innovative technology and systems research. Yet the most important strides forward will most likely come though true safety design and engineering, as opposed to overreliance on quality control or independent verification processes. This compelling logic of improved space safety engineering that comes from systems engineering thus derives from many sources. These include the very historical wisdom of Ockham's razor (i.e., to pick the simplest and least complex workable solution) up to the much more contemporary industrial research of Dr. Demming, which led him to create the key elements of the management system known as total quality control. Similar criteria for quality engineering and process control are found within the Baldridge prize competition or the six-sigma approach to quality design and management, etc. Some of these elements of quality control, system engineering, and analysis seem to be well ingrained in NASA's processes, but having its safety and quality processes divided among the various centers and various technology groups can diminish focus. In short, it would seem that NASA's safety programs and independent verification and validation (IV&V) processes could be substantially improved through integration and focus.

Likewise a NASA inspector's general office that clearly and resolutely recognized safety and integrity to be the organization's top goals would help to instill the type of culture that was found lacking when the CAIB conducted its review of NASA performance. At times one received the impression that at the top of NASA over the past 10 years "safety is job ten or eleven."

The shuttle experience should teach us many things. These lessons include a commitment to 1) eschew complexity; 2) avoid false economies; 3) avoid mixing incompatible technologies; and 4) emphasize modularity and the ability to update materials, technology, and subsystems. The closely related International Space Station (ISS) experience should teach us the following:

1) Prolonging and extending high-tech and complex projects add enormously to costs through inflation, lead to constant reengineering to adapt to emergency circumstances not identified in modeling and simulation exercises, create problems of access to replacement parts and equipment, and create a series of problems related to long-term maintenance of staff competencies, supporting test equipment, and facilities.

2) Basing the supply of key structural and life-support elements on a single launch system is unwise (and ultimately uneconomic). If you can use only one launch system and that system fails, the negative domino effect becomes huge.

3) Updating technologies through modularity and flexibility of design is highly desirable and can promote cost efficiency and safety.

4) Using reasonably tested off-the-shelf equipment in a redundant mode can in many cases make more sense than custom designing specialized components that have no backup.

5) Evolutionary systems that grow over time are most likely better to deploy than designing huge monolithic systems.

6) One should first design experiments and set program objectives and then afterwards begin to conceive hardware and software. In short, objectives first and hardware second is the right sequence and not the reverse.

In the overall initial design process, questions that should be explored include whether several smaller systems or free-flying robotic experiments might be better than one huge space facility?

Safety and Project Constellation

In all cases, new launch systems, space stations, and space exploratory craft must be designed from the bottom up with safety in mind to reduce risk and to provide better performance. The 11 study contracts that NASA undertook for the early planning of Project Constellation, plus its two internal studies, in many ways appear to have pursued such systems-level and goal-oriented planning. In short, these efforts were indeed directed at exploring the best way to achieve defined objectives. Several examples of this type of safety-led designing process can be identified in the Project Constellation design process.

The separation of heavy-lift vehicles from vehicles for the crew is clearly a safer, more cost effective, and logical way to proceed. This type of approach has been consistently identified in a number of studies, including the George Washington University space safety study in 2005. In close parallel with this approach is the idea of using robotics on space vehicles that do not require human crews to be onboard at all. This approach can provide for both cost and program efficiencies as well as enhanced safety. In this area, it is not clear that the Project Constellation design has leveraged the use of robotics to the maximum effect to save costs and reduce astronaut risk. Most of the missions to the moon to create infrastructure for a longer-term astronaut base, for instance, could be accomplished by robots that do not require life-support systems, eat food, drink water, or need to return to the Earth. The Italian project designed to construct a lunar observatory (as reported in Chapter 8) is conceived as being built by using robots to fit components together. If this project were to be built by astronauts, it would likely cost at least 10 times more and would, of course, risk many astronauts' lives.

Space exploration systems for the moon and Mars, however, can bring video and audio systems along so that humans can explore the moon "live via satellite." As far as the Mars mission is concerned, the reasons for a manned mission to the red planet, as opposed to continuing to explore via robotic systems, have not been made. Robotic camera systems and sensors could, for instance, be mounted on balloons designed especially for the Martian atmosphere. These systems could explore the entire Mars surface with great efficiency for extended periods of time. Humans, on the other hand, could not stay aloft for long-duration missions for reasons that include weightlessness and life-support systems.

NASA's Project Constellation is an ambitious program that has given the space agency new life. This undertaking will define the future of U.S. human-rated spacecraft for the next decade. It involves clear and specific guidelines related to performance, safety, and sustainability. Nevertheless there are also questions about plans for Project Constellation. These include issues concerning the specific plans for the crew launch vehicle, the escape module, the crew exploration vehicle, and even the unmanned solid-motor cargo-lift system. These questions include the currently compressed timetable for the development of these new crew vehicles between now and the end of 2012.

There are also questions about the viability of plans for the so-called spiral development of this program over a sustained period of time? In short, would several smaller undertakings be better than one large undertaking? Would competitive entrepreneurial projects with more limited government funding produce faster and more effective results? Are there parts of the program that should be internationalized, and should this be considered sooner rather than later? Would some more outside-the-box thinking that goes beyond the retro Apollo model for the Project Constellation ultimately be safer and more cost effective? Such options that might embrace electric ion propulsion from low Earth orbit to the moon, robotic missions to create human-rated lunar colonies, or even "space elevator" technology might be tested against a Project Constellation baseline in terms of performance, cost, and safety to see which perhaps five or six models truly produce the best results against test criteria. Outside review of such options would seem a prudent exercise before the United States fully commits itself to NASA's current $104 billion 13-year program.

One can question the extent to which current plans, projected to last at least through 2018, can be sustained effectively through many different presidential administrations to achieve longer-term space exploration goals as well as achieve the maximum degree of safety for future astronauts.

Designing the Launch and Crew Exploration Systems for Project Constellation

When Project Constellation first started, many people envisioned the crew exploration vehicle as very much like a minishuttle that would be a reusable craft that would sit atop a launch vehicle, much like the systems shown in the preceding chapter in Figs. 8.4 and 8.5. But the intensive planning process that followed the presidential vision for space exploration in January 2004 came to the conclusion that the reusable craft approach would neither be the most cost-effective nor safest approach to take. Years of experience have shown that an expendable capsule return was the safest and that building a system that would have to experience multiple returns into the Earth's atmosphere would be very expensive to design and build and that over time temperature and physical stresses on the craft would likely lessen its safety.

Thus, after study, the reusable crew exploration vehicle design was dropped. The other idea, to take an existing U.S. launch system such as Atlas, Delta, or Titan and upgrade its safety to a crew-rated reliability, was also discarded. The latest idea for the launch of the CEV is to take the highly reliable shuttle orbiter liquid-fuel engines and use a cluster of them to launch the crew exploration vehicle into orbit. It was also decided that the material and life-support systems needed for travel to the moon or Mars could best be launched by creating a vehicle with the solid rocket-fuel engines that are now used to boost the shuttle orbiter into space. In short, the idea is to use proven rocket engine technology from the shuttle program and reapply it in new ways. The crew exploration vehicle will

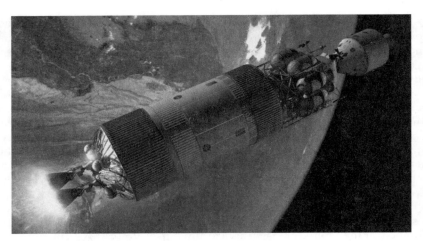

Figure 9-1 CEV capsule and landing system for the moon shown "mated" in Earth orbit (graphic courtesy of NASA).

then be able to go the ISS and return to Earth via a capsule return, just as is the case with the Soyuz vehicle.

Later versions of the CEV will be able to mate in orbit with cargo launched by a heavy-lift system that uses solid-fuel motors. The graphic in Fig. 9.1 shows the CEV mated with the lander system in Earth orbit before leaving on a trajectory to the moon.

There is considerable logic behind this plan in terms of taking a very conservative approach that does not have to develop much new technology. The shuttle orbiter motors have proven generally very reliable, although Appendix C does note some issues that should be addressed before final Project Constellation designs are adopted. These motors will be clustered to provide the needed launch thrust. In addition, there will be an emergency vehicle that could allow the astronauts to escape if there are problems with the liquid-fuel vehicle. Further, the NASA controllers can shut down the liquid-fueled vehicle by turning off the supply of oxygen to the motors if there is a problem in the launch engines. This design thus applies key lessons from the past in terms of full-envelope escape, use of proven technology, and avoidance of combining liquid-fuel with solid-fuel engines. The remaining issue is to develop a sound procurement and oversight process for the liquid-fuel motors plus sound IV&V for the production and test of these launch systems. Care must be taken to ensure that there is a reliable source of supply for all of the key elements of these launch systems as well as concerns about sole source production over the longer term.

The idea of using the solid motors from the shuttle program to lift "unmanned cargo" to orbit also makes sense in terms of historical experience. These solid-fuel motors are proven to be highly reliable. Safety issues have arisen by putting the solid and liquid-fuel motors together and problems with the foam heat insulation in between the two launch systems and the fragile ceramic-tile heat shield. If the solid motor systems should malfunction, then all that would be lost would be the cargo. Again there is an issue of sole source supply over the longer term (see Appendix C).

A final safety issue is that of the launch range facilities to support the Project Constellation operations. The Kennedy Space Center is now an antiquated facility that in some cases houses buildings and specialized equipment that is nearly 50 years old. Further, the area is subject to high winds, tropical storms, and hurricanes. It is near highly populated areas and high levels of security are not easily achieved. It has been recently revealed that urgent requests to update shuttle launch facilities and gantries were overruled under questionable circumstances [4,5].

Consideration might logically be given to creating a new launch site or colocating it with existing military launch facilities that are isolated from civilian populations, more secure and ultimately equipped with more modern equipment.

Historical Review

In the earliest days of human space exploration, starting with the Mercury program, the safety of astronauts was seen to be of utmost importance, and thus certain concepts evolved. These concepts were refined as the Gemini, Saturn/Apollo, and Skylab programs emerged over time. Key safety concepts, as identified over the last 40 years, include the following:

1) Create detection sensors that forewarn of major problems or malfunctions, and allow for an escape from the craft at all stages of the mission if possible.

2) Separate crew from cargo wherever possible.

3) Have a process to check and double check for reliability and performance, and correct all problems with as few waivers or exceptions to absolute safety as possible.

4) Recognize that it is not really possible to add or retrofit safety to a vehicle or spacecraft and that safety and safety margins must be designed in from the start.

5) Use robotics and automated systems to perform a mission or function rather than risking human life wherever possible.

6) Recognize that targeted and specifically designed programs with simplicity of design are likely to be safer than multipurpose systems that attempt to combine too many capabilities and involve too much complexity. (Again, this is what might be called the Ockham's razor approach to human-based space programs.) These early rules were evolved out of both design studies and real-world experience and served the early programs well. Of course none of these principles work well if there is not a universal safety culture at work within the NASA organization.

Over time, it appears that elements of "risk creep" and a form of over self-assurance have entered the space program, not only in the United States but in Russia as well. "Vigilant success" has tended to be replaced by the "assumption of success." The design and building of the shuttle violated a number of the rules because many high-level NASA management and governmental policy makers tended to see the shuttle as the equivalent of a modern airliner. After the *Challenger* accident, surveys of space shuttle engineers and NASA management and officials, for instance, clearly showed a widely differing view of the safety rating of these vehicles, with management and policy makers holding the view that the vehicle was many times safer than the assessment of the engineers. One cannot redesign the shuttle, but future systems such as those evolving under Project Constellation need to consider seriously the basic safety concepts just outlined. With the exception of more intensive use of robotics and automated avionics, this indeed largely seems to be the case.

Space Shuttle Safety

A number of steps can be taken to address the safety of the space shuttle and improve the chances that no more fatalities will come from the remaining shuttle launches. These steps are as follows:

1) Implement *all* of the CAIB recommendations. Most of the specific CAIB recommendations for upgrade of the space shuttle to detect, repair, and prevent damage to the TPS are complete. There remain several key issues that are unresolved. The most important of these are the ability to perform in-orbit repairs, to toughen the orbiter's outer skin, and to launch only after full safety precautions are fully verified and the foam-shedding issue fully resolved. It is important that NASA not be driven by budgetary and schedule pressures and to fully create the new independent technical engineering authority with full control over the approval of waivers. We feel that the minority report from the Stafford–Covey review panel should be taken seriously and all of their concerns fully resolved before STS-115 flies. Further there is danger that the CAIB report might be mistaken as a cure-all that would magically make the shuttle significantly more reliable. Although the shuttle orbiter might look the same as always (see Fig. 9.2), it has been upgraded and changed many times, and the safety review process must consider every potential failure mode.

There are more problems with shuttle safety than just the TPS, as noted in some detail in both Chapters 3 and 4 and Appendix C. Further it appears that the foam deflection (i.e., PAL) ramp as recommended by the CAIB might be a source of danger itself. The CAIB report must be considered as only one element in the shuttle safety enhancement program.

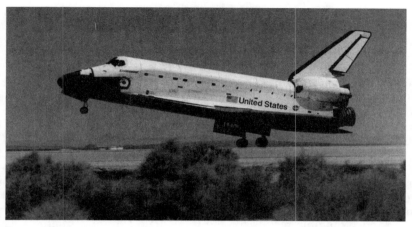

Figure 9-2 *Endeavor*, the youngest space shuttle orbiter, touching down at
Kennedy Space Center (photo courtesy of NASA).

2) Address the findings of the GW University Astronaut Safety Study
2005 and many deferred upgrades, especially of the environmental
systems (see Appendix C).

The first step in this process would be for NASA to prepare a report
that lists all upgrades, improvements that are in process or are currently
pending, deferred, or shelved. This listing would include all possible
upgrades that would improve the performance and/or safety of the shuttle. This report would address all of the areas of safety concern listed in
the summary charts of potential risks for the shuttle program, as listed at
the end of Chapters 3 and 4, as well as other pending safety upgrades recommended by NASA engineers or contractors (such as the pending work
on the PAL ramp). In short, it should include those explicitly identified in
this book as well as all pending shuttle safety upgrade activities. Such a
report should list the status and the cost of pending or alternative solutions, the time implications of making these upgrades, design changes, or
modifications, and what actions are deemed most appropriate as well as
those deemed to be of the highest priority. It should also indicate the
degree of risk associated with *not* implementing these safety improvements. Clearly NASA might be reluctant to respond for a variety of time,
cost, and policy reasons and especially for fear that it could delay the
return to flight of the shuttle even further.

It must be observed with some candor that if there is an effective and
comprehensive Space Shuttle safety program now in effect, then this data
and associated management/cost information would already exist in a
single place and the information should be readily available for briefing
acceptable sources. In light of the now over $2-billion, some 3 years and
the countless number of engineering and staff hours invested in returning

the Space Shuttle to flight-readiness, such an effort and a public disclosure of Shuttle safety information at least to Congress and oversight bodies seems essential.

3) Conduct shuttle review to consider the most important issues.

There are many aspects of shuttle safety to consider as just noted. A review of the most critical issues needs to be undertaken to see what could be done, either in upgrading shuttle safety prior to retirement as well as ensuring, if upgrades cannot be achieved now, that next generation systems can be so improved. Examples of these prime issues include the following:

a) *Escape capability*: For instance, can more be done to upgrade a launch-to-land full-envelope escape capability for the space shuttle than is currently the case? A specific review of escape options at all phases of a shuttle mission would be a useful exercise. Even if such an exercise did not produce tangible results for the immediate future, it might at least clarify options related to the CRL and CEV systems.

b) *Thermal protection system*: Is it impossible to replace the current 30,000-part tile and thermal layer TPS system with a better design? Could new metallic thermal protection systems or at least improved ceramic-tile designs (i.e., the simplified design found in the HL-20 program) be retrofitted to the shuttle? Should the PAL ramp be eliminated or redesigned? Can the toughness of the orbiter outside skin be further enhanced?

c) *Cargo/crew separation*: There is a need to separate the crew, together with their life-support systems, where and when possible. One concept would be to use the shuttle as a robotic-lift vehicle that might transport elements such as the Columbus space lab, the Japanese experimental module, or the Centrifuge accommodation module to the ISS and use the return as a way of bringing astronauts back from the space station. Operated in this mode, perhaps half of the remaining missions could be operated without crew, and the shuttle might actually carry more cargo.

d) *Waivers*: There is hard evidence that the Apollo fire, the *Challenger* and the *Columbia* accidents all have in common the granting of waivers as well as the override of safety officers or safety concerns of NASA engineers. The solution to shuttle problems should be found in solving the problems rather than granting exception to the difficulty. The basic process should be to identify the problem and fix it rather than simply granting waivers.

e) *Robotic operation of the shuttle*: There could be cost and safety advantages if one or more shuttle orbiters (see Fig. 9.3) were to be configured to operate entirely as a remotely controlled system. This capability already largely exists, except with regard to mating with the International Space Station.

Clearly there is a mystique surrounding the shuttle carrying astronauts into space. This is a signature role that is key to NASA's status as the premier space agency. At the outset in the 1970s, the shuttle

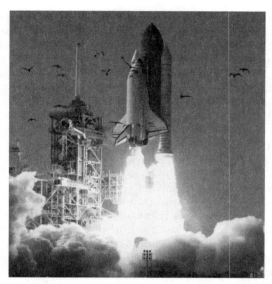

Figure 9-3   Could a shuttle mission operate robotically for a complete mission on a launch-to-land basis? (photo courtesy of NASA).

was "sold" to Congress on the premise that this vehicle would be very safe—like an airliner—and astronauts would ride into space with only very small risk. This basic initial misunderstanding has never been dispelled [6].

But if mystique ends up costing huge amounts of money and risking lives needlessly, then new options must be considered. Because there is crew already continuously in space onboard the ISS, there is no reason for NASA to insist that each shuttle be manned if this is unnecessary.

International Space Station

The ISS was designed with the idea that the shuttle would be the work-horse to transport the key structural elements of this experimental facility to space, repair critical components, and ferry astronauts to and from this unique habitat in space. No plan involving human life and safety should ever be agreed without a backup or contingency plan, but essentially the shuttle became the only means of transporting structural elements of the ISS into orbit, as well as critical components like the gyroscopic orbital stabilizers and the environmental control units [7].

Elements such as the Japanese experimental module (JEM), called Kibo, the centrifuge accommodation module (CAM), the Columbus laboratory, the Canadarm2 manipulator, etc. and other mission-critical elements of the ISS should have been redesigned in a more modular fashion, particularly after the *Challenger* accident in 1986. These elements, in short, should have been designed with contingencies to allow alternative launch and assembly options using expendable rockets. In fact, many of the ISS experimental programs might have been designed as a more modular system with the use of more free-flyer components such as the Spartan experimental platform [8].

There were two-and-one-half years lost in retrofitting the shuttle after the loss of the *Challenger* (from 1986 to 1988). The loss of shuttle flight capability after *Columbia* has essentially been from February 2003 through to late spring 2006 because the reflight mission in STS-114 in August 2005 only confirmed that key problems had not been fixed. The downtime for the shuttle therefore now amounts to more than six years. This, in turn, translates directly into the same number of years of downtime in constructing the ISS, and this is only one element of delay in the program. It is almost impossible to calculate the cost of the ISS program in terms of this six-year delay as reflected in inflation, in terms of the cost of supporting a vast standing army of engineers and technicians to support to the shuttle, and in terms of the lost time of highly paid professors and researchers planning for experiments on the ISS that might now never be realized. A conservative estimate would nevertheless place such costs in the range of $10–20 billion.

A launch program that separates human access to orbit from robotic cargo lifters might be too late to apply to the shuttle and the ISS. Likewise it is too late to redesign components of the ISS in a more modular fashion so that they can be deployed by alternative means, but these are key lessons that should be learned and applied for the future.

Beyond these issues and problems there are continuing concerns about ISS safety.

Reassessment of ISS Safety, Maintenance, and Operation

The operation of the ISS can be currently characterized as being little better than in crisis-management mode. Its operation with only two crew members was never intended. Further, there are questions concerning the total reliability and functionality of the environmental control systems (especially the oxygen generators and CO_2 and noxious gas monitors), the power systems, the space suits, and other life-sustaining elements of the ISS. The list of issues that represent some level of concern for astronaut safety which we are uncertain about (in terms of whether they may or may not have yet been fully rectified) includes the following: the gyro system; the availability of requisite boosting power to maintain the ISS orbit; the installation of a fire-fighting mist system; the illusive but apparent slow leak in the ISS atmospheric system; the lack, until recently, of video monitors at critical external locations; the limited IT and communications capabilities; the use of flash programming "fixes" that require operators to have knowledge of more and more programming anomalies; substantial

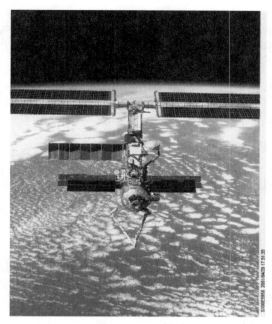

Figure 9-4   International Space Station represents a number of safety issues (graphic courtesy of NASA).

orbital debris; the need for emergency EVAs with no crew left onboard and thus requiring total control of the station from the ground; longer-term radiation exposure of the astronauts; and micrometeorite damage to the ISS and astronaut EVA concerns as a result of micrometeorites.

It was the view derived from the George Washington University study that it would be desirable for all of these issues and concerns related to ISS safety to have a thorough and independent assessment.

Most of all, there is the hugely ironic fact that the ISS (see Fig. 9.4), whose total cost might now be approaching $100 billion, is not really accomplishing its mission. The ISS was presumably designed and built to carry out a very long and demanding set of tests, experiments, and demonstrations, and yet the two-person crew can really only manage to maintain the station in orbit at this stage with very limited time for experiments. The once sizable American ISS experimental program has been cut in size, and European and Japanese experiments are not able to travel to the ISS. Their key experimental elements, as represented by the Columbus space lab, the JEM, and the CAM, have not even been deployed to the space station.

The most fundamental paradox thus becomes why are the United States and its international partners finishing something at tremendously high cost (in terms of money and risk to astronaut lives) when the reason for building it continues to erode [9]?

In short, the stated purpose of the ISS was to conduct space tests and experiments that have now been greatly reduced in scope. From a strategic planning perspective the ISS must be considered to have fallen far short of its mission goals.

Explore use of other expendable vehicles to complete the ISS as well as reassess the plans for the ISS final configuration and optimization for experimental programs

Once the basic issues of the ongoing operational strategies and objectives for the ISS are better determined, and when it is better known how the ISS can be safely operated and with what size crew, then reconsideration needs to be given to such issues as whether expendables, robotic shuttle orbiters, and/or "free flyers" could or should complete more of the key experimental mission objectives. Also, this process would address whether the international partners require the full ISS to be completed to achieve their most important goals. Given the fact that the ISS was planned in the 1980s, reconsideration of what makes the most sense for today's space programs seems essential. The announced new presidential vision does not indicate a need for the ISS beyond some degree of life testing. Such medical tests could presumably be completed with the ISS much as it is today. Billions of dollars and potentially a number of astronaut lives might be saved under newly redefined ISS program goals. Such a shift, however, clearly needs to be agreed to with the ISS international partners. It is recognized that significant obligations have been made to launch certain Japanese, Canadian, and European components, but there might be ways to meet international commitments and still reduce the scope of the ISS and lessen the number of shuttle launches.

Strengthening the NASA Organization

Measures to improve NASA's safety programs and to sharpen specific goals can be outlined as follows:

1) *Structure NASA for maximum efficiency and accountability.* NASA, in response to the CAIB and the Aldridge commission, has already been restructured. The new structure, which spreads responsibility for astronaut activities and operations and launch-vehicle development, does not appear to have anyone at the highest levels, that is, associate administrator, directly responsible for astronaut safety. It has now been revealed that there are questions as to whether the 200-person inspector general's office within NASA has fully discharged its duties with regard to safety regulations as well. The prominence of safety that was requested is not readily evident from the new structure, and the investigations of the IG's office only heightens the concern. Further, the relevance of NASA programs to

the greater benefit of the American public is likewise missing. A further improvement in the NASA structure might be considered in terms of having two prime units. One would be devoted to astronauts and safety, launch vehicles and robotics, and include the ISS and space exploration, while the other unit would address space sciences, applications, and education. This structure might even consider transferring aviation research and safety to the FAA and with it the Langley Research Center. Most importantly, we believe that the NASA Engineering and Safety Center and the NASA Independent Technical Engineering Authority need to be given prime responsibility for astronaut safety and true "say so" over waivers.

2) *Restructure NASA centers to achieve specific space transportation goals, and transfer certain tasks to private sector.* Today, major NASA centers and installations include Ames, Dryden, Glenn, Goddard, Johnson, Jet Propulsion Laboratory (JPL), Kennedy, Langley, Marshall, Stennis, and Headquarters. This represents a vast array of talented engineers and scientists engaged in a host of exciting and interesting operational and research projects. The total number of activities and programs has grown since NASA was created in 1958 in almost free-form style. These activities have expanded into a maze of projects based on the personal interests and capabilities of NASA personnel, plus the application of political power, and proliferation of technology and programs. In the process, NASA, in sharp contrast to virtually every space agency in the world, has evolved more and more towards exploring outer space and astronaut programs, with reduced emphasis on Earth-based space applications and science programs. The likelihood of NASA being able to accomplish space programs that are safer as well as ones that are considered more relevant by "John Q. and Jennie R. Public" would seem to be closely tied to focusing the work of its centers on clearly identified goals. This could involve transferring the various NASA centers to the status of federally funded research centers (as is now the case with JPL and as recommended by the Aldridge commission), transferring certain tasks to industry or universities and trying to focus on something like its top 10 goals. In the advice provided in the book called *Re-Inventing Government*, it might well be that NASA needs to do more "steering" and less "oaring" in managing the national space program. Thus a sleeker NASA with specific goal-oriented duties might be able to accomplish more. Today the various NASA centers, in various ways, appear to be "earmarks" by key local congressmen to bring home the "bacon" for their home states as political pork. This could perhaps be most significantly seen in the public statements of Representative Tom Delay whose jurisdiction included the Johnson Space Center in Houston, Texas. In comparison to the very large budgets of NASA centers, there is the startling example of Burt Rutan and Paul Allen achieving the successful development of the SpaceOne vehicle for a budget of $20 million. There is the parallel development by Elon Musk of a new rocket system via his small Space X company, which suggests that sleeker and more focused organizations might be able to accomplish more with less.

3) *Ensure a strong emphasis on safety, and in this respect ensure that the new Independent Technical Engineering Authority and the NESC have a clearly proactive research and risk-reduction role.*

This organizational concept of a sleeker and more goal-defined NASA, as noted earlier, is of prime importance to improved safety. The NESC requires a stronger mandate to be proactive in strengthening the design of human-rated space systems, given greater organizational and geographic cohesion and greater clout in NASA decision making. One option would be to grant to the new independent technical engineering authority responsibility for all safety matters and to move the NESC under this independent authority. Likewise the GAO, the ASAP, and even the FAA should be given increased authority for independent review of NASA space safety programs. This is because in many respects NASA internal review processes have not seemed to work and the inspector general's office is now under FBI investigation. In response to congressional and White House pressure, NASA (under both democratic and republican administrations) has found its astronaut programs strongly pressured by budget and schedule in a way that might well have adversely impacted safety concerns. Creating a new NASA culture of safety is important, but independent review and oversight might be a necessary part of achieving this goal. The preceding suggestion is only one possible option, but the main thrust is more organizational clout for space safety concerns and more oversight. This means more program say so in the safety programs and more independent review of NASA's success in achieving safety goals. Congress must face up to its responsibilities here and recognize that the CAIB report found that the latest shuttle failure "was that of national leadership" rather than of NASA management alone.

4) *Implement improved scheduling and budgeting process (recommendation 13 of CAIB).* The CAIB, in its recommendation 13, stated the need to create a realistic flight schedule and asked that NASA evaluate deadlines regularly to ensure that risks taken to meet the schedule are recognized, understood and acceptable. At this time, NASA is developing and perfecting a computerized manifesting capability in order to more effectively manage the schedule margin, launch constraints, and manifest flexibility so as to provide routine risk assessment and more room for changes and thus be able to make schedule and risk indicator data available in real time. The problem is that this process defines a schedule and risk assessment system as the solution. The real problem, in fact, is political or management override of safety concerns to meet deadlines. The improved system should be useful, but it does not solve the ability of safety officers' concerns to be overridden. This would be the prime safety value to be gained by the creation of the independent

technical engineering authority with oversight of safety and of the NESC. In short, the independent technical authority should assume responsibility for all safety activities including waivers, oversight of the NESC, etc. as follows:

a) Reduce granting of shuttle-related waivers, and solve problems rather than working around them (especially with regard to software, safety procedures established on the basis of historical precedent, and in response to risk creep).

The *Columbia* shuttle launch records, as reviewed by the CAIB, reported that there were some 5400 waivers granted by NASA officials. Many of these waivers were minor, but others were mission critical. Before the Apollo fire at Kennedy Space Center, a waiver was granted to allow combustible materials in the explosive pure oxygen atmosphere of the launch capsule. Before the *Challenger* launch, several waivers were granted related to the O-rings and the weather conditions allowable for liftoff. With the *Columbia* launch, the problem of foam debris shedding was routinely granted a waiver on the basis that "we have done so before." Previously granted waivers can thus be seen to be central to all three of these astronaut disasters.

b) Obtain specific funding for safety studies and lessons learned, and apply these findings to the CEV, CLV, and the solid-rocket-booster cargo rockets and other future programs. NASA might benefit from independent assessments with regard to safety practices, lessons learned, and exploration and evaluation of a range of program alternatives before deciding on the best way to proceed with the CEV, the CLV, the solid-rocket-booster cargo launchers, and other dimensions of its future programs. The minority report from the Stafford–Covey review committee that reported in August 2005 and February 2006 disclosure of the FBI investigation of the NASA inspector general's office with regard to issues involving safety violations seemed to show that NASA's "broken safety culture" does not yet seem to be fixed. It is absolutely imperative that NASA gets Project Constellation right if the space agency is going to survive in its current form.

Additional collaboration with other agencies such as the FAA, the Nuclear Regulatory Commission, as well as other international entities and government safety agencies, is recommended. AIAA-organized sessions that address "best practices" related to space safety would, for instance, be a desirable step.

Likewise a systematic search for relevant information about practices and safety precautions related to the chemical industries, the aviation industry, fire and combustion control research groups, hazardous waste, and radiation safety procedures would also be useful. The next phase of the effort would be to examine seriously how a new combination of robotic missions, robotically controlled heavy-lift vehicles, and reusable personal launch vehicles might be safer and more cost effective than a single-solution-type program.

Safety in Future Programs

The ability to predict the future is difficult for many reasons. Technological advances often come in unexpected spurts. Regulatory constraints or authorizations can also restrain or accelerate advances. Intervening variables and claims on resources from unexpected directions can dramatically impact programs such as space exploration that can often be seen as discretionary spending. There is clearly a need for a diversity of approach to R&D for longer-term human-rated space vehicles.

The lessons of history suggest that attempts to build very long-term programs in sectors with highly volatile technologies almost always tend to fail. Also history has shown that very often innovative and highly original new designs and technologies come from individuals or small teams as opposed to massive research programs. The examples run from the Wright Brothers and Von Braun to Burt Rutan and the SpaceOne vehicle. Certainly space research and development needs sophisticated teams of scientists and engineers and a large-scale aerospace industry, but it also needs to harness entrepreneurial genius. Improved safety practices and next-generation best ideas and best solutions might very well come from prizes and competitions to come up with outside of the box solutions. The Ansari X-Prize, the new Bigelow Prize, and other forms of competition that come from activities such as the NASA Institute for Advanced Concepts (NIAC) need to be among the tools to plan for a successful space future. To date, most prizes have been used to shoot for new rocket technology, but the same could be true for safety and risk reduction and alternative access to space technologies. The new John McLucas student research awards to promote space safety, sponsored by the Space Shuttle Children's Trust Fund and the Arthur C. Clarke Foundation, represent just one example. In this case, annual awards go the best student design efforts that come from the International Space University and the Universities Space Research Association (USRA) affiliated schools. In short, future space programs are most likely to become more efficient and safer if there is allowance for diversity of thought as well as active encouragement of innovation through entrepreneurial and competitive processes.

Entrepreneurial Approaches to Future Space Systems Development

One of the areas where surveys and interviews conducted by the George Washington University space safety study team showed remarkable consensus was in the view that private enterprise and entrepreneurial talent were key to future space program development. Virtually all those interviewed believed that private capital, private research, and private space programs were a necessary and desirable part of the future—especially when it involved new and entrepreneurial efforts. There was less consensus as to how such efforts might be regulated and controlled for purposes of safety, although many in the United States supported the FAA's initiatives as authorized by Congress to develop oversight regulations with regard to safety and private initiatives to access space. In future years, there will also likely be regulatory efforts within the United States and other countries toward meeting international requirements related to frequency assignments, control of debris, etc. Congress passed a new law that gave the FAA additional authority over private space initiatives in December 2004, and this was signed into law in January 2005. Most recently the FAA, in late December 2005, sent to Congress for comment an extensive report setting forth in detail how private flight into space by pilots, crew, and passengers will be regulated [10].

The success of the Space One flights has led to a new space tourism race among a number of entrepreneurial ventures. Most noted is Sir Richard Branson's initiative to proceed to commercial operations with Virgin Galactic. But Rocketplane Ltd. of the United Kingdom and the most recently announced Space Adventures project, with Middle Eastern investment backing and operating with Russian-built vehicles, have all indicated plans to start operations to take tourists some 60 miles or so into outer space around 2008 [11]. These new ventures, plus new FAA regulations concerning private spaceflight, have led to almost heady and very likely unrealistic expectations for private space initiatives. The safety concerns that these space tourism ventures give rise to are serious and numerous. Serious study of related safety, environmental, and regulatory issues must be conducted by competent entities as soon as possible.

Clearly the differences between spacecraft that operate at lower than hypersonic speeds (i.e., Mach 5 to 10) and those that operate at escape velocities (i.e., in the range of Mach 25 to 30) are significant. We still will need a NASA and other international space agencies for advanced R&D for many years to come, and private initiatives cannot replace state-of-the-art research capabilities.

The statement of Peter Diamandis, organizer of the X-Prize, likens the effort to create Space One by Burt Rutan and Paul Allen to be that of a new "furry mammal" as opposed to the "obsolete dinosaurs of the aerospace industry." Time will tell if we are indeed entering a new era of space exploration where private investment plays an ever more important role. Certainly we are in a time of transition, and the evolution will take time as well as effective public and private cooperation to succeed.

Nevertheless, private initiatives with private test pilots and private astronauts who are insured against risk (and their families provided for) add a new dimension of flexibility that government space agencies do not now have.

New entrepreneurial space programs know that failure means ruin for their program, whereas success means world acclaim. Private organizations such as Space X, Scaled Composites, SpaceDev, Bigelow Aerospace, Space Adventures, Rocketplane Ltd., etc. clearly have a different set of values and different types of incentive to succeed. The challenge for NASA is to find new and flexible ways to fuel these intellectual energies through diverse and competitive space research programs, to find better technology, better performance, and especially ways to create safer systems while also drawing on the talents and capabilities of traditional aerospace corporations [12].

Part of the challenge of the future will be not only to find new balance between private and public R&D in space but also to find the optimum human/machine interface so that astronaut crewed space programs will be focused on projects where humans are absolutely needed. NASA will need to find the areas where robotics, expert systems, artificial systems, and avionics can balance functions with those essential to human astronaut missions. This strategic division of functions will, of course, continue to change over time.

NASA and the Future of Space Safety

NASA is a great national U.S. resource, and the officials, scientists, engineers, and staff of this nearly 50-year-old institution have changed our view of space, the world, and our universe forever. There will be many who read this book and conclude that it does not fully recognize NASA's many positive contributions or sincere efforts to provide the highest level of safety support to its astronaut program [13].

We wish to state that despite our various findings that might imply criticism of NASA, or at least areas of concern with regard to NASA management, we indeed believe that NASA engineers, staff, and officials have in virtually all instances consistently made astronaut safety a high priority, made improvements in programs wherever possible, and reduced risks in a consistent manner. Although this book contains findings that seem "negative" or represent apparent critiques of NASA performance in this safety sector, this only represents a small percentage of NASA's overall space efforts. Some problems are inevitable when one is undertaking tremendously challenging tasks and developing totally new systems.

> Improvement can only come from honest assessment of problems and learning from the experiences of the shuttle, the ISS, and the various X-series development programs.

In short, it would not be possible to undertake a comprehensive review of any space agency and not identify comparable problems and issues. Improvement can only come from honest assessment of problems and learning from the experiences of the shuttle, the ISS, and the various X-series development programs. It is hoped that at least some of our observations and questions can be constructively and applied to the recently initiated crew exploratorn vehicle and crew launch vehicle for the moon and to other future space programs.

Finally, it should be recognized that there is a growing level of expertise around the world concerning the design of crewed vehicles and space safety processes and precautions. The new International Association for the Advancement of Space Safety (IAASS) has a growing body of knowledge and experience that can assist in the design of new vehicles and international space projects. To date, however, effective processes to use international expertise with regard to space safety within NASA have not yet been fully developed.*

This review of space safety has been undertaken in a serious vein. The intention has always been to discharge this undertaking in the form of an "honest broker" evaluating NASA's astronaut-related programs past, present, and future. Wherever possible, it is hoped that space safety problems can and will be redressed, safety standards and conditions improved, and space programs for astronauts improved in quality, concept, and safety. There is opportunity for improvement and safety enhancement everywhere: within NASA; within related U.S. governmental agencies, the White House, and Congress; within the aerospace industry; within related professional organizations, universities, and research institutes, within entrepreneurial organizations; and even within the aerospace trade press and the general news media that serve as a watchdog over the public interest. In short, improvements must come from far more than just NASA.

References

1 Schwartz, J., "Minority Report Faults NASA as Compromising Safety," *New York Times*, 18 Aug. 2005, p. A15.
2 "Mismanaging the Shuttle Fixes," *New York Times*, 19 Aug. 2005, p. A 20.
3 Gugliotta, G., "Foam Cracks May Delay Shuttle Launch," *Washington Post*, 2 Dec. 2005, p. A3.
4 Gigliotta, G., "NASA's Inspector General Probed," *Washington Post*, 3 Feb. 2006, p. A1, A8.
5 Leary, W. E., "Investigator at NASA Faces Inquiry over Safety," *New York Times*, 4 Feb. 2006, p. A9.
6 Heppenheimer, T. A., *The Space Shuttle Decision: NASA's Search for a Reusable Vehicle*, Vol. 1, NASA, Washington, DC, 1999, p. 245.
7 "Major ISS Components," *Aerospace Daily*, 12 Aug. 2004, p. 4, URL: http://www.aviationnow.com/avnow/news/cannel_aerospacedaily_story.jsp?id = news/par.
8 Berger, B., "NASA: Finishing Station With ELVs Would Cost More, Take Longer," *Space News*, Vol. 15, No. 32, 10 May 2004, p. 8.
9 "News: Space Station Partners Agree," *CoLab Aeronautics*, 27 July 2004, URL: http://216.239.51.104/search?Q=cache:VMVh42xsQtUJ:colab.rsnz.org/aero/+japan+space.
10 "Rules Proposed for Space Travelers," *Washington Post*, 30 Dec. 2005, p. A-5.
11 Schwartz, J., "More Enter Race to Offer Space Tours," *New York Times*, 18 Feb. 2006, p. B1–B7.
12 Tierney, J., "Go West, Young Astronaut," *New York Times*, 6 Dec. 2005, p. A31.
13 Berger, B., "NASA Credited with Making Progress Changing the Agency's Safety Culture," *Space News*, Vol. 15, No. 34, 24 April 2004, p. 3.

---

*Data available online at http://www.iaass.org.

Additional Reading

"Astronaut Mike Mullane Has Flown on the Shuttle Three Times and Would Go Again in a Heartbeat," *Reuters*, 19 Jan. 2006.

"Mismanaging the Shuttle Fixes," *New York Times*, 19 Aug. 2005, p. A20.

Mullane, M., Riding Rockets—The Outrageous Tales of a Space Shuttle Astronaut, Scribners, pp. 1–15, New York, 2006.

"NASA's Predicament," *New York Times*, 31 Dec. 2005, p. A30.

CHAPTER 10
A Better and Brighter
U.S. Space Program:
A New Vision for the Future

"The Earth is much too small and fragile basket for the human
race to keep all its eggs in."

—*Robert A. Heinlein*

On 29 December 2005 the FAA sent to Congress an extensive
123-page report outlining in great detail the rules and
regulations that it intends to put into effect with regard to
space tourism and other private space ventures involving
the launch of private vehicles with people onboard.

—*Rules proposed for space travelers,*
Washington Post, *30 December 2005*

NASA and the Past, Present, and Future of Space Exploration

This final chapter attempts to knit together the various topics addressed
throughout the book. Much of the first part of the book addresses the most
urgent issues of how NASA is going to restore the once again grounded
shuttle to flight, to build out the International Space Station, and to possibly
undertake the Hubble resupply mission. NASA has the difficult job of trying
to upgrade both the safety of the space shuttle and the International Space
Station to the best of its ability within a significant budgetary crunch. There
is also the added pressure of launching Project Constellation to explore the
moon, Mars, and beyond. NASA has chosen, consistent with the recommendations in the George Washington University safety study and a number of
others, to curtail the number of shuttle flights and reduce the scope of the ISS
build-out where and when practical [1]. NASA, at congressional urging, has
also advanced the date that replacement vehicles for the shuttle (i.e., the
CEV and private launch services to the ISS) are available to 2012, initiated
procurement action to acquire additional Soyuz vehicles to support the
ISS operations and provide escape capabilities, and issued an RFP to seek
private launch services to support ferrying astronauts to and from the ISS.
Beyond these NASA initiatives, however, some additional steps can be taken
to increase safety and mission success as outlined next.

The discussion of shuttle and ISS-related safety issues is followed by
an overview of future space launch technologies and systems that might

allow NASA in coming years to achieve its objectives with greater agility, flexibility, and safety. There are many exciting technologies, systems, and opportunities that deserve support. New options might allow NASA to accomplish more with less and in new and innovative ways that go beyond what and how NASA has done things in the past. In short NASA can achieve such new objectives by reinventing itself in terms of improved safety practices and culture, more efficient operations and structure, fuller involvement of the entrepreneurial community, and, in essence, by pursuing a new pathway to the future. At some point in time, the idea that the best way to send people into space is, in effect, to light an explosive chemical bomb under them will be seen as quite quaint.

Thus, the last part of this chapter returns to some very basic questions about what are NASA's objectives now and what they should be going forward. This final review addresses more than NASA and its pursuit of launch systems, space exploration, and space safety. This review asks what should be the core values of NASA's programs, its mission, and its very reason for existence? What might the U.S. space program and NASA hope to accomplish in the next 30 to 50 years? This concluding chapter even suggests that NASA cannot achieve true success and a fruitful and safe exploration program without a new vision. Thus this book ends with a five-point program that NASA might use to 'reenvision' its purpose and programs. This program is designed to go well beyond the last 30 years and "more of the same"; it outlines a course of action to engender new levels of public support. Indeed NASA, at the most fundamental level, needs to redefine its basic mission as being to sustain human existence both on this planet and beyond.

> This concluding chapter even suggests that NASA cannot achieve true success and a fruitful and safe exploration program without a new vision.

NASA and the Remaining Years of the Shuttle Program

There is broad agreement, both within and without NASA, that the shuttle program will at some point have to be phased out of operation and that this is likely within the next four to five years. It is the finding of this review and the George Washington University study that preceded this book that the permanent grounding of the shuttle should be done just as soon as possible. This is because the technology of this launch system is now aging and too complex, and there are basic design flaws such as the inability to provide launch-to-land escape capabilities. It is clear that new systems can be both safer and more cost efficient. Despite the extensive efforts to improve the safety of the shuttle in the current return-to-flight program, the basic design and enormous complexity of the millions of parts and tens of thousands of subsystems of the shuttle quite simply prevent any significant improvement in safety. The facts that the foam-shedding problem have proved so very difficult to solve and the ceramic tiles in the TPS are so difficult to protect are two strong indications as to why the shuttle ground-ing needs to be happen just as quickly as possible. The most recent discov-ery of cracks in the PAL ramp designed to keep foam debris from hitting the thermal protection system of the orbiter is yet another strong indication of why a new design and new launch system are both needed to provide a significantly safer ride to space.

The option of converting one or more of the shuttle orbiters to robotic control, or even building a new shuttle that is just for robotic operation, represents alternatives worthy of evaluation in terms of enhanced safety and providing a way forward to finish the ISS while reducing risk to astronauts. It has now been accepted by NASA, apparently, that curtailing certain elements of the ISS to reduce the number of remaining shuttle flights from 28 to 18 is a viable way to both reduce costs and improve safety. It is rewarding that NASA now seems embarked on this course that the George Washington University team examined in 2004 and formally set forth in February 2005.

In looking to the future, NASA must ensure the development of new and improved launch systems. Safety improvements now found in the design for Project Constellation include the use of the latest thermal pro-tection materials, having launch-to-land full-envelope escape capabilities, separation of crew from cargo until low Earth orbit is reached, improved propulsion systems (in terms of separating liquid-fuel systems from solid rocket booster), and atmospheric reentry in a capsule.

The current integral relationship between the continued operation of the space shuttle program and the International Space Station is tremen-dously strong. The prime reason to continue the shuttle program and undertake all but one of its launches is indeed to complete or service the ISS or provide an escape capability from it. If the space station could be completed with expendable launchers (Atlas V, Delta, Progress/Soyuz, ATV/Ariane 5, or ATV/H2A) or robotically controlled shuttle vehicles, or if the ISS were somehow rescaled in size and construction components reconstituted, the shuttle program could be phased out sooner. NASA has already agreed to a revised program for the next five years, which involves a reduced number of manned shuttle launches. This will also reduce costs and risks to astronauts. At the same time, the United States is bound by treaty obligations to its international partners—particularly Japan, Europe, Canada, and Russia—to honor agreements that have been made for many years, and thus these options are limited. The deployment of the Columbus space lab and the Japanese engineering module (JEM) and the completion of the Canadarm2 need to be given the highest prior-ity. Another important new option now underway is to contract out to a selected contractor the provision of astronaut transport and cargo supply to the ISS. This new NASA program is intended to fill the gap between the grounding of the shuttle and availability of the CEV, which will be around year end 2012 at the earliest.

Based on responses to the NASA RFP, a wide range of suppliers beyond the well-known Lockheed Martin and Boeing corporations is eager to provide these services. These "new kids on the block" include

Space X, SpaceDev, Inc., Constellation Services International, Inc., AirLaunch LLC, SPACEHAB, Inc., Andrews Space, Inc., Rocketplane Ltd., Universal Space Lines, and Bigelow Aerospace. NASA has allocated up to $500 million through 2010 to ensure these commercial services will be available [2].

Finally one tradeoff might be to turn the management and operation of the ISS over to international partners in exchange for restructuring the ISS design and mission goals. As part of this restructured international agreement concerning the ISS, a mechanism for the integrated control of ISS safety operations and escape procedures (rather than simply relying on the national franchises) is also considered to be another critical goal to enhance overall safety.

Fortunately most of these findings and recommendations are largely aligned with the strategic path that NASA now seems to be following.

NASA and Project Constellation

NASA has undertaken the ambitious Project Constellation initiative in response to the presidential mandate, now over two years old, to return to the moon and beyond. This effort was fueled by a number of study contracts undertaken in 2004. These studies developed the major design elements for the human-rated crew exploration vehicle (CEV) and a launcher system that can take cargo into space as well as lift the CEV into orbit. Under the urging of NASA's administrator in response to congressional requests, this program schedule has been accelerated, and instead of a "fly-off" between the two major competing aerospace teams the choice will now be made on prototype designs.

There are clear and specific guidelines related to performance, safety, and sustainability for Project Constellation, and the design requirements and performance concepts indicate that the launch systems and the CEV will provide for significant safety enhancements over the space shuttle systems.

Nevertheless, there remain questions about plans for the CEV and the new launch systems. These questions include the overall timetable for this development that is based on a more or less steady-state budget for NASA. This idea that one can stretch budgets to cover the continued flight of the shuttle, the completion of the ISS, the pursuit of a host of space science and astrophysics studies, the continued operation of the Hubble Space Telescope, and a variety of research institutes, remote sensing and monitoring projects, space applications, aeronautical research and educational programs, plus put together a new program to go the moon, has a very uncomfortable sense of *deja vu* about it. Ask NASA to do everything, and it ultimately becomes a recipe for failure.

It was indeed NASA's attempt, under congressional demands, to juggle the space shuttle, the ISS, the development of new space-plane technology, and a host of other programs that led the Gehman commission to conclude that the *Columbia* accident was a "failure of national leadership." In short, we do not seem to have learned from the *Columbia* accident the basic lesson that it is better to make hard choices and do some things well rather than to do all of them "stretched to the limits." Indeed the most recent indications are that NASA is at least $3 billion shy of the needed appropriations to fund the 18 shuttle missions that are currently projected as being necessary to complete the ISS [3]. This can reasonably be seen as not only NASA's problem of today but also of tomorrow. To put budgets and schedule on a collision course with astronaut safety is truly a failure of leadership.

> In short, we do not seem to have learned from the *Columbia* accident the basic lesson that it is better to make hard choices and do some things well rather than to do all of them "stretched to the limits."

There are likewise concerns about the newly adopted accelerated timetable for an early choice between the designs for the CEV and the launch systems as currently being developed by the two major design teams. There are also concerns about many of the development contracts in areas like avionics, information systems, and guidance systems going to extremely large teams of contractors to develop integrated systems, with NASA management trying to oversee how all of these complex systems integrate together (as discussed in Chapter 5). And there are further concerns about the viability of plans for the so-called spiral development of this program over a sustained period of time? One must question the extent to which the current plans for Project Constellation can be sustained through many different presidential administrations over the next 12 to 20 years to achieve both longer-term space exploration goals and the maximum degree of safety for future astronauts?

Previous attempts to design new launch capabilities to demanding objectives over the past decade have turned out to be more elusive than first anticipated. Projects such as the X-33, X-34, X-37, and X-43 were started full of hope, pursued with interest and vigor, but then, one after another, cancelled either because of the budgetary and resource claims of the space shuttle and the ISS or because of technical or management problems with these various projects. All of these designs looked good on paper and promised greater safety and cost efficiency, but once in actual production of hardware these programs were all cancelled. The NASA track record of making choices based on paper designs over the last 15 years is not encouraging.

There is a saying attributed to Yogi Berra, the New York Yankee, that goes, "If you come to a fork in the road take it." In the case of NASA and the U.S. Congress, this idea of trying to pursue many forks in the road at once with a very modest increase in the budget seems dangerous. This seems particularly true at a time when the U.S. overall national budget is experiencing record levels of red ink and an overseas war on at least two fronts is being pursued. Further, U.S. international trade deficits are at all time record highs, and "baby boomers" are set to begin retiring in droves, which will quickly put huge strains on government social service programs. The likelihood of sustaining needed funding for all of these programs seems low. Some choices clearly need to be made.

These new launch systems for Project Constellation are all conventionally propelled by explosive chemicals and bear a striking resemblance to an enhanced version of Apollo. The essential design involves a return to the use of expendable vehicles, just when Russia is going forward with a new reusable design. Indeed some critics of Project Constellation suggest that reusable vehicles to low Earth orbit and then on to the moon could carry less risk and would be far more cost effective. In particular one critic has suggested that a refurbished shuttle with ARMOR metallic head shields and an escape capability could provide more reliable access to low Earth orbit and that another vehicle (perhaps based on ion engines) could get crew to the moon. This critic suggests that an expendable system might cost $0.6 billion per launch while improved reusable systems could be more reliable and cost effective [4].

One must have confidence that these new launch systems for Project Constellation will be achieved on time and within budget, but past experience suggests otherwise. Although these new space systems will likely be safer than the space shuttle, there are no major technology strides forward that are being taken with Project Constellation—particularly noting that these systems will fly some three decades after the debut of the shuttle and some 40 years after the Saturn vehicle and the Apollo program. Just imagine a computer company saying we are bringing out a new project and it is very much "like UNIVAC on steroids."

There are thus a number of questions that seem reasonable to ask of NASA to ensure that its astronaut program remains as safe as possible and to restore public faith in its abilities.

Key Actions to Be Taken by NASA to Enhance Safety Now

The following questions seem reasonable to ask of NASA to ensure enhanced astronaut safety going forward.

1) *NASA should be asked by Congress and the OMB for a full accounting of all safety issues concerning the space shuttle.* This report should be as up to date as possible and rendered before another shuttle launch. It should address all pending or deferred efforts to make the shuttle safer since the *Columbia* accident and the reflight of *Discovery* in July/August 2005. This report would include the results of an independent assessment with regard to those concerns explicitly highlighted in this book as set forth in the figures at the end of Chapters 3 and 4 and in Appendix C to this book.

2) *NASA should be asked by Congress and the OMB to report on possible further curtailment of manned launches of the shuttle.* This should particularly reexamine current plans for the further build-out of the ISS. This report might explore how the ISS program could be completed either by use of expendable rockets, by converting some of the shuttle launches to robotic operation, or by further redesign of the ISS. The reasons as to why several missions of the shuttle could or could not be flown robotically should be explicitly addressed. Finally, one launch to refurbish the Hubble

Telescope, however, would appear to represent a reasonable risk and via a single mission would provide significant scientific returns.

3) *NASA should be asked to report on how its current approach to the launch and return of ISS crew could be strengthened.* This report would particularly address additional capabilities beyond the shuttle. Congress has indeed now authorized procurement of additional Soyuz vehicles. Such capability should be acquired to support emergency escape from the ISS by reviewing whether two Soyuz systems could be docked to the ISS at the same time and investigating whether new Soyuz's could be configured to accommodate up to three or more astronauts. Also in terms of supply capabilities to the ISS, there should be a report on the planned use of the European ATV capability or planned Japanese HTV capabilities.

4) *NASA should be asked to provide an explicit report with regard to how it has addressed the problem of granting shuttle and ISS-related waivers.* NASA should be asked about the extent to which it has instituted management training and safety-oriented values aimed at solving problems (including software issues) rather than working around them. As detailed in Chapters 3, 4, and 9, the *Columbia* orbiter records, and the CAIB report, there were some 5800 waivers granted by NASA officials prior to the *Columbia* launch. Many of these waivers were minor, but many hundreds should have been considered crucial.

5) *NASA should be asked to provide for an independent assessment of the safety of the ISS.* This assessment would include a review of remedial actions that might be needed after examining the issues noted in Chapter 5 of this book as well as in Appendix D.

6) *NASA should be asked to strengthen its safety program capabilities.* These actions should strengthen the organizational coherence of the NESC, simplify NASA extremely complex safety organization, and clearly assign safety as a prime and authoritative function to the shuttle independent technical authority. Also the U.S. government should refine and clarify the review process and oversight of NASA safety processes by the Government Accountability Office (GAO) and the Aerospace Safety Advisory Panel (ASAP). This is particularly so with regard to monitoring NASA's astronaut space operations and safety management programs. This might be done in conjunction with an independent assessment of how NASA manages its safety (and reliability assessment) programs in comparison to other organizations (both federal agencies and private enterprise).

7) *Additional steps would appear necessary within NASA and within its congressional oversight mechanisms to ensure a stronger emphasis on safety.* Action should be taken to ensure that the new independent technical engineering authority and the NESC have a clearly proactive research and risk-reduction role that goes beyond quality assurance and greater organizational and management say so. In short, safety is something that is designed in from the start and achieved through correcting problems rather than granting waivers when difficulties arise. Safety is much more than IV&V—it is a state of mind.

8) *Serious consideration should be given to restructuring NASA centers to achieve specific goals and transfer certain tasks to the private sector.* The major

Serious consideration should be given to restructuring NASA Centers to achieve specific goals and transfer certain tasks to the private sector.

NASA centers and installations house a vast array of talented engineers and scientists. Their activities have expanded since 1958 into a maze of projects and diverse undertakings. The likelihood of NASA being able to accomplish space programs that are safer as well as being considered more relevant by the general public would seem to be closely tied to focusing the work of its centers on clearly identified goals. Some NASA centers could be transferred to the status of federally funded research centers (as is now the case with JPL and as recommended by the Aldridge commission). Certain tasks could be transferred to industry or universities (just as the University of California has won a contract to oversee the Sandia Labs in New Mexico). The objective would be to focus NASA on its top goals, so that NASA does more steering and less oaring in directing the national space program [5].

9) *NASA needs to implement fully an improved scheduling and budgeting process as set forth in recommendation 13 of the CAIB report.* The CAIB stated the need to create a realistic up-to-date flight schedule and asked that NASA "evaluate deadlines regularly to ensure that risks taken to meet the schedule are recognized, understood and acceptable." At this time NASA is developing a "computerized manifesting capability" in order "to more effectively manage the schedule margin, launch constraints, and manifest flexibility" so as provide "routine risk assessment." This would allow NASA management to understand the status of programs quickly and accurately. It would allow NASA leadership to understand the ramifications of changes and be able to make schedule revisions and see risk-indicator data in real time. This process needs to be strengthened and even more importantly protected against political and management pressure overrides.

10) *NASA should be asked to prepare a report on how it defines safety objectives and risk-reduction measures.* This report should cover lessons learned from the Mercury, Gemini, Apollo, shuttle, and ISS programs through the various development programs it has started and cancelled, including the HL-20, the X-38, the X-33, X-34, X-37, and X-43.

11) *NASA should be asked to assess, rate, and prioritize the value of all of the various future launch systems.* This should cover the access to orbit options listed later in this concluding chapter (as well as other realistic or promising options not covered). This evaluation and rating of future systems should be provided in terms of assessing longer-term launch options based on their projected cost efficiency, pollution factor, safety and overall viability, and also based on their possible deployment in 2015, 2025, or later.

Future Programs for Space Exploration and Enhanced Astronaut Safety

The ability to predict the future is difficult for many reasons. Technological advances often come in unexpected spurts. Regulatory shifts or authorizations can also restrain or accelerate advances. Intervening variables and

---

Ten Year Time Horizon: Improved Propulsion Systems

❑ **Improved Chemical Propulsion**
   - Scramjet technology and X-Series follow-ons (Dreamchaser, Space Dev et al)
   - More cost effective conventional launch systems (i.e. Space X)
   - Throttle-able solid rockets or Hybrid systems
   - Other chemical propulsion systems (plus the launch of "robotic fuel generators" advanced but small scale advanced robotic systems on Moon/Mars)
❑ **Electric Propulsion Systems**
   - Conventional Ion engines to LEO or from LEO to the Moon.
   - Advanced Ion propulsion systems with much greater efficiency & safety than chemical systems
❑ **Gravity Gradient "Slingshot" Acceleration**
❑ **Nuclear Propulsion Systems**
   - Various forms of NEP-NTP nuclear ionization, plasma and heated propellants

---

Figure 10-1 New term advancements in space propulsion.

claims on resources from unexpected directions can dramatically impact programs such as space exploration that can often be seen as discretionary spending.

Figure 10.1 recaps some of the promising new and alternative ways forward in space launcher systems that could evolve to maturity in the next decade or so. Further, Fig. 10.2 summarizes longer-term systems that

---

Longer Range Systems for Access to Space

B. Medium Term Systems (10 to 20 years)

- **Nuclear Propulsion** - Advanced nuclear ionization and heated plasma propellants
- **Tether Based Launch Systems** – Use of tethers to lift vehicles to higher orbits

C. Longer Term Future (15 to 50 Years in the Future)

Mass Drivers and Rail Guns

- **Mass driver systems on moon** -Potentially very safe on the Moon
- **Rail or "Coil" Gun Systems** - For robotic systems or inert "non-manned" systems. Again might be used on the Moon

Space Elevator

Space Elevator: - Based on new nano-tube carbon/fullerene technology) plus robotic climbers. (Materials must be 70 to 200 tensile strength of steel)

Solar Sails

Solar Sail Power Craft - Based on mylar materials and micro-porous materials

---

Figure 10-2 Longer term methods for more cost effective and safer access to space.

might represent breakthrough capabilities in terms of efficiency and safety. All of these approaches must be actively pursued in the context of not only increased economic or propulsion efficiency but also in terms of increased safety.

It is because of the speed of technological obsolescence, based on historical precedence from all high-technology industries, that caution must be raised concerning NASA's stated intention to define the future in terms of a single program, such as a spiral development of the CEV program with a 20-year timeline. Such a single-minded approach, as opposed to a multisystem and more modular approach based on a combination of launch systems and technologies, could well retard innovations, especially with regard to launch systems safety. The development of the space tourism business might ultimately help derive a better and more cost-effective program for deep-space exploration that might also be safer and with less risk.

The modular design conceived by Boeing for a CEV design that could in theory be used in a spiral development to mount a mission to Mars some 20 years hence seems technologically sound today (see Fig. 10.3). But this design, it must be recalled, is very reminiscent of the designs for the spaceship going to Jupiter developed for *2001: The Space Odyssey*, a Hollywood picture that was made in 1968.

We have already seen from both the space shuttle and the International Space Station that space systems designed to last 20 years into the future end up being obsolete not only from a technical and systems viewpoint, but sometimes in terms of the need or utility of such facilities. One only has to look at EPCOT as it is today or the 1939 New York World's Fair and its World of Tomorrow exhibits to see how fast technologies overtake futuristic forecasts.

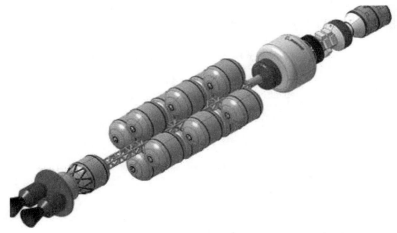

Figure 10-3   Boeing modular spiral development CEV design for future Mars mission (photo courtesy of Boeing from NASA Web site).

Innovative Space Safety Research

It is especially desirable for new programs to be started by NASA and other space-related entities and university programs in the United States and abroad to stimulate competitive research programs in launch system and space system safety. To this end the International Association for the Advancement of Space Safety (IAASS), at its first conference held in Nice, France, in October 2005, devoted a part of its program to organizing closer coordination of organizations interested in space safety around the world and to stimulating new and innovative research in this field. Discussions within the academic committee of the IAASS conference are now considering such issues as those set forth in Fig. 10.4.

It is hoped that these points will also be discussed within the International Astronautical Federation (IAF), the International Academy of Astronautics (IAA), and by others such as the International Space University and other universities around the world.

Those involved with the new international space safety research initiative should consider that today's problems and assessments of space risks can and will change over time. There is good reason to believe that one or more of the concepts for advanced propulsion systems, as noted earlier, will be successful in coming years and that these systems will not only be more reliable and cost effective, but also offer astronauts a much greater margin of safety. In short, the longer-term safety issues will find that "exploding chemical rocket motors" as a safety concern might some day become as antiquated as broken axles on a covered wagon. The future of space exploration and safety is thus foreseen as focusing on issues such as those presented in Fig. 10.5.

A final observation on safety in the aerospace industry is that although NASA and related industries have undertaken a great deal of research and placed great stress on astronaut safety, overall safety standards and performance in the aviation, air transport, and aerospace

---

Designing in Safety: International Programs and Safety Research:

❑ Consider needs for greater agreement between US, Russian, Japan, Canada and Europe as to safety guidelines, procedures and "acceptable risk limits" with respect to current and future space programs. (e.g. with regard to EVAs, collision avoidance, redundancy, crew escape and staffing requirements, remote health & medical standards, radiation guidelines, etc.)

❑ Develop international approach to exploration and colonization of Moon and Mars and remote off–world transport systems with uniform or at least coordinated safety standards.

❑ Develop plan for longer-range launch systems and develop relevant associated future safety standards. Funding for such efforts should be provided by NIAC and international affiliates of the IAASS. (In essence "safety" must be "planned" into future space vehicles and systems).

Figure 10-4   A longer term agenda for space safety research.

MAJOR FUTURE ASTRONAUT CONCERNS BEYOND PROPULSION

❑   Radiation, Solar Flares and Cosmic Energy
❑   Medical and health problems occasioned by living in a low gravitational environment
❑   Debris, Micrometeorites, Comet Systems
❑   Sustainable colonies (and related concerns about food and water production, medical
    care, microbes and pandemics, genetic damage and mutation, etc.)
❑   Psychological aspects of living and working in outer space and sense of isolation

<u>Key Finding</u>: Longer-term risk elements will not be with launch vehicle propulsion systems
as we move beyond Chemical fuels to more reliable and safer system to access outer space.

Figure 10-5   Longer term space safety concerns.

industry do not necessarily compare well with what many consider high-risk professions such as mining as shown in Fig. 10.6.

Thus future efforts that address safety standards should also address ways in which scientists, engineers, technicians, and test operators can also be exposed to lesser risk and improvements in safe working conditions.

Entrepreneurial Approaches to Future Space Systems Development

One of the areas where surveys and interviews undertaken in the George Washington University studies on space exploration and safety showed remarkable consensus was in the view that private enterprise and entrepreneurial talent was key to future space program development. Virtually all of those interviewed believed that private capital, private research, and

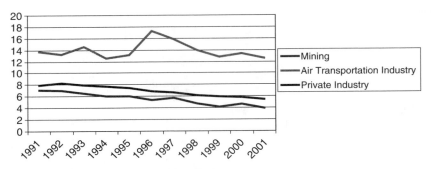

BLS Reportable Injuries/100 Workers

Figure 10-6   Bureau of Labor statistics reports on industry injuries in the United States.

private space programs were a necessary and desirable part of the future. There was less agreement, however, about how such efforts might be regulated and controlled for purposes of safety. Congress did pass a new law that gives the FAA additional authority over private space initiatives as of December 2004, and congressional hearings on this subject were carried out in February 2005.

On 29 December 2005 the FAA sent to Congress an extensive report outlining in great detail the rules and regulations that it intends to put into effect with regard to space tourism and other private space ventures involving the launch of private vehicles with people onboard [6]. The FAA regulations, now out for public comment as published in the Federal Registry, are expected to be finalized by the end of June 2006. Despite the length of the proposed rules, the requirements are not particularly onerous. The operator of a space tourism business would only be required to 1) have a pilot with an FAA pilot certificate, and each crew member would need a medical certificate issued within a year of the flight; 2) train the crew and pilot to ensure that the vehicle would not do harm to the public even if abandoned; and 3) inform all participants of the associated risks and have them sign a consent form. Physical examinations for passengers would be recommended but not required unless a "clear public safety need is identified" [7].

In the wake of the success of the SpaceOne flights, there is today almost heady and very likely unrealistic enthusiasm for private space initiatives. Clearly the differences between spacecraft that operate at lower than hypersonic speeds (i.e., Mach 5 to 10) and those that operate at escape velocities (i.e., in the range of Mach 30) are significant. The statement of Peter Diamandis, organizer of the Ansari X-Prize, likens the effort to create SpaceOne by Burt Rutan and Paul Allen to being that of a new "furry mammal" as opposed to the "obsolete dinosaurs of the aerospace industry." Time will tell if we are indeed entering a new era of space exploration where private investment plays an even greater role than before. Certainly we are in a time of transition, and the evolution will take time as well as effective public and private cooperation to succeed. One of the key issues is whether the U.S. government and NASA ultimately abandon all space efforts in low Earth orbit and below to private enterprise and concentrate all of their activities to space exploration and science to areas related to the moon, Mars, and beyond.

Certainly, this much is true. Private initiatives with private test pilots and private astronauts who are insured against risk (and their families provided for) add a new dimension of flexibility and risk management that government space agencies do not now have.

New entrepreneurial space operators know that failure means ruin for their programs whereas success means world acclaim. Private organizations such as Space X, Scaled Composites, SpaceDev, Bigelow Aerospace, etc. clearly have a different set of values and different types of incentive to succeed. The challenge for NASA, in its role of space explorer and developer of new launch systems, is to find new and flexible ways to fuel new intellectual energies, find better technology, and create safer space systems and yet do this through conventional governmental processes.

Drawing on the talents and capabilities of traditional aerospace corporations might not be sufficient to succeed in this quest. NASA might indeed find that it must be able to capture the entrepreneurial talents of inspired innovators to achieve its goals.

> NASA might indeed find that it must be able to capture the entrepreneurial talents of inspired innovators to achieve its goals.

There are other unique challenges that NASA faces. It will likely also be critical to find not only a new balance between private and public R&D in space but also to find the optimum human/machine interface. Robotically controlled launch and exploration systems might represent the best way forward in many cases. It is not sufficient for NASA to embark on missions that put humans at risk when in fact they are absolutely not needed—and also add billions of dollars to program costs.

In short, NASA will need to find the areas where robotics, expert systems, artificially intelligent systems, and avionics can balance astronaut capability or even assume responsibilities of certain space exploration, mining, or colony-building functions. This balance will, of course, continue to shift over time. Such a shift can save costs, extend exploration efficiencies, and enhance astronaut safety.

NASA is a great national U.S. resource, and the officials, scientists, engineers, and staff of this nearly 50-year-old institution have changed our view of space, the world, and our universe forever. There will be many who will read this book and conclude that it does not fully recognize NASA's many positive contributions or sincere efforts to provide the highest level of safety support to its astronaut program and its ardent commitment to explore space and discover the hidden mysteries of outer space. Despite our various findings that might imply criticism or at least areas of concern with regard to NASA, it important to note we have sought to identify problems rather than extol strengths. In short, we believe that NASA has consistently made astronaut safety a high priority and striven to improve programs and reduce risks wherever possible. Some problems are inevitable when one is undertaking tremendously challenging tasks and developing totally new systems. Indeed, it would not be possible to undertake a comprehensive review of any space agency and not identify comparable problems and issues. Improvement can only come from honest assessment of problems and learning from experience from the shuttle, the ISS, and the various X-series development programs. We hope that at least some of our observations and questions can be constructively applied to the recently initiated Project Constellation, the crew exploration vehicle, and the new launch systems for the moon, Mars, and beyond exploration program.

Even if only some of our findings prove to be useful and can be practically implemented and thus save the lives of astronauts in future space programs, then this book will have served its intended purpose. We see the opportunity for improvement and safety enhancements within NASA, as well as the need for changes within related U.S. governmental agencies, the White House, and Congress. Improvements can also be made to improve safety practices within the aerospace industry as well as by updating the best practices approaches supported by related professional organizations, universities and research institutes, and even within the aerospace trade press that serves as a watchdog over the public interest. Finally, a great deal can be learned from all of NASA's manned space programs up to this date that should be applied to Project Constellation in creative and innovative ways. The preceding findings and recommendations thus seek to identify the best opportunities for improved space exploration programs going forward.

Future Direction of NASA Space Exploration and Research Programs

Sir Arthur Clarke once said, "Predictions are difficult, especially about the future." This is another way of saying that critiques of the past are much easier than setting forth wise new directions for the future. Yet in the case of the U.S. space program and NASA, the past tells us a great deal. A review of NASA and U.S. aerospace history, especially over the past three decades, reveals a number of successes as well as documents a number of mistakes and even some failures.

On the positive side NASA could certainly be commended for 1) continuing an active and scientifically rigorous planetary, solar, and deep-space astrophysics research program; 2) active promotion of science, technology, engineering, and math (STEM) educational programs in the United States (although these programs now seem to be in danger of being cut back); 3) sustaining the Chandra, the Hubble Space Telescope, and other new space telescope programs; 4) undertaking a number of successful international cooperative space research projects; 5) pursuing a wide range of remote-sensing programs that have studied the Earth's oceans, atmosphere, and land masses and told us a great deal about the biosphere in which we live; and 6) pursuing a number of innovative programs to study pathways to the future such as the NASA Institute for Advanced Concepts (NIAC), new challenge prizes to seek new space solutions, and the new nuclear propulsion research initiative in Idaho.

Under the category of mistakes one might include the following: 1) overpromoting and overestimating the safety, utility, and cost efficiency of the space shuttle and then continuing its operations past a point of diminishing returns without developing a suitable replacement (as recommended by the Roger's commission in 1986); 2) creating a complex internationally interwoven design for the International Space Station that was too elaborate, too expensive, and totally shuttle dependent before first trying out more modest scientific missions and commercial applications in low Earth orbit using much smaller and flexible free-flying facilities; 3) putting the future of NASA, for the last 30 years, into a basket largely marked "astronaut program totally dependent on LEO-constrained chemical-based launchers that essentially can only go back and forth to the ISS"; 4) pursuing numerous failed X-series vehicles that all ended prematurely without success; 5) not developing a cost-efficient and reliable heavy-lift capability that could go to either LEO or into deep space; 6) failing to research the cost-effective deployment of new efficient space power technology and systems (to make affordable space solar-power systems feasible); 7) not focusing more heavily on more creative use of robotics as an alternative to manned space exploration; and 8) failing to explore more creative partnerships with private enterprise, innovative entrepreneurs, and creative genius to approach the whole space enterprise in new and perhaps more rewarding, cost-effective, and safer ways.

These past accomplishments and various concerns tell us much. The highs of Project Apollo and the lows of the two shuttle failures can both serve to suggest new pathways forward. How? A review of NASA's last three decades can help us define a new vision for space exploration and space safety. This can only start with a clear vision of where the United States and the planners of space exploration around the world are seeking to go in the decades and even centuries ahead.

One cannot have a clear vision about astronaut safety without first asking the right questions about the goals of Project Constellation and NASA's space exploration plans for the future. Dan Goldin, NASA's longest-serving NASA administrator, spent over a decade at NASA trying to reorganize its centers, attempting to eliminate "mom and pop" operations, and seeking to use corporate models to create a NASA that could develop space programs that were "better, faster, and cheaper." Instead, Administrator Goldin and other NASA leaders should have been asking: "What is it that NASA should be doing and seeking to achieve in the decades ahead? What can we be doing more creatively, differently, and with a longer-term vision of what space research and exploration really mean?" Because NASA space programs are in a very real sense big business with employment targets, expenditure levels to maintain, and large multiyear contracts to carry out, fundamental questions about purpose, change, and vision are extremely difficult to explore—especially with congressional funding and politics playing a big role in where the money goes. NASA's vision statement and strategic plans are slick, glossy, and very attractive, but they end up looking like a laundry list of multiyear programs to be funded.

The world's educational systems, just like NASA, place great stress on students knowing the right answers rather than encouraging a "curiosity process" that can lead to whole new lines of thought and inquiry [8].

If one were to try to simplify what NASA's vision might be in the form of a few questions, the result might be along the following lines:

1) How can we use space systems and technology to make the Earth's biosphere more sustainable so that *homo sapiens* and other species of fauna and flora can survive for the longer term?

2) How can we use space—and most likely space solar-power systems—to provide the Earth with reliable, long-term, cost-efficient, and environmentally safe sources of energy when petrochemical, coal, and other supplies of energy are exhausted?

3) How can we best plan—in terms of safety, cost efficiency, and innovative science and technology—to use the resources of the solar system to sustain Earth and its inhabitants for eons into the future as well as increase our knowledge of the universe?

4) Can we deploy space systems to prevent the destruction of human civilization from the impact of asteroids, meteorites, comets, or other near-Earth objects (given the possibility of a major impact (by Asteroid 2004MN4) coming in the 2029–2036 time period).

The interesting thing about such questions is that if one takes a longer-term view of things it suggests that the U.S. goals for the future and those of all of the inhabitants of Planet Earth (i.e., all flora and fauna) are closely intertwined. Second, it suggests that goals like sending astronauts to the moon in 12 years or so and to Mars at some future date with a conventional set of chemical rockets seem like "one-off" events rather than a true vision for the future. A longer-term goal of, say, colonizing the moon or Mars or creating a permanent space elevator complex to offer long-term and low-cost transportation to outer space would, for instance, suggest that we probably should be reevaluating our objectives. Is it possible to devise low-cost and reasonably reliable launchers to send highly capable robotic missions to the lunar surface over the next decade to prepare a safe habitat for astronauts? This habitat would perhaps, over time, become equipped with radiation shielding, water and oxygen generators, and material processors that could sustain astronauts for the longer term.

A longer-term vision for NASA might consider restructuring its space exploration plans along the lines of a five-point program as outlined in the following section. This would lead to a new NASA that would undertake a U.S. space program which would be more focused on immediate planetary needs (i.e., saving the planet's biosphere, providing access to clean, cheap energy and enhancing the provision of low-cost educational and health-care services to a world community that seemingly sees the United States as the enemy rather than as a caring friend); developing a more cost-effective and longer-term strategy for going to the moon and Mars (using a more complex mix of astronauts and robots) to stay there for the long haul rather than for a short-term stay with limited payoffs; and creating a NASA that is more goal driven, more agile, more entrepreneurial, more cost effective, and more innovative at finding ways to achieve big payoffs with millions of dollars rather than billions of dollars.

Five-Point Program for Reenvisioning NASA, Space Exploration, and Astronaut Missions

These five pathways to the future would include the following:

1) Reenvision NASA's programs and its international cooperative space programs to ensure a better balance between and among space science, space applications, and space exploration. Not too surprisingly, the

average Joe (or Josephine) taxpayer would like to think that NASA expenditures go in some good part to developing new space applications related to saving the Earth from life-threatening near-Earth objects, or supplying low-cost, clean, and nonpolluting energy to the planet or otherwise making the everyday lives of humans better or safer. The man or woman in the street would be more interested in NASA if it could be demonstrated that space programs could at least in part assist in generating new jobs, helping tame hurricanes, reducing pollution, supplying clean energy, making global educational and health programs lower in cost (and thus help to blunt efforts to recruit new terrorists from the ranks of the young), or perhaps even saving the Earth from destruction from asteroids and comets. This new NASA would thus help to identify and make better use of scarce resources and use space science and technology to make life here on Earth safer, more rewarding, and more sustainable. [This would include programs to address global warming and to carry out research with regard to detecting and diverting near-Earth objects (NEOs) from cataclysmic collisions with our planet [9,10].] If the public perceived that there is a "new NASA that is working for you," there might be more support over the longer term for exploration of outer space, scientific research, and space colonization.

2) Restructure NASA. As described earlier, the first step might well be to make all of the NASA centers into federally financed research and development centers (FFRDCs). This would allow these research centers to better assist in the overall national research programs (not just NASA). Further, these restructured centers would have clearly defined "center of excellence" goals and objectives. Thus there might be one center that works with industry and academia to develop new and creative launch systems (chemical, electrical/ionic, nuclear, space elevators/tether systems, solar sails, gravity gradients, etc.). There might be another center to focus on missions to planet Earth (atmospheric monitoring and pollution reduction, ocean and land-mass research, innovative space applications such as for solar energy, space robotics, and pollution control, etc.). Then there might be yet another to undertake planetary, solar, and deep-space research. The space exploration program might indeed remain at Houston, but its focus would perhaps shift to address such issues as strategic planning for permanent space colonies on the moon and Mars, which would be shielded from radiation and built by robots [11]. This type of effort would be perhaps much less focused on recruiting and training hundreds of astronauts who would never go into outer space, but much more concerned with the use of robots, radio telescopes on the far side of the moon, and developing lunar-based mining operations, as well as moon-based solar-power systems and information networks so that most lunar operations might indeed be carried out from control centers in Houston.

3) Downsize NASA in order to make it more agile, adept, and better focused on clearly defined objectives of national and strategic importance in space and to become more agile. This might mean that aeronautical research would be moved to another agency and shorter-term tasks perhaps also

handed off to industry, other federal agencies, or perhaps even universities. The new NASA would focus on longer-range scientific and technology issues, extremely complex engineering tasks, and facilitating innovations of critical importance to a sustainable planet.

4) Reenergize the U.S. space program. This objective could be achieved by active encouragement of small entrepreneurial aerospace entities through challenge prizes (like the Ansari X-Prize), through small business administration incentives, or other ways to stimulate "geniuses" to find new ways to think outside the box. This might be done by further extending the scope of NIAC or by other small and low-cost units. Teams made up of people from Space X, SpaceDev, the Space Elevator Corporation, the International Space University, and other academic entities could be asked to help the new NASA to achieve its newly defined goals. This new NASA would address issues such as to how we can use robots cheaply or new types of launchers to accomplish a more exciting and comprehensive set of goals. Again, the average citizen is skeptical of large governmental bureaucracy and the huge megacorporations. In a nation that celebrates innovative heroes such as the Wright Brothers, Samuel Morse, Alexander Graham Bell, and Thomas Edison, it is indeed just possible that the next great idea might likely come from the workshop garage or the lab of an eccentric than a multibillion-dollar laboratory. We need to look to people like Paul Allen, Elon Musk, Burt Rutan, Robert Bigelow, Peter Diamandis, Brad Edwards, and other innovative thinkers of our times to identify new targets. This new vision for U.S. space would identify new goals that are achievable in space exploration and research, astronaut safety, robotic systems, space applications, and even space colonization and tourism. The new NASA would have the mandate, the will, and the opportunity to truly address longer-range objectives covering the next 30 to 50 years. The new NASA would anticipate not only ways to do things more efficiently and through entrepreneurial talent, but would have the creativity and will to generate truly new technology, software, and systems that could not only help us save our world but take us to other worlds faster and hopefully more safely.

5) Revitalize entrepreneurial access to space programs, and generate new partnerships. There would be new hands-off, user-friendly, and incentive-based programs that would allow smaller enterprises to develop entrepreneurial programs in space tourism, space habs, or space applications (including private mission to planet Earth incentives that would be driven more by innovative thinkers than large contracts). Such initiatives could be geared to stimulate new approaches to solar-power systems in space and especially to allow new synergism to occur between space applications, space science, and space exploration. (The programs designed to sustain life on the moon might indeed help us sustain power generation, mining, or material processing here on Earth.) In this new environment we can find that we might only need 10 to 20 astronauts rather than the army of 240 astronauts in training we have today. We might be able to design totally new types of spacecraft that are more than just marginally safer but perhaps 100 to 1000 times more reliable and secure.

Ultimately one must ask what the $104-billion investment in Project Constellation will provide in longer-term payoffs, in terms of fundamentally new launch technologies or in terms of space safety or new technology that will help sustain our species? Currently there is not a great deal of "bang for the buck" in this program. We really do not seem to envision important new astronaut discoveries or technological breakthroughs in a program that will largely recreate the accomplishments of Project Apollo.

Before we are completely committed to developing in small increments only marginally new technology with conventional chemical rockets and landing capsules that are in many ways like those used in Mercury and Gemini, it seems wise to explore what a truly alternative and visionary space exploration program might deliver to U.S. citizens through a smaller, smarter, restructured, and goal-oriented NASA that dares to ask the truly big questions about what do we want out of our space program. The Project Constellation planning has, in many ways, learned from the past, and it has delivered much of what it was asked to accomplish. There is a separation of crew and cargo in the most dangerous parts of the mission. The return to a capsule design for atmospheric reentry of astronauts is probably the safest design. The plan to provide a complete launch-to-land escape capability for astronauts is a key point that the George Washington University and other studies have emphasized. Also the decision to design an expendable launch system based on shuttle motors rather than trying to modify and requalify an existing launch vehicle like the Atlas or the Delta or the Titan will also likely pay safety dividends. Further, there is historically proven merit in designing the CEV on the basis of a spiral concept, which allows for modularity and thus the flexible addition of new technology over time. These are all points that NASA's Project Constellation design teams seem to have learned from past astronaut safety studies and recommendations from space safety panels.

Yet, the potential of implementing fundamentally new technology that would take us beyond the basic danger of chemical rockets is really not a part of Project Constellation although this program is envisioned to span decades. This is not surprising in that the industrial architects of the Project Constellation launch systems are experts in building chemically fueled launch vehicles. Because we are in many ways looking 10 to 20 years ahead, it seems reasonable to give serious consideration to totally new launch systems that can be better, safer, more cost efficient, and promote some breakthrough technology. Project Constellation is a space program that started as a presidential mandate in January 2004 [12]. This program, as with many space programs before it such as Project Apollo and the space shuttle, was stimulated by a presidential call for advancement.

Project Constellation is a program that was defined in only a matter of a few weeks under the constraints of a presidential deadline rather than open forum of competitive ideas. It is not too late for a broader and more open process to take place. Rather than millions of dollars being spent on design studies by aerospace contractors—leading ineluctably to a multibillion dollar construction program—the intellectual review effort proposed here should be a wide-open competitive effort among the best and most innovative thinkers of our time. This exercise could be carried out within universities, research centers, or perhaps conducted under the tripartite auspices of the American Astronomical Society, the AIAA, and the Institute of Electrical and Electronics Engineers or the National Academies of Sciences and of Engineering. In short, totally new space launch systems and space safety of a fundamentally different nature can only come from a willingness to look afresh at the entire space exploration agenda—and this would include at least a reappraisal of Project Constellation. The worst that can happen from such an open competitive review would be to find that the Project Constellation planning is fully vindicated and the currently accepted program is reendorsed.

As we find ourselves halfway through the first decade of the 21st century, the sky is no longer the limit. Our only limits are those that we place on our imaginations. For human civilization to sustain itself for the long term, it must strive to exist at least on two planets and for the very long term within two star systems. We have a very long way to go.

References

[1] *Space Safety Study: Vulnerabilities and Risk Reduction in US Human Space Flight Programs*, George Washington Univ., Washington, DC, 2005.
[2] Klotz, I., *Space Updates Astro Expo*, 7 Dec. 2005, URL: www.astroexpo.com/neus/
[3] "NASA's Predicament," *Washington Post*, 31 Dec. 2005, p. A30.
[4] General Accounting Office, "Crew Exploration Vehicle and Crew Launch Vehicle," GAO Report, Washington, DC, Jan. 2006, URL: www.nasaproblems.com.
[5] Osbourne, D., and Gaebler, T., *Re-Inventing Government*, Plume Books, New York, 1993.
[6] "Rules Proposed for Space Travelers," *Washington Post*, 30 Dec. 2005, p. A-5.
[7] "Required Reading for Space Travelers," *Washington Post*, 2 Jan. 2006, p. A-15.
[8] Gelb, M. J., *How to Think Like Leonardo da Vinci*, Bantam Dell, New York, 2004.
[9] Friedman, L., "Update Letter on near Earth Objects," The Planetary Society, Jan. 2006, Pasadena, California, p. 1.
[10] Schweikart, R., "We Must Decide to Do It," *The Planetary Report*, Vol. XXV, July/Aug. 2005, Pasadena, California, pp. 1–2.
[11] Mendell, W., "Meditations on the New Space Vision: The Moon as a Stepping Stone to Mars," paper IAC-04-IAA 3.7.1.01, International Astronomical Congress, October 2001.
[12] "The Vision for Space Exploration," NASA Publications, NP-2004-01-334-HQ, Washington, DC, 2004, pp. 1–22.

APPENDIX A
Key Background Facts in Space Flight

Table A.1 Chronology: Some Key Dates in Manned Spaceflight

Date	Milestone
1957—October	First Soviet Sputnik launched
1958—November	NASA is created.
1961—April	Soviet cosmonaut Yuri Gagarin is the first man to orbit the Earth.
1961—May	First Mercury manned space flight within the U.S. space program
1961—May	President John F. Kennedy sets U.S. target to reach the moon before the end of the decade.
1962—February	John Glenn becomes the first U.S. astronaut to orbit the Earth.
1965—June	Gemini-4 astronauts undertake first EVA.
1967—June	Three astronauts killed in Apollo launchpad accident.
1968—December	Apollo spacecraft orbits the moon.
1969—July	First Apollo moon landing; Neil Armstrong first man on the moon
1970—April	Apollo-13 near disaster
1972—December	Apollo-17 is the last manned spaceflight to the moon. Astronaut Gene Cernan was the last of the Apollo explorer's to leave the moon.
1977—May	Skylab launched
1981—April	First flight of the space shuttle
1986—January	Loss of Space Shuttle *Challenger* with seven astronauts aboard
1988—September	Return to flight of the space shuttle after 2.5 years
1998—April	First modules of International Space Station launched
1999—June	First shuttle docked with ISS
2003—February	Loss of Space Shuttle *Columbia* (STS-113) with seven astronauts
2003—October	First manned spaceflight by China
2004—January	President George W. Bush announces new space vision to explore "the moon, Mars, and beyond."
2004—October	SpaceOne wins the Ansari X-Prize for commercial spaceflight.
2005—July/August	Shuttle Orbiter *Discovery* (STS-114) returns to flight, but the fleet is again grounded when foam-shedding problem reoccurs.

(continued)

Table A.1 Chronology: Some Key Dates in Manned Spaceflight

Date	Milestone
2005—September	NASA announces broad design features for Project Constellation.
2005—December	NASA issues RFP to industry seeking to lease commercial services to ferry supplies and astronauts to the ISS.

Table A.2 International Launch Services[1]

Launch service provider	Rocket	Launch site
Arianespace of Toulouse, France	Ariane 44	Kourou, FG
Arianespace	Ariane 5	Kourou, FG
Boeing	Delta	Cape Canaveral AS, FL, and Vandenberg AFB, CA
China Great Wall	Long March	Xichang
Daimler-Benz and Kurichev of Russia	Eurorocket	Still under development, but will be available shortly
International Launch Services (subsidiary of Lockheed Martin)	Atlas II	Cape Canaveral AS, FL, and Vandenberg AFB, CA
LS in partnership with Russia	Proton	Baikonur, Khazakhstan
Indian Space Research Organization	Heavy-life ISRO vehicle	Bangalore, India
Japan, Rocket System Corp.	H-2 and H-2A	Tanegashima, Japan
Orbital Sciences Corp.	Pegasus®/ and Taurus®	Wallops Island Flight Facility, VA, and Vandenberg AFB, CA
SeaLaunch (consortium headed by Boeing)	Modified Zenit	Pacific Ocean platform
Yuzhnoe (Ukraine)	Zenit 2	Baikonur, Khazakhstan

Table A.2 shows a summary of launchers available worldwide that can lift reasonable-sized satellites and experimental missions to Earth orbit. By 2008 or so a number of new commercial ventures such as Rocketplane Ltd., Space Adventures, and Virgin Galactic have indicated plans to offer commercial flights to LEO space.

Reference

[1] Pelton, J., *Basics of Satellite Communications*, 2nd ed., Professional Educational Services, Chicago, IL, 2006, p. 146–47.

Appendix B
Glossary

ACRV	= astronaut crew return vehicle
AERCam	= autonomous extravehicular robotic camera
AI	= artificial intelligence
AIAA	= American Institute of Aeronautics and Astronautics
ALTV	= approach and landing test vehicle
ARC	= NASA Ames Research Center
ARMOR	= adaptable robust metallic operable reusable (a new design for a thermal protection system)
ASAP	= Aerospace Safety Advisory Panel or Astronaut Safety Advisory Panel
ASIC	= application specific integrated circuit
ASIS	= abort sensing and implementation system
AT&T	= American Telephone and Telegraph
ATO	= abort to orbit
ATV	= automated transfer vehicle of European Space Agency
BBC	= British Broadcasting Corporation
BET	= best estimated trajectory
BFS	= backup flight system
BST	= Bio Systems Technology, Inc.
CAIB	= *Columbia* Accident Investigation Board
Canadarm	= original crane-like manipulator arm used on the shuttle for special repair or rescue missions.
Canadarm 2	= crane-like manipulator arm being installed in the International Space Station
CDMA	= code division multiple access
CEV	= crew exploration vehicle
CFD	= computational fluid dynamics
CNES	= Centre National d'Etudes Spatiales (France)
COL-CC	= Columbus control center for the European Space Laboratory on the ISS
Constellation	= name of the project to develop new launch systems and the CEV to send astronauts to the moon
COSPAS–SARSAT	= international search and rescue satellite system
COTS	= commercial off the shelf
CRL	= Communications Research Laboratory of Japan (now merged with other research agencies and is known as NICT)

CRV	= crew return vehicle
CSA	= Canadian Space Agency
DCU	= digital computer unit
DFRC	= NASA Dryden Flight Research Center
DOD	= U.S. Department of Defense
EADS	= European Aeronautics Defense and Space Company
ELM	= experimental logistics module
ELT	= emergency locator transmitter
ELV	= expendable launch vehicle
EMU	= extravehicular mobility unit
ESA	= European Space Agency
ESTEC	= European Space Research and Technology Center
ET	= external tank on the space shuttle
EVA	= extravehicular activity
FAA	= Federal Aviation Administration
FFRDC	= federally financed research and development center
FY	= fiscal year
GAO	= General Accounting Office
GCNR	= gas core nuclear rocket
GEO	= geosynchronous orbit (This is also referred to as GSO or geostationary orbit as well as the Clarke orbit after Arthur C. Clarke.)
GPC	= general-purpose computer
GPS	= geopositioning satellite
GRC	= NASA Glenn Research Center
GSE	= ground-support equipment
GSFC	= NASA Goddard Space Flight Center
GSOC	= German Space Operations Center
HAL/S	= high-order assembly language
HL 20	= a NASA prototyped design for a crew return vehicle that was cancelled.
Hypergolic fuels	= tonic fuels that provide explosive force when mixed together
ICBM	= intercontinental ballistic missile
ICS	= interorbit communications system
IMU	= inertial measurement unit
INS	= inertial navigation system
ISPR	= international standard payload racks
ISRO	= Indian Space Research Organization
ISS	= International Space Station
ISTP	= integrated space transportation plan
ISU	= International Space University
ITA	= independent technical authority (recommended to be established within NASA)
ITAR	= international traffic in arms regulations

IV&V	= independent verification and validation
JAXA	= Japanese Aerospace Exploration Agency (This was formed as NASDA was merged with other space research agencies.)
JEM	= Japanese experimental module
JIMO	= Jupiter icy moons orbiter
JPL	= Jet Propulsion Laboratory
JSC	= NASA Johnson Space Center
KSC	= NASA Kennedy Space Center
Ku-Band	= 14/12-GHz satellite frequencies
L/D	= lift/drag ratio
LEM	= lunar excursion module
LEO	= low Earth orbit
LFBB	= liquid fly-back booster
LH$_2$	= liquid hydrogen
LOX	= liquid oxygen
LRC	= NASA Langley Research Center
LTMCC	= large throat main combustion chamber
MAGR/S	= miniature airborne GPS receiver/shuttle
MBS	= mobile base system
MEC	= master event controller
MEO	= medium Earth orbit
MER	= mission evaluation room
MMS	= mobile servicing system
MMU	= manned maneuvering unit
MPD	= magnetoplasmadynamic
MPLM	= multipurpose logistics module
MSBLS	= microwave scan beam landing system
MSFC	= NASA Marshall Space Flight Center
NAA	= North American Aviation
NACA	= National Advisory Committee on Aeronautics
NASDA	= National Aeronautical and Space Development Agency (This organization after merger with other entities is now known as JAXA.)
NASP	= national space plane Development program (USA)
NEP	= nuclear electric power
NERVA	= nuclear engine for rocket vehicle application
NESC	= NASA Engineering and Safety Center
NEXIS	= nuclear electric xenon ion system
NIAC	= NASA Institute for Advanced Concepts
NICT	= National Institute for Information and Communications Technology of Japan (a new Japanese research institute formed by the merger of CRL and TAO)
NOAA	= National Oceanic and Atmospheric Administration of the United States
NSTS	= NASA Space Transportation System

NTP	= nuclear thermal power
NTR	= nuclear thermal rocket
OMB	= Office of Management and Budget
OMS	= orbital maneuvering system
OSP	= orbital space plane
OSTP	= Office of Science and Technology Policy of the United States
PASS	= primary avionics software set
PDGF	= power data grapple fixture
PEM	= proton exchange membrane
PLB	= personal locator beacon
PLS	= personal launch system
PLSS	= portable life-support system
PM	= pressurized module
PPS	= precise positioning service (GPS receiver)
PSAC	= President's Science Advisory Committee
RCS	= reaction control system
RLV	= reusable launch vehicle
RMS	= remote manipulation system
R-O-F	= recommendations, observations and findings of the CAIB
RSA	= Russian Space Agency or Russian Federated Space Agency (now known as Roskosmos)
RTG	= radioisotope thermoelectric generator
RTLS	= return to launch site
S-Band	= 2–4-GHz band used for mobile satellite and government satellite services
SEDS	= small expendable deployer system; also Students for the Exploration and Development of Space
SIAT	= shuttle independent assessment team
SIGI	= space integrated GPS inertial system
SIP	= strain isolator pad
SNAP	= space nuclear auxiliary power
SPAN	= spacecraft analysis room
SRB	= solid rocket booster
SSC	= NASA Stennis Space Center
SSTU	= single stage to orbit
STE	= special test equipment
STG	= space task group
STS	= space transportation system (more commonly known as the space shuttle)
TACAN	= tactical air navigation unit
TAL	= transatlantic abort landing
TAO	= Telecommunications Advancement Organization of Japan (This organization merged with CRL to become NICT.)
TDRS	= tracking and data relay satellite

TPS	= thermal protection system
TTC&M	= tracking, telemetry, command, and monitoring
UE	= user equipment
UHCL	= University of Houston–Clear Lake
USRA	= Universities Space Research Association
WAAS	= wide area augmentation system
X-Prize	= $10-million award for the first successful commercial spaceflight (This prize was won by Burt Rutan and Scaled Composites for the flight of SpaceOne; this is also known as the Ansari X-Prize.)
X-Series	= series of experimental vehicle developments undertaken by NASA (Those experimental vehicles covered in this report include the X-38 crew return vehicle and the X33, X-34, X-37, and X-43 reusable launch vehicles.)

Appendix C
Detailed Technical Review
of Shuttle Vulnerabilities

Chapter 3 provided an overview of technical concerns related to the space shuttle program. Table 3.1, in particular, presented a summary of the safety concerns related to the space shuttle, the degree of seriousness for each concern, the extent to which there has been flight experience with this type of problem, and short suggestions as to how these problems might be addressed. This appendix provides greater detail with regard to each of these issues.

General Problem of Aging

A number of studies and congressional testimonies have addressed the issue of shuttle safety and aging. These date from at least 1999 and continue with new data developed in the context of the *Columbia* accident review. These studies show issues with not only the shuttle orbiters but also serious infrastructure concerns. These studies have raised serious questions about the effect of age on the reliability of the space shuttle program. These reviews and key documents underline the extent to which the shuttle program could now be considered obsolescent as a result of the wear and tear on the orbiters over time, the difficulty of sustaining over long periods highly trained NASA maintenance and refurbishment staff technicians, in addition to the many outmoded design features of the shuttle. Elements such as hydraulics, wiring, brittle bolts, gearing systems, and even structural elements subject to salt-water corrosion are all components within the space shuttle orbiter that must be considered risk factors as a result of aging.

Age and obsolescence, when considered together with a reduced NASA and contractor workforce for maintenance and refurbishment and reduced funding for the shuttle program, combine to raise serious questions as to whether space shuttle program safety remains in jeopardy despite the estimated $2 billion in direct and indirect expenditures associated with the return-to-flight activities that NASA has undertaken in response to the CAIB report. In short, will sustained safety improvements and contractor and NASA support for shuttle refurbishment continue not only for the next few launches but for the next 10 to 20 launches that will take us some six years into the future?

In a June 1999 letter to the White House, NASA Administrator Daniel Goldin declared that the nation faced a "space launch crisis." He then reported on a NASA review of shuttle safety which indicated the budget for shuttle-related effort in fiscal year 2000 was "inadequate to accommodate upgrades necessary to yield significant safety improvements [1]." Yet only modest budgetary increases ensued after this urgent plea.

On 23 September 1999, space shuttle safety hearings were held before the House Science Committee's Subcommittee on Space and Aeronautics. These hearings were called to allow the subcommittee to be briefed on recent events in the space shuttle program that had raised safety concerns. STS-93 problems prompted this hearing. U.S. House Subcommittee Chair Representative Rohrabacher applauded NASA's decision to halt flights, thoroughly investigate, and fix the problems associated with bad wiring, which has since been found in all four space shuttles. Rohrabacher repeated a long-standing personal concern that budget cuts and contract milestone incentives might be having an impact upon maintaining a sufficient level of safety assurance in the space shuttle program. Despite Rohrabacher's comments, monies for major refurbishment for the shuttle were not forthcoming.

After malfunctions during STS-93 in July 1999, NASA Administrator Daniel Goldin established a shuttle independent assessment team (SIAT) chaired by Harry McDonald, director of NASA Ames Research Center. Among the team's findings, reported in March 2000, were the following:

1) SIAT had a major concern that "safety of the Space Shuttle Program is being eroded." The major factor leading to this concern "is the reduction in allocated resources and appropriate staff .... There are important technical areas that are one-deep." Also, SIAT felt "strongly that workforce augmentation must be realized principally with NASA personnel rather than with contractor personnel." Despite these findings, the money for shuttle refurbishment shrunk, and the recruitment and training of a new workforce to replace the aging workforce at Kennedy Space Center did not occur.

2) The SIAT was concerned that the "Space Shuttle Program (SSP) must rigorously guard against the tendency to accept risk solely because of prior success." Yet it would appear that "prior success" allowed conditions just noted to continue without remedial action.

3) The SIAT was very concerned with what it perceived as "Risk Management process erosion created by the desire to reduce costs ...."

4) The shuttle independent assessment team report also stated that the shuttle "clearly cannot be thought of as operational in the usual sense. Extensive maintenance, major amounts of specialized labor and a high degree of skill and expertise will always be required." However, "the workforce has received a conflicting message due to the emphasis on achieving cost and staff reductions, and the pressures placed on increasing scheduled flights as a result of the Space Station [2]."

5) Senator John McCain, R-Arizona, requested a GAO study in August 1999, a few weeks after the STS-93 mishap. The subsequent report in August 2000 from the GAO, a congressional investigative body, stated, Workforce reductions are jeopardizing NASA's ability to safely support

the shuttle's planned flight rate. Reduced to 1800 employees, the shuttle program has many unfilled positions and current employees (show) signs of overwork and fatigue." The report stated, citing numerous internal NASA studies, "workforce reductions are jeopardizing NASA's ability to safely support the shuttle's planned flight rate." The GAO report noted that serious staffing challenges will remain in the future, as the shuttle program has more than twice as many workers over 60 years of age than under 30. Even after the *Columbia* accident, these issues have still not been redressed as the return-to-flight activities have focused on the primary recommendations that involved making the shuttle fleet less vulnerable to TPS failure, but no substantive redress to the KSC staffing and training issues appears to have been made.

At its March 2001 meeting, NASA's Space Flight Advisory Committee advised that "the space shuttle Program must make larger, more substantial safety upgrades than currently planned ...a budget on the order of three times the budget currently allotted for improving the shuttle systems" was needed [3].

In April 2002, Richard Blomberg, former chair of the Aerospace Safety Advisory Panel (ASAP)—an independent review group to NASA—testified before the House Subcommittee on Space and Aeronautics, raising his concerns about an aging shuttle fleet:

1) In all of the years of my involvement, I have never been as concerned for space shuttle safety as I am right now. That concern is not for the present flight or the next or perhaps the one after that. In fact, one of the roots of my concern is that nobody will know for sure when the safety margin has been eroded too far. All of my instincts, however, suggest that the current approach is planting the seeds for future danger.*

2) Blomberg said that, because of budget shortfalls, many already planned and engineered improvements to the space shuttle system have had to be deferred or eliminated. Some of these would directly reduce flight risk. Others would improve operability or the launch reliability of the system and are therefore related to safety.

3) "Moreover, the current plans and budgets are not adequate even to retain the present Space Shuttle risk levels over the entire likely service life of the system," Blomberg stated.

4) Unfortunately, as systems continue to age, they tend to change. Some of these changes are predictable. Others, however, are subtle and often unpredictable. As components and subsystems age beyond their design lives, they may fail more often and with new and unanticipated failure modes. Thus, the well-established characterization of the system is no longer fully valid. The Aerospace Safety Advisory Panel believes that the Space Shuttle is heading in this direction.

---

*Data available online at http://www.space.com/missionlaunches/
sts107_fleet_030201.html.

The problems that arise with an aging complex system can be exacerbated if critical skills are lost. Even with the best documentation and succession planning, some expertise is lost as experienced personnel retire. In the case of the space shuttle, repeated Government and contractor hiring freezes during its operating life have led to a lack of depth in critical skills. Thus, it is reasonable to assume that the ability of the space shuttle workforce to anticipate new problems and to mount innovative efforts to maintain safety will inevitably diminish.[†]

Specific Problems with Aging

There are a number of specific problems caused by aging. These issues include wiring that resulted in specific life-threatening issues for STS-93, ceramic tiles, and other elements of the TPS, main engine wear-out components, heat exchanger coils, hydraulics, brittle bolts, safety and performance standards that need to be adjusted over time, space shuttle refurbishment and maintenance infrastructure and equipment, and shuttle component corrosion.

Wiring Problems

NASA grounded the entire shuttle fleet when a short circuit shut down a critical engine controller on the *Columbia* (STS-93). After a complete inspection of the shuttle fleet, technicians found wiring defects on other shuttles that could have caused major problems or even loss of a vehicle and crew [4]. The intricacy and the sheer size of the shuttle wiring suggests that despite the refurbishment that has occurred wiring deterioration could still be considered a safety risk, and manual inspection should be undertaken prior to the next shuttle launch.

Tile Problems

The issue of the tiles and the fragility of the thermal protection system remains at the most critical level of concern, and thus this subject is addressed elsewhere. See the following for a more detailed review and recommendations regarding the shuttle thermal protection system.

Main Engine Components with Accelerated Wear-Out

The shuttle main engine was designed by the Marshall Space Flight Center and Rocketdyne, and it has performed well over time. Nevertheless, the

---

[†]Data available online at http://www.space.com/missionlaunches/ sts107_fleet_030201.html.

William P. Rogers Report on the *Challenger* accident in 1986 clearly indicated that there were components of the main engine that constituted elements of risk because they "degrade more rapidly with flight use than anticipated" as demonstrated in "extensive 'hot fire' ground tests." Clearly these problems are endemic to the shuttle design, and although protective actions can and have been taken, the lifetime limits for a shuttle main engine have never been definitely established [5]. It would be desirable to undertake a lifetime performance analysis of the main engines of all of the remaining shuttles to verify that each of the orbiter engines is judged to be capable of extremely reliable operation for up to 15 launches.

Heat-Exchanger Coil

The heat-exchanger coil is key in that its failure could allow the leakage of hydrogen into the liquid-oxygen fuel tanks and potentially lead to an explosion that would destroy the vehicle and result in the loss of the crew. The wear-out of one of these units could thus lead to a category 1 failure. Replacement and extensive testing of these components remain a critical part of the refurbishment and retrofit program [6,7]. The George Washington University study found that it would be desirable for the reliable performance of the heat-exchanger coil to be recertified prior to reflight of the shuttle in terms of wear-out and replacement standards.

Hydraulics

Another concern with wear-out, expressed very early on in the shuttle program, is the operational hydraulics associated with the shuttle. Any system that depends on a mechanical or hydraulics system that is exposed to great g-force stress and thermal extremes over a period of decades could thus be considered a risk factor. The particular failure mode could result in many different results, but clearly there are conditions where a category 1 failure could occur.

All of the shuttle hydraulic systems should therefore be recertified prior to reflight of the shuttle in terms of updated standards for wear-out and extended performance.

Safety Margins and Performance Design Margins over Time

One of the consistent messages found in the Apollo program, the *Challenger* accident report, the *Columbia* accident report, and in the surveys and interviews conducted for this study is the need for substantial safety and design margins. Regardless of whether one is talking about wear-out concerns expressed with regard to the early human-rated launch systems, the space shuttle, the construction and operation of the ISS, or the design of new launch systems for the future, those with substantial experience in the space industry call for extra caution and safety margins. They urge that very substantial margins (i.e., 30 to 40% above and beyond a 100% design goal) be applied to the stress testing of all major active aspects of launch systems and that they be operated below 100% nominal levels as well. Passive systems should also have reasonable performance and wear-out margins, but these need not be as great as for the active systems.

In short, full dynamic, acoustic, and thermal loads need to be considered in the application of safety standards that take into account aging and structural deterioration and stress over time. It would be desirable for the NASA structural handbook to be reviewed and updated as appropriate to ensure that more than adequate testing standards are applied and that aging factors are applied for additional margin.

There is thus concern that NASA, because of the urgency of completing the deployment of the ISS on time and within budget, might be driven in the direction of lifting the maximum amount of cargo with each future flight so as to complete its overall mission with heavy loads and with less margins than might be appropriate for good safety. This approach to shuttle operation with 100% of lift obviously puts greater stress on units that might be subject to wear-out stress or end-of-life failure (as represented by the bathtub curve of failure events observed in in-orbit systems [8]).

Space Shuttle Infrastructure

The issue of wear-out extends beyond the shuttle hardware to the support infrastructure critical to the overall systems operation. In 2000, NASA identified 100 infrastructure items that demanded immediate attention. NASA briefed the Space Flight Advisory committee on this infrastructure revitalization initiative in November of that year. The committee agreed in its report that "deteriorating infrastructure is a serious, major problem" that must be addressed. When the committee toured several Kennedy Space Center facilities, they declared them to be "in deplorable condition." NASA subsequently submitted a FY 2002 request for $600 million to fund the infrastructure initiative. Congress provided only $25 million for vehicle assembly building repairs. NASA has reallocated limited funds from the shuttle budget to the most pressing infrastructure repairs and intends to take an integrated look at infrastructure as part of its shuttle service life extension program. Nonetheless, both space shuttle upgrades and Kennedy Center infrastructure revitalization has been mired by the uncertainty surrounding the shuttle program's lifetime. If it is indeed national policy that the shuttle will continue to fly for many years to come, then "NASA, the White House, and Congress alike now face the specter of having to deal with years of infrastructure neglect [6]." The damage from the 2004 hurricane season in Florida has, of course, further intensified this problem with less than requested monies provided to deal with this latest infrastructure concern.

Richard Blomberg, former chair of the ASAP, cited as an example of failing shuttle support infrastructure the collapse of a weld in a fuel line during the launch count for STS-110. The mobile launch platform (MLP) on which the line was mounted was originally designed and built for the *Apollo* program and then refurbished for the space shuttle (emphasis added). Blomberg argued that it is not reasonable to expect the MLPs and similar vintage infrastructure to continue to support space shuttle operations well into the future unless significant effort is expended on renewal, upgrade, and life extension. The weld rupture in the MLP for instance had no immediate safety consequences, but it did delay the launch and could have resulted in significant damage to the shuttle. He added that the "program may not be so fortunate in the future [9]." The study concluded that there appears to be a need for all infrastructure, support facilities, and test and measurement equipment that support the shuttle to be independently reviewed and reported on as soon as possible, looking to an operating schedule that extends at least through 2010. This report should cover the current status of these facilities with a prioritized list of remedial action and projected costs associated with these upgrades.

Shuttle Corrosion

Approximately 90% of the shuttle structure can be inspected for corrosion, but corrosion in the remaining 10% can remain undetected for the life of the vehicle. Moreover, the risk of undetected corrosion can increase as other inspections are undertaken and subsystems removed to create new levels of exposure or if intervals between inspections are extended because of reduced staffing.

Removing and replacing thermal protection system tiles sometimes results in damage to the anticorrosion primer that covers the shuttle's sheet metal skin. Tile replacement often occurs without first repriming the primed aluminum substrate. This problem also can occur with regard to repriming of the external tank when repairs are required during manufacture, but assurance has been given that this issue is covered by new quality control and verification (QC&V) processes now in place at Lockheed Martin. Prior to STS-107 corrosion was found in the *Columbia* on the lower forward fuselage skin panel and stringer areas. Other corrosion concerns focus on the area between the crew module and outer hull, which is a difficult area to access for inspection and repair. There is also concern that unchecked corrosion could progress from internal areas to external surfaces through fastener holes, joints, or directly through the skin.

It would seem that updated standards need to be set, especially for QC&V procedures covering such aspects as corrosion and wear-out assuming each orbiter might be launched as many as 15 times more before it is retired.

Brittle Bolts

A total of 88 A-286 steel bolts were used on *Columbia*'s wings, and, of these, 57 were recovered. Of those 57, a total of 22 had brittle fractures. Investigators determined that liquid metal embrittlement caused by aluminum vapor created by *Columbia*'s breakup could have contributed to these fractures, but the axial loads placed on the bolts when they separated from the carrier panel/box beam at temperatures approaching 2000°F likely caused the failures.

Findings of the CAIB report regarding these brittle bolts included the following:

1) The present design and fabrication of the lower carrier panel attachments are inadequate. Bolts can readily pull through the relatively large holes in the box beams.

2) The current design of the box beam in the lower carrier panel assembly exposes the attachment bolts to a rapid exchange of air along the wing, which enables the failure of numerous bolts.

3) Primers and sealants can accelerate corrosion, particularly in tight crevices.

4) The extent to which all of these issues with regard to bolt embrittlement have been addressed is not clear and thus remains an area of concern.

Vulnerabilities Caused by Retrofit

Numerous experts have testified or reported about concerns over lack of timely retrofits. Two of these are summarized next:

1) In testimony of September 2001 [10], the GAO reported that NASA has started to define and develop some specific shuttle upgrades, which had been recommended in a 2000 GAO report. For example, requirements for the cockpit avionics upgrade had been defined, and phase I of the main engine advanced health monitoring system was in development. Nevertheless, NASA had not yet fully defined these planned upgrades. The studies on particular projects, such as developing a crew escape system, have not led to specific action to achieve such capability, and indeed both the HL-20 and X-38 have been cancelled. Moreover, previous GAO concerns with the technical maturity and potential cost growth of particular projects have proven to be warranted. For example, the implementation of the electric auxiliary power unit has been delayed indefinitely because of technical uncertainties and cost growth. Also, the estimated cost of phase II of the main engine advanced health monitoring system has almost doubled, and NASA has cancelled the proposed development of a block III main engine improvement because of technological, cost, and schedule uncertainties.

2) In a statement before the House Subcommittee on Space and Aeronautics, Richard Blomberg, former chair, Aerospace Safety Advisory Panel, indicated serious concerns over logistics and funding for the remaining life of the space shuttle program. This is because not only are retrofits and design improvements deferred, but support capabilities to make such retrofits are deferred as well. *For example, some of the shuttle special test equipment (STE) still employs vacuum tubes* (emphasis added).

Much maintenance and improvement of this infrastructure has already been deferred to conserve resources for current operations. As a result, there is a large backlog of not only restoration but upgrade work as well. If restoration continues to be delayed, it will reach a point at which it may be impossible to recover.

We believe this last statement is likely an exaggeration, but nevertheless, in light of extremely tight budget constraints that are in effect, proper restoration and maintenance of the ground support systems must be viewed as an important element contributing to overall flight safety. It would be desirable to have a comprehensive safety report on the status of all retrofit work and all primary launch support equipment associated with the test of retrofit operations prior to the next shuttle launch.

Other Areas of Vulnerability

Vulnerabilities at Liftoff

Many space missions have had problems during countdown, but generally these problems are cleared after some delay either because of a correction of the problem or by the issuance of a variance if the problem is judged to be inconsequential. The first flight of the space shuttle was delayed by a subtle timing error, which was traced to an improbable condition in the flight control software [11].

Since that first flight, many problems with software quality control in the space shuttle program have been reported. In one such assessment, a recommendation was made that NASA should upgrade its workforce and management practices to make it a leader in software engineering and software quality. Although NASA has areas where there is outstanding ability with regard to software engineering and systems engineering quality, this is not uniformly the case, and in the shuttle program there are special concerns that are addressed in later sections of this report.‡

This same report also recommended that "NASA should maintain as much in-house capability as possible to reduce its dependence on contractors and to provide proper assurance that contracted work is done on time and with as much attention to safety and other qualities as future systems require and deserve." There are other reports such as the Aldridge commission, however, that make alternative recommendations to move towards more contractor effort and to sharpen NASA's role to improved oversight capabilities.

We feel that as far as safety oversight is concerned NASA and NASA-related FFRDCs (with a special mandate given to the new ITA/NESC) should have control of technical and safety oversight. For the design of new manned flight systems, new and flexible relationships with entrepreneurial

---

‡Data available online at http://books.nap.edu/books/030904880X /html/index.html.

organizations, smaller research centers and universities might be able to allow new, simpler, and ultimately safer designs to emerge. Dominant control by the largest aerospace contractor (at least based on DOD experience) can produce more complex systems that often lead to higher costs and longer production schedules and more demanding operating systems.

The buildup of ice on the fuel tanks has been a problem in some launches. Because of the vulnerability of the heat shields, NASA guidelines are to launch with no ice on the fuel tanks to avoid having anything that would fall off because of the vulnerability of the tiles. Nevertheless, variances can be granted to launch when the risk is judged to be extremely small [12].

Debris affecting launch can come from several sources: ice that accumulates on the shuttle assembly, insulation from the external tank or solid rocket boosters, or debris on the ground or launch equipment.§ Even woodpeckers have done damage to the foam insulation of the external fuel tank.¶

Clearly the most critical element at launch has been the susceptibility of the space shuttle to tile damage. These problems are fundamentally caused by the design and installation of the tiles themselves. In a 1994 report on tile vulnerability, one conclusion was that "it was clear at the onset of the study that some management problems affected the quality of the tile work." During some operations, it was found that a few tiles had no primary bond with the shuttle; they were held in place only by the friction of the gap fillers.

This report recommended "that NASA inspect the bond of the most risk-critical tiles and reinforce the insulation of the external systems (external tank and solid rocket boosters) that could damage the high risk tiles if it de-bonds at takeoff." Only a small percentage of the tiles constitute high risk. Damage to those tiles during launch has always been a significant concern. As observed in the 1994 report, "de-bonding of insulation on the external tank (an event of minor concern) could damage critical tiles on the shuttle, eventually causing the loss of the vehicle and crew." Unfortunately, this statement proved to be prophetic in the case of *Columbia*'s last mission. The corrective actions in this respect, however, have been fully set forth in the CAIB report and addressed in depth in the return-to-flight program.

The other critical element is the escape capability for the astronauts at the point of liftoff. Currently the astronauts only have the option of a slide escape system, which is very likely to represent too slow of an exit path in case of a large-scale explosion of the rocket fuel. The design of the shuttle

---

§Data available online at http://www.spacedaily.com/news/fischbeckShuttle.pdf5.

¶Data available online at http://www.pao.ksc.nasa.gov/kscpao/status/stsstat/1995/jun/6-05-95s.htm [cited 5 June 1995].

does not allow for an explosive ejector system that would allow egress with a much higher chance of survival. Currently only the design and operation of a totally new personal launch system would solve this problem of complete mission escape capabilities. (This is one of many reasons why the Rogers' commission and various reports on safety that followed have urged the development of a new manned launch capability to replace the shuttle.)

Because there is no viable escape capability for the space shuttle during launch for the first two minutes and limited options for repair of the shuttle in orbit, there are limited safety options to explore except for better planning for new vehicles. The current safety options related to the shuttle come down to such alternatives as the reexploration of developing a robotically controlled shuttle, use of expendable vehicles, and/or reducing the scope of the fully deployed ISS.

Liftoff Through Orbital Insertion

During this stage, vulnerabilities are present for the space shuttle. Two malfunctions occurred on STS-93 during the just-described orientation process. This resulted in an improper orbital insertion and resultant safety hazards. Further upgrades to the orbital maneuvering system (OMS) and reaction control system (RCS) would be desirable, primarily with respect to the propellants used, to achieve more efficient operation and maintenance of the shuttle. More importantly such changes would reduce the safety risks associated with these two of the shuttle's attitude control subsystems.

In hearings before the House Science Committee's Subcommittee on Space and Aeronautics on 23 September 1999, two events that occurred during STS-93 mission were reviewed because of the safety concerns they raised. The two problems occurred during orbital insertion. First there was an electrical short in the wiring system. As a result, a liquid-oxygen-level (LOX) sensor in the main engine detected a low level resulting in early shutoff of the main engines. The electrical short occurred in one of the electrical distribution power circuits that provide power to the main engine controller. The short took place 5 s after liftoff and lasted for 400 ms. It resulted in the shutdown of two digital computer units (DCUs); these were the primary DCU for engine #1 and the backup DCU for engine #3. The redundant systems of the shuttle that were in place had taken over, and no abnormality in operation of the main engines occurred [13]. The second event, the lower than normal reading of the LOX sensor, resulted in the improper orbital insertion of STS-93. Because of the reading, all three main engines shut down 0.15 s early, and the shuttle had a speed of 15 ft/s lower than planned. It was determined that a hydrogen leak on the interior of the nozzle of one of the main engines caused an increase in the amount of oxygen to maintain the proper mixture. Propellants were thus used earlier than expected. This in turn resulted in an underspeed of the shuttle during the final stages of its orbital insertion. The orbit achieved was seven miles lower than the planned altitude. This did not ultimately seriously impair the operational objective of STS-93's mission, because the delivery of the Chandra X-Ray Observatory was still successful. Nevertheless potential for much more severe results was clearly present [13].

The events that occurred during the orbital insertion of the STS-93 serve to highlight the connectedness of the sequence of events, which begins at the launchpad and ends when the shuttle achieves its final orbit. The short in the electrical system did not affect the operation of the main engines because of the redundancies of the system, and after this mission NASA took several steps to ensure the proper maintenance of the wiring system on all of the shuttles even though questions about wiring maintenance as already outlined still persist. However, had the hydrogen leak occurred earlier, or had it been a larger leak, the final orbital insertion might have been more of a problem.

In upgrades proposed to the space shuttle in the report by the Committee on space shuttle Upgrades, the OMS/RCS subsystems were discussed to increase the safety and efficiency of their operation. The OMS/RCS systems currently use monomethyl hydrazine fuel and a nitrogen-tetroxide oxidizer. These are both highly toxic substances. These two propellants are hypergolic, so that no source of ignition is required because they in effect explode on contact. The OMS and RCS subsystems currently have separate propellant tanks to support their operation. The proposed upgrades would modify the OMS/RCS systems to use engines that operate on liquid oxygen and ethanol, two nontoxic propellants. In addition to the engine replacements proposed, the two subsystems would use a central propellant storage area [14].

Using nontoxic propellants would in general reduce hazards although new fuels that require an oxidizer would create new costs and difficulties. In addition to being nontoxic, the proposed propellants are less corrosive than the ones currently in use, which would result in a reduction in maintenance costs [14].

The proposed modification could also improve the performance of the engines in orbit, and the engine's source of liquid oxygen could be used as a redundant life-support system for the shuttle.

The proposed OMS/RCS upgrades do pose some difficulties. The new system would require additional tanks, insulation, and thermal control to operate the engines, which would make these two subsystems more complex. Also, the fuels are not hypergolic, and so an ignition source would be required that could potentially reduce reliability. In short, because of the cost, complexity, and schedule, these upgrades and the uncertain risk reduction they offer do not lead to a clear course of action [14].

One of the critical elements in the telemetry, command, and control of the space shuttle during its launch into low Earth orbit is the advanced tracking and data relay satellite network. This network allows real-time communications from the shuttle during launch and after deployment in LEO via a network of geosynchronous-based satellites and is key to the safe operation of the shuttle as well as the ISS. The advanced TDRS system has increased bandwidth and enhanced performance, but there are several questions about the extent to which further redundancy as well as security precautions against terrorist or hacker attacks against the system would be advisable in systems upgrade or third-generation designs for the next system. An increasing number of shuttle and ISS operations are being automated and often require continuous telemetry command and control operations to make continuous real-time communications with NASA ground control, which increases the importance of noninterrupted links being sustained.

Continuing safety and reliability review is desirable both of TT&C operations in general and the advanced TDRS system in particular. Such upgrades should take into account cost, performance, safety margins, and potential application to future NASA or other space programs as new manned space systems are designed and built.

Vulnerabilities Through On-Station Operations

Many of the critical phases during a shuttle mission are automated processes controlled by the onboard computers, which can be taken over by the crew and executed manually if it is deemed necessary. The docking of the shuttle to the ISS, however, is only initially computer controlled, as the final step of mating the two is a completely crew-controlled operation. The launch of the shuttle is also carefully timed in order to place the shuttle on a direct course for the ISS as it orbits the Earth. Two vulnerabilities exist during the docking of the shuttle with the ISS. The first vulnerability is the possibility of a docking anomaly as a result of control mechanisms or if being manually docked as a result of pilot error. The second key concern is a launch anomaly that could place the shuttle in an improper orbit that would not allow or make much more difficult the proper mating with the ISS. Software malfunctions, either onboard the ISS or on the shuttle, could also complicate the proper mating between the two systems. Beyond the vulnerabilities related to the mating process, the delivery of cargo payload also represents issues of vulnerability.

Docking Between the Shuttle and the ISS

When the shuttle is near 2000 ft from the ISS, the commander moves to a flight station in the rear of the crew cabin and takes control of the vehicle. Through careful manipulation of the shuttle's thrusters (and only those thrusters facing away from the ISS solar arrays to avoid damaging them), the commander must mate the two surfaces within an error of

3 in. to allow the seal on the shuttle and ISS docking rings to form an airtight seal.**

Mission specialist Mary Ellen Weber who has docked with the ISS aboard Atlantis said, "I don't know if most people realize how complex an effort this is," when referring to the docking process. Pilots train for over a year in NASA simulators, and human pilots control an enormous amount of government aerospace operations. Although risks are involved, pilots trained by NASA and other government agencies are extremely well qualified to manage these risks, and accomplish their mission's objective. Nevertheless an improved laser guidance and alignment system designed for close quarter maneuvers and improved venier thruster system could certainly be designed for a new personal space launch system as would undoubtedly be the case with the Crew Exploration Vehicle or Crew Return Vehicle. If the shuttle were to be converted to complete robotic control, the docking process would likely be the area where the greatest attention would need to be directed.

Launch Anomalies That Could Insert the Shuttle into Improper Orbit

If an anomaly during launch or orbital insertion occurs, as has been the case on several occasions, then the shuttle might be placed on an improper course to meet with the ISS to perform a proper docking. This would require the shuttle to change its orbit altitude before it comes close to the ISS or in the worst case abandon the mission.

As the shuttle closes in on the ISS, the crew closely monitors the vehicle as the computers fly it. In addition, a handheld laser is used to double check the range and closing-rate data. During this phase of the docking process, the vulnerability exists, as during any portion of the several computer-controlled phases of a shuttle mission, for a software error to execute improper commands to a hardware system, or to fail to handle or detect a hardware system failure properly. (See the Computer and Software Vulnerability section for a more detailed discussion of the software-related issues and vulnerabilities.)

Other Concerns Related to Shuttle and ISS Docking Operations

ISS software malfunctions are also a source of vulnerability during on-station operations, including the docking operations. These issues with regard to the ISS are discussed in Chapter 5 and further in Appendix D.

Also, delivery of cargo from the payload section of the shuttle once docking has been achieved can lead to safety risks. The rail cart system was designed some two decades ago and is not optimized for delivery of

---

**Data available online at http://www.space.com/missionlaunches/missions/
sts101_docking_dodont_000421.html.

large and sensitive cargo items. A new system for loading cargo onto the ISS should clearly be designed as part of any new launch system.

Vulnerabilities in Orbital Flight and EVAs

There are several vulnerabilities for the space shuttle during orbital flight. One of these safety concerns in low Earth orbit is orbital debris. This includes both meteorites and man-made objects in space. There are, of course, also the effects of shuttle subsystem failure such as failure of life-support systems, control thrusters, etc. during orbital flight, but these are addressed in other sections. Another possible hazard is that of radiation. Shuttle missions do not expose the crew to any natural radiation hazards that are different than previous space missions. In fact risks from radiation are reduced compared to the Apollo missions, and measurement techniques are greatly refined over those used in earlier missions. The crew wears dosimeters, and dosages are monitored on an ongoing basis [15]. Risk factors related to radiation, cosmic waves, or other such hazards are addressed in the International Space Station section. In many ways the orbital debris and micrometeorite hazard is not only the most significant but also the one that is increasing over time.

According to a recent study [16] there have not yet been any confirmed incidents in which collision with orbital debris has severely damaged or destroyed a spacecraft, but there have been a number of spacecraft malfunctions and breakups that might have been caused by impacts with debris. Smaller debris particles have certainly pitted windows of the U.S. space shuttle, as well as the Salyut and Mir space stations.

Since the late 1970s, studies of the debris population using modeling techniques have predicted that the hazard from orbital debris is likely to grow in time unless deliberate actions are taken to minimize the creation of new debris. This predicted increase in space debris hazard will force spacecraft designers and operators to take countermeasures against the threat of debris or to face a heightened risk of losing spacecraft capability as a result of impacts. Projected future increases in the debris hazard have already had an effect on the design of low-Earth-orbit spacecraft (such as the International Space Station). In short, any large spacecraft with long projected functional lifetimes have a significant probability of colliding with damaging debris, and this likelihood increases with over time.

Thus concern about the orbital debris hazard has grown in the last decade. A number of events, including the breakup of several rocket upper stages and the replacement of shuttle windows after impacts by small particles, certainly increased awareness of this problem. NASA models of the space environment now suggest that "meteoroids and orbital debris pose a significant threat to the shuttle."[++] Four factors

---

[++]Data available online at http://books.nap.edu/books/0309059887/html/4.html#pagetop.

determine how the space debris environment affects space systems operations: time in orbit, projected cross-section area, orbital altitude, and
orbital inclination. The first three are the dominant factors, but orbital
inclination can still be a concern because debris buildup is different at different orbital inclinations. Beyond these four factors there is, of course, the
possibility of a deliberate attack on a shuttle or the ISS. Terrorist concerns
will be addressed later in Appendix C.

Effects of Orbital Debris and MicroMeteorites

Large debris objects are typically defined as objects larger than 10 cm in
size. Such objects are capable of being tracked, and orbital elements are
maintained. During the course of missions, shuttles have executed collision-avoidance maneuvers in order to avoid catastrophic collisions with
these large debris objects.

Small debris objects (smaller than a few millimeters in diameter) have
already caused some damage to operational space systems, and in calcu-
lating potential damaging impact one must consider not only the size of
the debris but also the relative velocity of the debris to the shuttle or the
ISS. These impacts have had no known effect on mission success, but as
noted earlier the probability of adverse results are mounting over time as
debris in low Earth orbit continues to increase despite efforts to reduce
orbiting "space junk" through due diligence procedures. The effects of
small debris have included damage to the shuttle windows; damage to
the Hubble Space Telescope (HST) high-gain antenna; severing of the
Small Expendable Deployer System-2 (SEDS-2) tether; and damage to
other exposed shuttle surfaces. One such source of small debris involves
the flaking of small paint chips as a space object ages under the influence
of solar radiation, atomic oxygen, and other forces. Paint, which is used
extensively on both spacecraft and rocket bodies for thermal control reasons, can deteriorate severely in space, sometimes in a matter of only a
few years. The potential magnitude of the problem was not fully recognized until the 1983 flight of the STS-7 mission. On this flight an impact
crater on a shuttle window resulted from a paint chip smaller than a milli-
meter in diameter. Subsequent analyses of spacecraft components
returned from LEO have confirmed the presence of a large population of
paint particles, even though the orbits of individual particles decay quite
rapidly.

To protect crews from debris during flight, operational procedures
have been adopted. In the case of the space shuttle, it is often oriented
during flight, with the tail pointed in the direction of the velocity vector.
This flight orientation was adopted to protect the crew and sensitive shuttle systems from damage caused by collisions with small debris.
Operational restrictions have also been adopted for extravehicular activities (EVAs). Whenever possible, EVAs are conducted in such a way as to
ensure that the EVA crew is shielded from debris by the shuttle orbiter,
but a further review and update of operational safety policies in this

regard could likely provide some further risk reduction. This concern is address again in the findings section because it represents an even greater hazard for ISS operations [17].

Modeling of the Space Debris Environment and Risk Assessment

Risk assessments have been routinely performed on LEO spacecraft since the 1960s. Calculation of the probability of an impact from space debris requires a meteoroid/space debris environment model, a spacecraft configuration, and a mission profile. One such prediction is shown in Fig. 3.2. Calculation of the probability of a penetration and/or a failure caused by space debris requires detailed knowledge of the spacecraft configuration. (Tables C.1, C.2, C.3, and C.4 show results of risk analysis for shuttle components, during an EVA, and total risk of critical failure.)

Risk assessments have proved invaluable in ensuring the safety of shuttle operations. Shuttle missions are operationally reconfigured whenever a preflight risk assessment indicates that the risks of space debris are at an unacceptable level. Care must be taken to adjust risk calculations for both the shuttle and the ISS as the hazard level grows over time. In this respect, the clearer definition of safety standards and risk analysis should desirably be undertaken by the NESC and in time by the ITA if this is formed.

Mitigation of the Effects of Debris

One aspect of debris mitigation is to avoid the generation of debris under normal operation. Approximately 12% of the present catalogued space debris population consists of objects discarded during normal satellite deployment and operations. It is normally relatively easy, both technically and economically, to take mitigation measures against these objects under

Table C-1 Damage Thresholds for Shuttle Components [17] (Likely Implications of Collision with Orbital Debris or Micrometeoroid)

Effect on the Orbiter	Diameter of debris
Required replacement of window	0.04 mm
Penetration of a space suit	0.01 mm
Penetration of a radiator tube	0.5 mm
Penetrate leading edge of wing	1 mm
Penetrate crew cabin aft bulkhead	2 mm
Penetrate thermal protection system tiles	3 to 5 mm
Penetrate crew cabin's (average surface)	5 mm
Active collision avoidance if possible	10 cm or larger

Table C-2   Predicted Number of Impacts on Shuttle [17] (Probability of Impact During Space Shuttle Missions in Low Earth Orbit)

Diameter of Meteor or Debris	Ten-Day Mission	400 Ten-Day Mission
>0.04 mm	700	300,0000
>0.1 mm	100	40,000
>0.5 mm	1	400
>1 mm	0.09	35
>2 mm	0.008	3
>3 mm	0.002	0.8
>5 mm	0.0005	0.02
>3 cm	0.000004	0.002

Table C-3   Predicted Risks to Astronauts Associated with Debris [17] (Risks to Astronauts from Debris Associated with EVA)

Length and Type of EVA	6-h EVA	180 EVAs
Probability of no penetration	99.98% (1/4,800)	92.7% (1/14)
Probability of no critical penetration (hole >4 mm)	99.997% (1/31,000)	98.9% (1/91)

Table C-4   Total Calculated Risk of Critical Failure [17] (Cumulative Probability of Critical Accident on Shuttle Mission)

Risk Conditions	Ascent	Reentry	Debris collision	Total
Without risk of collision with debris considered	Mean score probability of 1 out of 219	Mean score probability of 1 out of 356	Not applicable	Mean score of 1 out of 131
Risk with debris and meteoroid considered	Mean score probability of 1 out of 219	Mean score probability of 1 out of 356	Mean score probability 1 out of 200	Mean score of 1 out of 79

standards now in place. For example, clamps and covers can be retained by parent bodies. Tethers can become space debris if they are discarded after use or if they are severed by an impacting object (man-made debris or meteoroid). New multistrand tether designs can reduce the risk of being severed. At the end of missions, tethers can be retracted to reduce the possibility of collision with other objects. Other mission-related particles can be generated unintentionally, as in the release of slag (up to several centimeters in diameter), during and after the burn of solid rocket motors. Fragmentations of upper stages and spacecraft can represent a significant amount of space debris larger than 5 cm in diameter, and these are harder to prevent. Incidents of abandoned upper-stage components have affected a wide range of launch vehicles operated by the United States, Russia, China, and ESA.

Protection strategies for manned missions such as the space shuttle can incorporate both shielding measures and in-orbit repair of damage caused by penetrations. Current shield designs offer protection against objects of reasonable size. Because it is impossible to protect completely, even from debris smaller than 1 cm in some cases, the probability of no penetration (PNP), as shown in the preceding tables, is the main criterion for shield design. During a mission, inspection of damage from debris can be done by an EVA or by the remote manipulator system (RMS) cameras, if the RMS is onboard (about 80–90% of missions). Based on the recommendations of the CAIB, there are now plans to use enhanced imaging capability at the ISS that could inspect the shuttle for impact damage while docked at the ISS.‡‡ Crewmembers engaged in EVA need protection from natural and man-made debris. Current space suits have many features with inherent shielding qualities to offer protection from objects of sizes up to 0.1 mm. By properly orienting their spacecraft, astronauts might be able to use their vehicles as shields against the majority of space debris or direct meteoroid streams.

Collision Avoidance

Current space surveillance systems do not reliably track objects in LEO with a radar cross section of less than 10 cm in equivalent diameter. For space objects large enough to be tracked by ground-based space surveillance systems, collision avoidance during orbital insertion and in-orbit operations is technically possible. As a part of its reassessment of operating procedures after the *Challenger* accident and the Roger's commission report, NASA developed a collision-avoidance procedure for the space shuttle. Before the launch, analysis is performed of the expected location of catalogued debris for the first few hours of the mission to determine if any will pass close to the shuttle.

When the shuttle is in orbit, the Space Surveillance Network (SSN) will notify NASA if a catalogued object is predicted to pass within a box measuring 2 km by 2 km by 5 km. If the predicted distance closes to 2 km in a radial position or 5 km along the track, the shuttle will perform a collision-avoidance maneuver if it does not compromise either primary payload or mission objectives.

---

‡‡Data available online at http://news.bbc.co.uk/1/hi/sci/tech/3283507.stm.

The shuttle requires 45 min warning to plan and perform a collision-avoidance maneuver [18]. From 1989, when this procedure was implemented, through February 1994, the shuttle received four notifications and performed three collision-avoidance maneuvers according to the NASA JSC report of [19]. Further research in such collision-avoidance techniques for both the space shuttle and the ISS could produce further improvements in operating procedures as well as noting optimum times for EVAs. Such research could also improve the safety design of future human-rated vehicles, especially with regard to the design of window systems.

Another example of mitigation is the design of a mission so that a sensitive component faces the rear, rather than in the direction of motion. Figure C-1 illustrates how orbital attitude changes the number of expected impacts on U.S. space shuttle windows. Space shuttle rule 2-77 states that the shuttle should use the orientation which causes the least number of window impacts unless it compromises mission objectives [20]. The space shuttle also uses orbits believed to have a lower flux of debris whenever possible. According to the flight rules referenced in Fig. C.1, shuttle orbital altitudes below 320 km are thus often used when this is possible and when this does not compromise high-priority objectives [20].

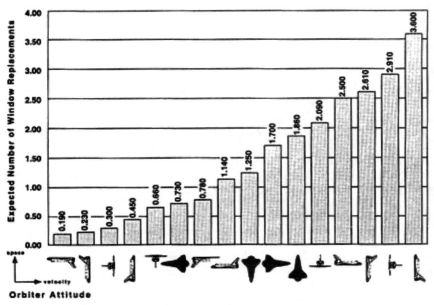

Figure C-1 Expected number of window replacements for U.S. space shuttle at various orbital attitudes (Source: NASA Johnson Space Center).

Without mitigation of the debris environment or operational changes, the growing number and total cross section of space debris would increase the likelihood of collisions, which in turn could generate new debris. Placing spacecraft into disposal orbits with limited orbital lifetime (e.g., 25 years or less) can have a particular effect on curbing the growth of the debris population by the elimination of mission-related debris generated before mission termination. Further research and coordination by NASA with the United Nations (U.N.) Committee on the Peaceful Uses of Outer Space, the ITU, the other space agencies, and the International Association for the Advancement of Space Safety is recommended to see how debris minimization and control can be advanced.

Vulnerabilities of Space Suits

This section explores the basics of space-suit design and safety considerations for the space shuttle program as well as looks to future space-suit design. Space suits, from their earliest designs to those envisioned for Mars, provide environmental protection, reliability, and redundancy. Vulnerabilities of space suits are considered small compared to other vulnerabilities covered in this report.

Exploration in space requires human beings to take their environment with them because there is no atmospheric pressure and no oxygen to sustain life. Inside a spacecraft, the atmosphere can be controlled so that special clothing is not needed, but when outside humans need the protection of a space suit. Above about 60,000 ft, humans must wear space suits that supply oxygen for breathing and maintain a pressure around the body to keep body fluids from boiling.

During the Gemini program, when the first American stepped into space, oxygen was fed to the space suit by a 25-ft umbilical to a chest-mounted pressure regulator and ventilation assembly. For the Apollo missions, exploring the moon required independence from the spacecraft. A portable life-support system (PLSS), worn as a backpack, provided oxygen, filters for removing carbon dioxide, and cooling water, giving Apollo crewmen the independence they needed.

The PLSS supplied oxygen while circulating cooling water through a garment worn under the space suit. Lithium-hydroxide filters removed carbon dioxide from the crewman's exhaled breath, and charcoal and Orlon filters sifted out odors and foreign particles from the breathing oxygen. An emergency supply of oxygen was mounted atop the PLSS, together with communications equipment for talking with fellow crewmen on the lunar surface and with flight controllers in Houston. Additionally, the communications systems relayed back to Earth biomedical data on the crewmen.

The Apollo lunar surface space suit and PLSS weighed 180 lb on Earth, but only 30 lb on the moon because of the difference in gravity.

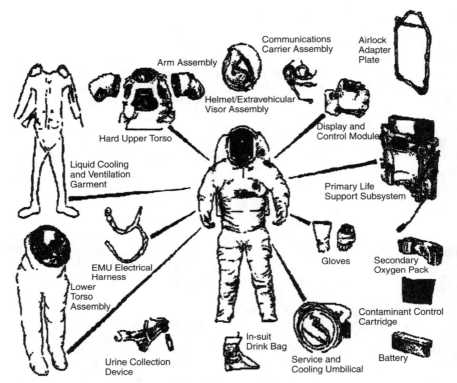

Figure C-2   Components of shuttle space suits.

Space Shuttle Space-Suit Design

Space suits used in the Apollo and Skylab programs were custom manufactured for a specific astronaut. Suits for the space shuttle[§§], however, are
composed of separate components that can be assembled to make space
suits to fit almost anyone. Several sizes of each component are manufactured and placed on the shelf for future use. Components are selected to
fit an astronaut's size and assembled into a complete space suit. Figure C.2
below provides a sketch of the various interchangeable parts.

Suits are approximately 3/16 in. thick, with 11 layers of materials
including orthofabric, aluminized Mylar®, neoprene-coated nylon,
Dacron®, urethane-coated nylon, tricot, nylon/spandex, stainless steel,
and high-strength composite materials. Suits are designed to last for up to
15 years and to be used on many missions. Suits are white to reflect heat
in space, where temperatures in direct sunlight in space can be over 275°F.
Because the shuttle suit is designed only to work in zero gravity, it can be

---

[§§]Data available online at http://history.nasa.gov/spacesuits.pdf.

much heavier than the Apollo suit, which, including the life-support backpack, weighed about 180 lb. The shuttle suit, including the life-support system, weighs about 310 lb. The suit itself weighs about 110 lb.

Once the astronaut is fitted, a training suit is assembled using duplicate sized components. The actual flight suit is assembled later using the same size components, and the astronaut will check out this suit during chamber testing and other test events. Just before a shuttle mission, the suits designated for flight are tested, cleaned, and stowed on the shuttle. After each flight the suits are returned to the contractor for postflight processing and reuse.

Astronauts have more than one wardrobe for spaceflight, and what they wear depends on the job they are doing. During ascent and entry, each crewmember wears special equipment consisting of a partial pressure suit, a parachute harness assembly, and a parachute pack. The suit, consisting of helmet, communication assembly, torso, gloves, and boots, provides pressure. This suit is designed to protect against exposure in the event that the crew must parachute from the shuttle.

Suits for Extravehicular Activity

The PLSS, when combined with the space suit, becomes the extravehicular mobility unit, or EMU. The PLSS consists of a backpack unit permanently mounted to the hard upper torso of the suit and a control-and-display unit mounted on the suit chest. The backpack unit supplies oxygen for breathing, suit pressurization, and ventilation. The unit also cools and circulates water used in the liquid-cooling ventilation garment, controls ventilation gas temperature, absorbs carbon dioxide, and removes odors from the suit atmosphere. The secondary oxygen pack attaches to the bottom of the PLSS and supplies oxygen if the primary oxygen fails. The control-and-display unit allows the crewmember to control and monitor the PLSS, the secondary oxygen pack, and, when attached, the manned maneuvering unit.

The manned maneuvering unit (MMU) is a one-man, nitrogen-propelled backpack that attaches to the space suit. Using hand controllers, the crewmember can fly with precision in or around the shuttle cargo bay or to nearby free-flying payloads or structures. Astronauts wearing MMUs have deployed, serviced, repaired, and retrieved satellite payloads.

The MMU propellant, consisting of noncontaminating gaseous nitrogen stored under high pressure, can be recharged from the shuttle. The reliability of the unit is guaranteed with a dual parallel system rather than a backup redundant system. In the event of a failure in one parallel system, the system would be shut down, and the remaining system would be used to return the MMU to the shuttle cargo bay.

During an EVA, the astronaut has about seven hours, plus or minus a half-hour, to complete his or her work. This time is dependent on the rate the astronaut is using the available air and water from the backpack. The harder the astronaut works the faster the air and water are used. The secondary air supply provides 30 min of air that can be used in an emergency to get the astronaut safely back inside the shuttle. There are nevertheless upgrades to the design of these suits as discussed next.

Future Space Suits

A new generation of spacesuits is under design for use during activity in space. The Mark III suit, a combination of hard and soft elements, is being developed at the NASA Johnson Space Center (JSC) in Houston, Texas. The AX-5, a hard, all-metal suit, is being developed by the NASA Ames Research Center (ARC) in California. Both suits are being designed to be easy to get into and out of, be comfortable to wear, allow adequate mobility and range of motion for the jobs to be performed, and fit different size astronauts.¶¶ In addition to the usual protection from radiation, micrometeoroids, and man-made debris, both suits have been designed to operate at a pressure of 8.3 psi. Current space shuttle space suits operate at 4.3 psi and require a time-consuming prebreathing operation prior to the beginning of any space walk or escape operation. Astronauts in the space station will be able to prepare for outside activity in much less time, and this would be critical in the event of an emergency escape maneuver.

NASA's JSC has also been exploring more flexible suits designed for Mars. Such a suit would be filled with biosensors that would provide constant feedback of an astronaut's vital signs to mission planners back on Earth. The suit would be mobile and lightweight, but yet able to provide mechanical counterpressure to offset the low atmospheric pressure on Mars. These suits would also include two-way audio and video capability.

A suit filled with biosensors would need a way of communicating all of the data it gathers. Researchers at NASA's Jet Propulsion Laboratory are working on a small, wearable communication device that could link biosensors, as well as chemical and radiation detectors, to a base station on Mars or even to Earth. These investigations include the possible use of wireless networking equipment that is also being provided to the public in commercial components, systems, and networks.*** Sensors have been used since the days of Mercury flights, when astronauts were connected to myriad electronic sensors to monitor their vital signs. Nanotechnology is being used to create biosensors that will make spacecraft like the space shuttle simpler, safer, and more efficient. Sensors can be shrunk to about $20\,\mu$, and astronauts could even swallow the inexpensive sensors [21].

¶¶Data available online at http://history.nasa.gov/spacesuits.pdf.
***Data available online at http://www.space.com/businesstechnology/technology/spacesuit_sensors_010827-1.html.

Escape from Shuttle

In the event that the crew must parachute from the shuttle, the space suit has inflatable bladders that fill it with oxygen from the shuttle. These bladders inflate automatically at reduced cabin pressure. They also can be manually inflated during entry to prevent the crewmember from blacking out. Without the suit pressing on the abdomen and the legs, the blood would pool in the lower part of the body and cause a person to black out as the spacecraft returns from microgravity to Earth's gravity. The partial-pressure suit and equipment will support a crewmember for a 24-h period in a life craft in case of an egress over water. Failure of the suit's inflatable bladders could jeopardize the life of a crewmember.

Effects of Nitrogen

Current-generation spacesuits for the space shuttle era are not highly pressurized. Before leaving the shuttle to perform tasks in space, an astronaut has to spend a period breathing pure oxygen before proceeding into space. This procedure is necessary to remove nitrogen dissolved in body fluids and thereby to prevent its release as gas bubbles when pressure is reduced, a condition commonly called "the bends." Prebreathing allows the astronaut's body to adapt to the difference in pressure between the spacecraft cabin and the suit. As just noted, the next generation of suits, by operating at a higher pressure and thus matching that of the space station, will reduce or eliminate the need for prebreathing and the threat of the bends.

Environmental Dangers

The space suit can at least to some degree protect the astronaut from deadly hazards. Besides providing protection from bombardment by micrometeoroids, the space suit insulates the wearer from the temperature extremes of space. Without the Earth's atmosphere to filter the sunlight, the side of the suit facing the sun can be heated to a temperature as high as 250°F; the other side, exposed to darkness of deep space, can get as cold as −250°F.

Clearly it is desirable to continue an active R&D program for space-suit development to support both the shuttle and the ISS. Research is particularly recommended for flexible suit systems, improved nitrogen/oxygen mixes, improved radiation and micrometeorite protection, and electronic sensors. This R&D should be pursued with the objective of implementation as soon as adequate testing of these systems is complete.

Review of Shuttle Thermal Protection System and Its In-Orbit Repair

The TPS is arguably the most important and yet most vulnerable element of the space shuttles. For the completion of a shuttle mission, the TPS is as crucial as other systems such as the avionics, structure, and propulsion because of its vital function of protecting the shuttle from temperatures as low as −250°F in orbit, to temperatures close to 3000°F during reentry. The crews' safety relies on the ability of the TPS to withstand such temperature ranges. Failure in any area can result in complete disintegration of the shuttle as seen in the *Columbia* disaster of February 2003. The TPS consists of approximately 24,000 tiles and 2300 flexible insulation blankets in a variety of sizes, shapes, thicknesses, and materials. Table C.5 outlines the approximate temperature capabilities and location on the shuttle of the different materials used in the TPS.

The tiles that make up the TPS are delicate and have to be protected from the stresses on the shuttle's structure during flight. During launch, the shuttle's overall structure bends and shifts from the aerodynamic forces, vibration, and acceleration.

While in orbit, the shuttle shrinks slightly because of the −250°F temperatures and reexpands during the heat of reentry. To prevent damage, the tiles are bonded with a silicone adhesive to strain isolator pads (SIP) of felt Nomex, which are in turn bonded to the shuttle's surface. The purpose of the SIP is to allow the tiles to "float" very slightly to limit damage during the stresses of launch and reentry. Despite these efforts, returning

Table C-5 Materials Used in TPS Systems, Capabilities, and Locations

Material	Maximum Surface Temperature, °F	Location on Shuttle
Felt reusable surface insulation (FRSI) blankets	350–700	Payload bay doors and inboard sections of upper wing surface
Low-temperature reusable surface insulation (LRSI)	700–1200	Upper surface of fuselage around cockpit
Advanced flexible reusable surface insulation (AFRSI)	700–1200	Majority of upper surface of shuttle
High-temperature reusable surface insulation (HRSI)	1200–2300	Lower surface, edges of vertical stabilizer, and around forward windows
Fibrous refractory composite insulation (FRCI)	1200–2300	Penetrations and leading-edge areas
Toughened unipiece fibrous insulation (TUFI)	1200–2300	Base heat shield (around engines) and upper body flap
Reinforced Carbon-Carbon (RCC)	2300–2960	Nose cone and wing leading edges

shuttles almost always have damaged or missing tiles. Damage can occur from a variety of sources throughout the mission such as ice and foam strikes during launch and meteoroids and orbital debris during orbit.

The amount of damaged/missing tiles is crucial to a safe reentry for the shuttle. Too large a breakdown in the integrity of the TPS will allow superheated air to affect the aluminum structure of the shuttle during reentry. This was displayed in the *Columbia* disaster of February 2003 where a piece of insulating foam that struck *Columbia* during launch was believed to have caused a breach in a reinforced carbon–carbon panel on the leading edge of the left wing. This breach allowed superheated air during reentry to weaken the structure resulting in failure of the wing and ultimately the breakup of the shuttle.

The vulnerability of the TPS is not only a result of the complexity of the system but also the maintenance required to upkeep its reliability. Each of the 24,000 plus tiles as well as the insulation blanket system must be manually checked to see if it is cracked or damaged. The adhesive bond of each tile is checked by a "wiggle" test, where the bond of the tile to the shuttle is checked to see if it would withstand launch and reentry. If a damaged tile is found, it either has to be patched or replaced with a one-of-a-kind numbered tile that is specifically shaped for that position on the shuttle. This wiggle test that is carried out by a crew of six is highly subjective and can lead to errors of judgment and certainly adds greatly to the cost of the program because there is a tendency to use an abundance of caution. The installation of the tile itself leads to many vulnerabilities. It was found in formal review processes, as reported in the articles cited next, that installers in some instance had used saliva spit on the bonding surface to speed up the epoxy adhesion process—a dangerous act that reportedly can weaken the longer-term holding power of the epoxy [22].

The TPS also has to be rewaterproofed after each flight because of the waterproofing material burning off at a temperature of 1100°F. Without the waterproofing the TPS could be exposed to water absorption that again could affect its integrity. The fact that these processes rely mostly on human interpretation increases the susceptibility of the TPS. The lack of a foolproof method of tile repair and reinstallation has been a leading safety concern for the life of the space shuttle program largely because the process must be done largely by hand. With tens of thousands of tiles to handle and reinstall, the hazard factor associated with this reconditioning process is enormous.

In 1980, prior to the first shuttle launch, NASA Administrator Robert Frosch addressed top NASA officials about the problems with the thermal protection system and the possibility of developing a tile repair kit for astronauts. A quarter of a century later the feasibility of such repair in space remains elusive although progress is being made in this respect [6,7].

As of July 2004, NASA reported that its latest attempt to devise in-orbit repair capabilities might allow holes, cracks, or gouges in the shuttle wings as large as 4 in. in size to be addressed while docked to the ISS, but large-scale problems could still not be addressed. Further, if in-orbit repairs required very extended EVAs then the risk of the repair activity would itself become a safety issue [23,24]. Although the tile configuration of the TPS requires such stringent maintenance, it has shown its effectiveness over the past 23 years. NASA is investigating the composition of future TPS for possible shuttle improvements or a completely new reusable launch vehicle (RLV).

NASA researchers are developing a new adaptable, robust, metallic, operable, reusable (ARMOR) TPS, as a potential system for future NASA spacecraft. The ARMOR TPS promises a greater level of safety as it has similar thermal capabilities to ceramic tiles and it reduces the amount of maintenance required to keep the TPS intact. ARMOR panels are larger than the ceramic tiles, do not require waterproofing, and attach directly to the underlying structure by means of mechanical fasteners. This reduces the complexity of the TPS because it is easier to inspect/replace the smaller quantity of panels. At present however these panels still weigh more than current tiles, and there are no plans to use this technology on the space shuttle.

Advanced ceramics, improved thermal blankets, and "hot" structures are also being looked at to increase the effectiveness and safety of future RLV TPS. Even more advanced metallic thermal protection systems have been developed and appear to be very promising.

In-Orbit Repair

In the wake of the *Columbia* disaster, in-orbit repair of the shuttle TPS has become a major focus in returning the shuttle to flight status. The future of the shuttle program could rely on the ability to inspect and repair the TPS, both in orbit and when docked with the ISS. Reliable techniques are needed for inspecting the TPS for damage, gaining access to all possible damage sites, and perfecting tools and materials needed to patch over cracked, eroded, or missing tiles. The *Columbia* Accident Investigation Board addressed the subject of inspection and repair of the shuttle's thermal protection system. Their observations included the following:

1) For non-Station missions, develop a comprehensive autonomous (independent of ISS) inspection and repair capability to cover the widest possible range of damage scenarios.

2) Accomplish an in-orbit thermal protection system inspection, using appropriate assets and capabilities, early in all missions.

3) The ultimate objective should be a fully autonomous capability for all missions to address the possibility that an ISS mission fails to achieve the correct orbit, fails to dock successfully, or is damaged during or after undocking.

NASA's in-orbit repair strategy began to emerge after STS-107 and includes at least the following considerations: defining the critical damage size, that is, the damage threshold that would trigger some sort of space-walk inspection and/or repair attempt; techniques for inspecting a shuttle for damage; the materials and tools needed to repair such damage; and the space-walk access required to implement any such repairs. Subsequently this approach to in-orbit fault detection and repair has been further refined, based on the CAIB findings.

There are now various ways that the shuttle can be examined for damage. The use of spy satellites or other imaging systems to view shuttles in orbit could help assess damage before attempting reentry. If such methods had been adopted on the 2003 flight, the extent of damage to Columbia's leading edge might have been assessed and possible alternative plans made for the return of the crew. The remote manipulator system (RMS) has been used in the past to obtain an external view of the shuttle by having a camera attached to the end and steered to see certain parts of the vehicle. Unfortunately Columbia was without the RMS during its critical last mission, and, even if it had been installed, its ability to view out-of-the-way locations such as the underside of the wing is restricted. The use of astronauts' EVA is another option to inspect and repair the shuttle in orbit, but this was not done either.

In the near term, missions to the ISS will require approaching space shuttles to perform a pirouette maneuver approximately 400 ft below the station. This will allow the ISS crew to take photographs of the shuttle's underside with telephoto lenses. Once docked, cameras on the shuttle's RMS and the station's mobile Canadarm2 should provide coverage needed to spot any significant damage. The critical factor of determining the depth of any tile damage might not be possible without a space-walk inspection or development of some new scanning technology. Powerful spy satellites can also be used to detect problems with the shuttle as recommended by the CAIB, but their accuracy in terms of damage detection is unknown at this stage.

Engineers have not yet settled on what sort of caulk-like patch material is best suited for repairing broad areas of tile damage. Issues include the viscosity of the material, which astronauts must be able to apply and then spread or mold to some degree, and the time needed for any such material to cure. Tests will also be required to ensure any such material can stand up to worst-case reentry temperatures and conditions. Techniques for repairing damage to a shuttle's RCC panels pose a much more difficult challenge and will take longer to develop. The panels play a critical role in the creation of a boundary layer as the shuttle reenters through the region of maximum heating. The boundary layer provides a natural insulating effect, limiting entry temperatures to under 3000°F. Any repair option would have to not just plug a breach but also ensure the smooth airflow needed to set up an insulating boundary layer.

These techniques can only be used for missions servicing the ISS at this time. Hubble servicing mission 4, originally scheduled for 2005, has been cancelled as in-orbit repair away from the ISS has been designated by the NASA administrator during 2004 as being too dangerous, despite National Academy of Sciences' advice to the contrary. If the Hubble repair mission continues on the basis of using robotic devices for this mission, the technology could conceivably be applied to future repair capabilities related to either the space shuttle or the ISS, but this remains a number of years away from any practical application.

One system, AERCam-SPRINT, has already been tested in 1997 on shuttle mission STS-87. AERCam (autonomous extravehicular robotic camera) is a small, hand-deployed, and captured remote-controlled inspection tool. It carries its own avionics and nitrogen-gas propulsion. The surface of the ball-shaped robot is covered with cushions to prevent damage in case of collisions with other space hardware. It weighs a little less than 38 lb, and is outfitted with two cameras, position lights, and a floodlight. The AERCam is designed to fly very slowly, just less than ¼ ft/s. Although its flight was restricted to the cargo bay during flight STS-87, the AERCam demonstrated that free-flying cameras can be easily controlled and provide detailed external views of the shuttle. David Akin, a leading space robotic expert at the University of Maryland in College Park, said, "There are concerns about loss of signal...but with some modifications to the shuttle communications systems, or better placement of dedicated antennas, it should be possible to do remotely-controlled close inspections of the tiles."[+++] With continued research and development it might be possible that a system like AERCam could be equipped to spray-in-place ablative materials, but whether this might be used for actual shuttle repair cannot be clearly answered at this time.

The capability to repair damaged tiles in orbit will dramatically increase the safety of a shuttle mission. The integrity of the shuttle's TPS will be able to be determined before attempting reentry. If effective, this should significantly reduce the possibility of the TPS failing during reentry.

Vulnerabilities During Reentry

The *Columbia* disaster on STS-107 took place during the reentry of the shuttle. The *Columbia* Accident Investigation Board reported the physical cause of the accident as follows: a piece of insulating foam that came from the left bipod ramp of the external tank struck the carbon–carbon panels of the left wing of the shuttle. This resulted in a breach of the thermal protection system that allowed superheated air to penetrate and melt the aluminum structure of the left wing leading to the breakup of the shuttle [6, p. 49]. This disaster took place during reentry, but the events that led to the breach of the thermal protection system took place 81.9 s after liftoff. This underscores the possibility that the vulnerabilities which exist during any phase of a shuttle mission might very well have had its cause originate in an earlier phase of the mission.

The preceding section presented information about vulnerabilities with respect to the heat shield and the thermal protection system. In short, the integrity of the heat shield is critical during the reentry of the shuttle as temperatures reach super hot levels, and this represents the primary vulnerability during this phase of the mission. Thus the protection of the

---

[+++]Interview of Professor David Akin, University of Maryland, by Peter MacDaron, Jan. 11, 2005.

heat shield during the preceding mission phase is critical to reducing the vulnerabilities to the shuttle during reentry.

The process of reentry begins when the shuttle is rotated to a nose-first position. The orbiter is positioned differently when in orbit to avoid the possibility of space debris hitting the cabin or leading edges of the wing [6, p. 3]. The OMS and RCS are used to make the attitudinal adjustments to prepare for reentry. The shuttle then flips over to enter the atmosphere wings up. Before the entry interface, leftover fuel is burned from the RCS engine, as this area will encounter an enormous amount of heat during reentry. The shuttle's descent through the atmosphere is controlled by the OMS system until the flight-control surfaces become effective. The shuttle reentry is primarily computer controlled [6, pp. 63–67]. Because the system is computer controlled, the software flying the vehicle is a source of potential vulnerability.

The shuttle's approach for landing begins at 10,000 ft and Mach 9. The approach is controlled by the guidance system using the TACAN and MSBLS subsystems. The primary vulnerabilities that exist at landing are damage to the tires/wheels, execution of a change in landing site, or delays caused by weather.

While *Columbia* was in orbit, the damage to the left wing caused by the foam strike was being analyzed. After the debris analysis team concluded the strike was not a safety risk to flight, engineers considered the possibility of landing-gear damage that could result if the gear doors were damaged from the foam strike. When referring to two engineers who were considering possible scenarios that could result if the landing gear were damaged, the CAIB report states, "Both engineers felt that the potential ramifications of landing with two flat tires had not been sufficiently explored." To address this, a simulation was performed at Ames Research Center, and the tests concluded that it was a "survivable but very serious malfunction." In the initial considerations of a bailout vs a belly landing, Bob Daugherty, the engineer who performed the simulation, said the following in an e-mail: "Think about the pitch-down moment for a belly landing when hitting not the main gear but the trailing edge of the wing or body flap when landing gear up...even if you come in fast and at slightly less pitch attitude...the nose slap down with that pitching moment arm seems to me to be pretty scary...so much so that I would bail out before I would let a loved one land like that" [6, p. 164]. All of the options in the case of two flat tires pose a serious vulnerability to the crew.

If the primary landing location at Kennedy Space Center is not available because the weather there is below NASA guidelines, the shuttle can then either divert to Andrews Air Force Base in California or remain in orbit until the weather meets the landing requirements. If the shuttle is kept in orbit, there are extra fuel and supplies onboard to last several days past the planned date of reentry.

If a serious anomaly occurs during the shuttle's launch, then one of several abort sites can be used to land the shuttle, depending upon where in the ascent the problem occurred. The options are as follows: 1) return to launch site, 2) East Coast abort landing, 3) transoceanic abort landing, 4) abort once around, and 5) abort to orbit. The weather at these landing sites is checked to be within guidelines, and the sites are staffed by NASA, contractor, and DOD personnel [25]. Certainly a serious vulnerability to the shuttle can occur in the case of an anomaly during ascent in the sense that the failed component itself could interfere with the glide to landing.

Vulnerabilities at Touchdown and the Shuttle Braking System

The most perilous part of the shuttle's return to Earth is caused by extreme heating to temperatures in the range of 2000–3000°F created by friction against the atmosphere. These issues are addressed in the preceding section on reentry and the section on the shuttle's thermal protection system. There remain risk issues even after orbital reentry for a lifting body without active control capability. These risk elements include atmospheric conditions during reentry and landing, the parachute system, and the active braking capability.

It remains quite important that shuttle touchdowns occur during reasonably calm atmospheric conditions, that the deployment mechanism for the parachutes be carefully checked for each mission, and that margin is maintained so that all parachutes need not deploy to allow the shuttle to come to a safe stop. The most serious difficulty recently noted is with the shuttle braking system. This problem is addressed next, but its serious implication is that inadequate x-ray screening of the shuttle has been carried out for some time. This x-ray screening has far wider implications and remains an "alarm signal" as to the quality of NASA refurbishment and testing processes for the entire program.

In the early part of 2004, a serious problem was discovered in the braking system on the space shuttle *Discovery*. Some gears situated in one of four actuators used to move the two-part rudder on the *Discovery* were found by x-ray examination to have been improperly installed at the time of original manufacture. During return-to-flight checks, NASA engineers discovered that one gear in the actuator was installed backward. These gears are only slightly asymmetric, and as a result they are able to fit into the actuator assembly both ways. When installed incorrectly, the actuators would not be able to withstand the excessively high forces experienced by some sections of the rudder; however, it just so happened that the faulty actuators were not installed in these sections. A failure of the actuator would lead to the rudder being jammed, and this could lead to serious consequences in the landing process.

NASA has since removed four spare actuators it had installed in *Discovery's* rudder and found that another actuator also had its gear installed backward. They have launched an investigation into why the critical equipment had never been examined despite major overhauls every three to four years. New actuators for the entire fleet have been ordered from the manufacturer, Hamilton Sundstrand Space Systems. Currently the new actuators are now being installed, and the status of this work can be found on the NASA Web site.

Perhaps the most serious issue remaining is why postflight checkout of shuttle systems after each flight would not have detected such a problem in the braking system on the *Discovery* many years ago?

No further safety upgrades appear necessary in this area based on the GW team review. Nevertheless, one of the tasks that the new NASA Engineering and Safety Center (NESC/ITA) should be assigned is a review of postflight checkout procedures including the more extensive use of x-ray and other sensing technologies to detect safety problems and hazards before relaunch. This review should include not only the review and test procedures themselves but also the development of a detailed management checklist review of all procedures and activities. The update of quality control and verification procedures for the refurbishment and retrofit of the space shuttle as well as the training and management procedures for shuttle restoration seem as important as the physical improvements to the shuttle recommended by the CAIB. Finally in the design of future systems care should be taken to avoid some of the installation, detection, and maintenance problems encountered with the shuttle.

Fuel Tank Vulnerabilities

The space transportation system design includes solid-fuel rockets plus liquid-hydrogen and oxygen-driven motors. The solid rocket system was initially chosen because of its reliability, but these systems once ignited cannot be turned off or shut down. Further, there have been many changes and consolidations in the suppliers of solid-fuel rockets over the last 40 years. With the most recent consolidations, only two suppliers of solid-fuel rockets remain in the United States.

The liquid rocket system was chosen for the orbiter when it was originally designed because these rocket systems are reusable, throttleable, and can be shut off on command. The problem is that both liquid hydrogen and liquid oxygen are very hard to maintain in a steady state because of the need for cryogenic cooling. For this reason leakage from the tanks is very difficult to control. There have been at least two launches where fuel leaks have occurred in the orbiter. Further, the O-ring problem with the solid rocket booster for the *Challenger* resulted in catastrophic failure, and the foam insulation from the SRB also was the cause of the *Columbia* failure. Although there have been many improvements in the H_2-O_2 engines since the original shuttle motors were designed, the fuel tanks, fuel pumps, and especially the seals that prevent leakage of the cryogenic fuels remain of concern with regard to the safety of the shuttle system.

The interview process, which has involved talking to several dozen selected individuals with in-depth space backgrounds, has found that virtually everyone consulted believes that it is not possible to design a "total mission escape" capability for the shuttle system. This is especially true during liftoff where solid rockets with continuous burn are present. Those consulted believe that the current H_2-O_2 fuel tanks, fuel pumps, and fuel line seals constitute a higher level of risk than should be present in a 21st-century human-rated launch system. Further there is the belief that SRBs should not be used in future systems because of the inability to shut down the system or provide escape capabilities during liftoff without fundamental design innovations.

Escape Planning for the Space Shuttle in the Pre-Challenger Era

Early designs of the space shuttle assumed that it would be operational much like a commercial airliner, so that a shuttle crew escape system was considered unnecessary. From the initial design stages, however, the space shuttle was designed to provide a complete rescue capability for stranded astronauts. This included sufficient cabin space to allow the rescue up to seven stranded members of the crew. Because rapid response of the rescuing vehicle is essential for a rescue mission, it was initially thought it that it might be able to launch a second shuttle within 24 h of notification. In the popular image presented to the public in such media as the James Bond movie *Moonraker*, this concept of rapid liftoff and ultrareliable operation was widely accepted.

Rescue of stranded astronauts in space is still a possibility and can be accomplished via the docking of two space shuttles with crew transfer accomplished in a pressure-controlled environment, or if docking is not possible, transfer is done using EMUs [9]. But even from the first test flights, NASA has been exploring other crew escape options. Crew ejection seats, crew extraction systems, and a crew compartment/capsule escape system have been considered. Although crew escape systems have been discussed and studied continuously since the shuttle's early design phases, only two systems have been incorporated: one for the developmental test flights and the second current system installed after the *Challenger* accident. Both designs have extremely limited capabilities, and neither has ever been used during a mission [6].

The first design for rapid emergency egress of the crew used ejection seats for the two pilot positions. These ejection seats were installed on the shuttle test vehicle *Enterprise* and tested in 1977 ([19] found in [6]). The same system was installed on *Columbia* and used for the four orbital test flights during 1981–1982. Even though this system was designed for use during first-stage ascent and in gliding flight below 100,000 ft, there was considerable doubt about the survivability of an ejection that would expose crewmembers to the solid-rocket-booster exhaust plume. After the developmental test-flight phase was completed with STS-4, *Columbia*'s fourth flight, the ejection seat system was deactivated. All space shuttle missions after STS-4 were conducted with crews of four or more, and no escape system was installed until after the loss of *Challenger* in 1986.

Post-Challenger

The fact that a crew escape system was not included in the shuttle design was severely criticized after the loss of *Challenger*. The Rogers commission ([20] found in [6]) recommended that NASA "make all efforts to provide a crew-escape system for use during controlled gliding flight" and "make every effort to increase the range of flight conditions under which an emergency runway landing can be successfully conducted in the event that two or three main engines fail early in ascent."

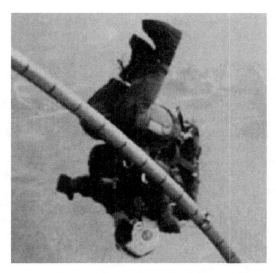

Figure C-3   Demonstration of the pole bailout system.

In response to these recommendations, NASA developed a second escape system, the current "pole bailout"system for use during controlled, subsonic gliding flight (see Fig. C.3). The system requires crew members to vent the cabin at 40,000 ft (to equalize the cabin pressure with the pressure at that altitude), jettison the hatch at approximately 32,000 ft, and then jump out of the vehicle. The pole allows crew members to avoid striking the shuttle's wings.

In April 2002, the Aerospace Safety Advisory Panel (ASAP) reported to NASA that "a satisfactory crew escape system could be a major source of risk reduction if the space shuttle is to be flown for an extended number of years [22]."

To date, no truly viable launch-to-land escape system is available for the space shuttle and our team interview process identifies this as a major ongoing safety concern.

Vulnerabilities in the Electrical Power System and Environmental Control and Life-Support System

The ability for astronauts to survive and operate the space shuttle during a mission is the result of the electrical power system (EPS) and the environmental control and life-support system (ECLSS). These systems provide the flight crew with a habitable environment and the power required to complete their mission. They have proved highly reliable in the past, but failure could result in lack of power, water, temperature control, or breathable air within the shuttle, which could have devastating consequences.

A failure in a fuel cell led to the emergency return of Apollo 13 to Earth because of an inadequate oxygen supply. Most recently in early September 2004 the main oxygen generator for the ISS failed because of a blockage in the generator lines. Clearly, careful review of oxygen generator safety needs to be maintained although the shuttle system is different from the Russian-designed system onboard the ISS [26].

The EPS consists of three subsystems: power reactant storage and distribution (PRSD), fuels cells, and electrical power distribution and control (EPDC). The PRSD subsystem stores cryogenic hydrogen and oxygen in supercritical conditions in double-walled, thermally insulated spherical tanks in the midfuselage of the shuttle. It then supplies these reactants to the three fuel cells, which through an electrochemical reaction generates all onboard electrical power from launch until landing. Heat and water are produced as byproducts of this electrical power generation, and thus this process supplies temperature control and usable water to the shuttle's crew. The generated electrical power is controlled by the EPDC and distributed to all of the shuttle systems necessary for successful completion of the mission, including the solid rocket boosters and external tank during launch.

ECLSS maintains the livable conditions for the crew within the shuttle. It controls all aspects required to keep the astronauts alive and comfortable. Breathable air, carbon-dioxide levels, pressurization, temperature control, and water supply and regeneration are all controlled by the ECLSS.

The safety and reliability of these systems are of great importance. They have many redundancies built in that allow the systems to keep operating effectively in the event of minor failures. For example, a single fuel cell is sufficient to provide enough power and resources to insure safe vehicle return for the shuttle. The resultant safety concern is therefore minor because of the demonstrated reliability of the system with over 99.99% availability being demonstrated for each of the three cells. However, the upkeep for these highly reliable fuel cells cost approximately $15 million per year at present for maintenance and repair, and unfortunately these fuel cells do not currently live up to their proposed operational life. Two distinct upgrades are being considered to replace the current cells—longer-life alkaline and proton-exchange-membrane (PEM) fuel cells. Longer-life alkalines are similar to the current fuel cells except that they would operate at reduced reactant temperatures and would be designed to resist corrosion and improve reliability. PEM fuel cells use a moist polymer membrane as the electrolyte in the electrochemical reaction. The benefits of the PEM cells could include large savings in operations costs, improvements in safety through the use of nontoxic electrolytes, and an increase in power for the shuttle. However, the PEM cell upgrade would require an expensive and potentially open-ended technology research program and might pose a slightly increased risk of failure to the shuttle until significant flight hours have been logged by the new powerplant.

Onboard sensors constantly check and display life-support system vitals to both the crew of the shuttle and NASA personnel back on Earth. This allows any factors that could jeopardize the safety of the crew to be recognized early and hopefully solved before it escalates into a hazardous situation.

NASA delayed the launch of the *Endeavor* STS-113 in November 2002 because of a detected leak in the system that sends oxygen to the space suits worn by astronauts during launch and reentry. This leak was fixed before launch, but if the problem had arisen after launch the shuttle's breathing air supply could have been affected and thus would have led to safety concerns for the crew. It is such occurrences that indicate remaining serious concerns of these power and environmental control systems.

The greatest problems with environmental control systems or power systems actually apply to the ISS rather than the space shuttle. As improvements to the environmental control systems for the ISS are developed, these should be also applied to the shuttle to the maximum extent possible.

Propulsion

The propulsion system of the shuttle comprises the space shuttle main engines (SSME), solid rocket boosters (SRB), the orbital maneuvering system (OMS), and the reaction control system (RCS). The three SSMEs and two SRBs are used to launch the shuttle into low Earth orbit before the OMS inserts the shuttle into the correct orbit. The OMS and RCS were discussed earlier in the context of docking maneuvers and docking safety and will not be addressed further here.

The space shuttle main engine is the most advanced liquid-fueled rocket engine ever built. Its main features are variable thrust, high performance, reusability, and total redundancy. Safety concerns arise with the SSME because of the sheer complexity of the engine that took over 10 years to develop and also because the engine requires the use of volatile cryogenic fuels. Liquid oxygen has to be kept at temperatures below $-298°F$ to avoid returning to a gaseous form, whereas liquid hydrogen has to be kept below $-423°F$. This makes both the liquid oxygen and liquid hydrogen quite difficult to store over long periods of time.

The SSMEs were developed in the 1970s and are constantly being upgraded to increase their safety and reliability. One such upgrade is the incorporation of the large throat main combustion chamber (LTMCC) to further improve the reliability of the engines by reducing the system operating pressures and temperatures. George Hopson, manager of the space shuttle main engine project at Marshall said, "With this design change, we believe we have more than doubled the reliability of the engine." NASA has also been investigating a new channel-wall nozzle to replace the current nozzle that has far fewer parts and welds. This will reduce the complexity and vulnerability of the engine. As with the channel-wall nozzle, a second cooling apparatus could be upgraded. The water membrane evaporator is being considered as a replacement for the shuttle's flash evaporator system, which cools the shuttle during launch and reentry and also provides supplemental cooling in orbit. The current flash evaporator is experiencing corrosion, which creates a risk of freon leaks.

Upgrades such as these will continue to increase the reliability and safety of the SSMEs.

The two SRBs used during launch consist of four segments filled with a mixture of solid-form chemicals that burn at a rapid rate, expelling hot gases from a nozzle to achieve thrust. Solid propellants as used in the SRBs are stable and can be easily stored making them much safer than liquid rockets before launch. Safety concerns arise however as once the SRBs are ignited they will burn until all propellant is exhausted. This is a large vulnerability to the safety of the shuttle as the SRBs cannot be throttled or turned off during launch. NASA is investigating the addition of a fifth segment to the SRB that would modify the nozzle and insulation and alter the grain of the solid fuel to provide a more risk-tolerant thrust profile. The use of liquid boosters has also been considered as a possible upgrade to the two SRBs. NASA estimates a proposed liquid fly-back booster (LFBB) will experience a catastrophic failure every 1520 launches, which is an unprecedented level of reliability for a new, highly complex booster. NASA, however, has no plans at this time to replace the SRB on the shuttle at this time.

Auxiliary Power Unit

Each shuttle has three APUs, which are used to power the vehicle's hydraulics during launch and reentry. The APUs use hydrazine propellant to drive a high-speed turbine that produces hydraulic power. However, the hydrazine fuel is toxic. Further, during the *Columbia* mission STS-9 in 1983, two out of the three APUs caught fire during landing. NASA is studying an electric system to replace the APUs that would include ultracapacitors and batteries to provide energy storage and power supply. These systems would be less toxic and reduce the risk using hazardous fuels. Again budget limitations would appear to limit the introduction of these innovations even though these systems might prove to be vital to the safe completion of a shuttle mission. Continued inspection, maintenance, and upgrades of the existing APUs will reduce the susceptibility of these systems to failure and ultimately make the shuttle missions safer. Replacement of the APUs as soon as possible would appear to be highly desirable. A NASA report on the feasibility of such APU replacement is considered to be of importance to an overall shuttle safety review.

Computer and Software Vulnerability

The space shuttle is a fly-by-wire vehicle with redundant computer systems and extremely sophisticated software capable of entirely controlling the shuttle during many phases of a mission. The computer can do so, for example, during reentry and ascent. The critical element of mission operation where fly by wire is currently not available is during docking and separation operations.

Five general-purpose computers (GPCs) control the shuttle's data-processing system. These computers vote to determine if one has failed and provide redundancy in case of a failure. Four of the five computers run the primary avionics software set (PASS), and the fifth is a backup flight system (BFS) capable of performing most of the important functions of PASS. Two magnetic tape mass memory units (MMU) store the large amounts of data produced during a mission, and a computer data bus network allows for serial digital communication to systems on the shuttle and back to the GPCs.[†††]

PASS is composed of the operating system software and the application software, which are capable of controlling the shuttle and are divided into operation sequences that control different phases of the mission. The application software is divided into overlays and loaded from the MMUs when the phase of flight it controls is reached. The software is written in high-order assembly language (HAL/S), which is a language specifically designed for real-time flight control software.[†††]

From this brief description of the flight computers, it can be seen that there is enormous complexity to this system, and the software controlling it is a source of vulnerability for shuttle missions. The following section will briefly discuss the software development process, sources of software errors, and incidents of software malfunctions that can or have previously created safety hazards during a mission. Also there will be some consideration of the security of the software system with respect to possible hacker attacks or intrusion on ground station computers. Next, this section will discuss the shuttle's communications and navigation system hardware and review incidents of failures within each system.

In January 1992 the Aeronautics and Space Engineering Board (ASEB) assembled a committee to review the space shuttle software development process, from initial requirements to the final stages of loading the object code onto the GPCs. The findings of this committee were presented in an ASEB report entitled *"An Assessment of space shuttle Flight Software Development Processes* [27]." The committee was initially charged with determining whether the independent software verification and validation process (IV&V) being used by NASA should continue (in addition to the embedded V&V process done by NASA and its development contractors). The report defines the objectives of IV&V as follows: 1) "demonstrating the technical correctness, including safety and security, of the system/software"; 2) "assessing the overall quality of the system/software products"; and 3) "ensuring compliance with the development process standards" [27, p. 29].

The committee recommended that NASA should continue the IV&V process because it believed that such an independent check is necessary to maintain NASA's quality and safety requirements [27, p. 17]. IV&V certainly aids in the process of developing safe software in a complex

---

[†††]Data available online at http://science.ksc.nasa.gov/Shuttle/technology/sts-newsref/stsref-toc.html.

development process. Figure C.4 outlines the software development process for a single operational sequence, which underscores the complexity involved.

In addition to the preceding recommendation, the committee's report defines the two ways a software problem can affect the safety of the shuttle system it is controlling: 1) "the software can fail to recognize or properly handle a hardware failure that it is required to control," and 2) "the software can issue incorrect or untimely outputs that contribute to the system reaching a hazardous state" [27, p. 63]. The source of these errors that can lead to hazardous system operation can be logic errors in the software. Logic errors occur when either the requirements definition is incorrect, but the implementation of the requirements is correct, or when the requirements definition is correct, but the implementation of them is not [27 p. 64].

There are three approaches that could be applied to deal with software errors. The first is to have a correct requirements definition and a correct implementation of them. The second is to use redundancy. This is already accomplished in the shuttle, which uses the five GPCs as just described, and the BFS uses a different version of the software. The third method is to follow

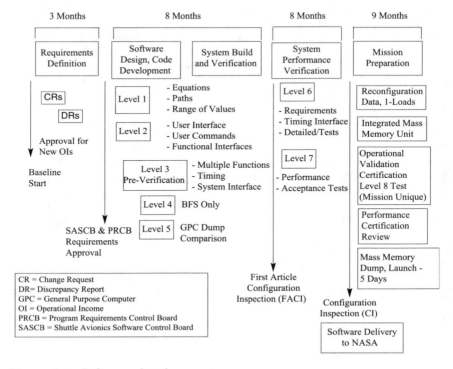

Figure C-4   Software development process.

the system-safety engineering approach. This is done by identifying potential system hazards and placing the software module in control and the requirements definition used in its creation under special analysis. This approach also uses software fail-safe mechanisms to attempt to generalize failures in order to handle ones that might not have been foreseen [27, pp. 64, 65].

Some software errors, for instance, were detected during the prelaunch inspections on STS-78. An unusual reading from one of the master event controllers (MEC) was detected the day before the scheduled launch. The MEC has many important functions including the arming and ignition of pyrotechnics to separate the SRBs and the external tank from the shuttle. Software errors were determined to be the cause, and after being analyzed they were found to be not critical to the mission. Software errors or computer hardware failure can in many instances trigger category one failures. This is because processors at one time or another control virtually all of the critical aspects of a space shuttle mission; thus, software problems need to be seen as vital infrastructure whose functions must be constantly monitored and reviewed. This means that any upgrade or change to software must always be checked and double checked.

Communications Subsystem Vulnerability

The shuttle's communications system is made up of the following primary subsystems: S-band system, Ku-band and UHF system, payload communications system, and an audio system. As the following examples will show, these subsystems are vulnerable to hardware failures.

On two separate missions aboard the *Discovery*, the Ku-band communications system failed. In June of 1998, *Discovery* was on its way to docking with the Space Station *Mir*. The shuttle lost the ability to transfer high rates of information as well as TV pictures to document the docking operation with Mir [28].

The Ku-band system also acts as a rendezvous radar system during docking operations. On this mission the radar system continued to function. Another Ku-band failure occurred in October 2000, also aboard the *Discovery*. The shuttle was preparing to dock with the ISS when the Ku-band system failed. During this anomaly, the rendezvous radar system as well as communications through the subsystem were affected. The shuttle was still able to accomplish the docking operation using laser range finders and star trackers, but this made the process more complex and certainly raised the risk level for this operation because the shuttle's commander had to use the laser range finder to orient the shuttle during docking.‡‡‡ The space shuttle navigation system is made up of three inertial measurement units (IMUs), three tactical air navigation units (TACAN), two air data probes, a microwave scan beam landing system

---

‡‡‡Data available online of http://spaceflightnow.com/Shuttle/ sts092/001011kuband/.

(MSBLS), a star tracker system, and two radar altimeters.§§§ The three
IMUs provide inertial attitude and velocity data to the navigation control
software onboard the shuttle. The three TACANs provide the bearing of
the shuttle to a TACAN VOR station. This system is used to navigate to
the landing site during reentry. The MSBLS is used on final approach to
the landing site. The air data system provides information on the move-
ment of the shuttle in the atmosphere to be used during reentry once
flight in the atmosphere has been established. It is stowed during other
phases of the mission to be protected by heat shields. The star trackers
provide navigation information during rendezvous if needed. The star
trackers also provide information to collaborate the three IMUs, and the
radar altimeter provides the AGL altitude data. Any of the just-described
subsystems are vulnerable to hardware failures as well. When a hardware
failure does occur, it can be difficult to determine which component failed
while in orbit. In December of 2001, one of the IMUs aboard *Endeavor*
failed while the shuttle was docked to the ISS. The operation of the unit
was restored within 45 min of its failure. However it was still labeled as a
failed unit because the reason for its failure could not be determined at the
time.¶¶¶

NASA flight rules state that if two IMUs fail special precautions must
be taken. In this case, although the safety of the *Endeavor* or ISS crew was
not at risk, further IMU failures could have posed a risk to the reentry
phase of the mission.

One of the current strengths of shuttle safety in terms of crew training
for operation is the shuttle Avionics Integration Laboratory (SAIL). This
training and testing lab features a complete set of shuttle avionics. This
allows for end-to-end testing and verification of shuttle software for all
missions. SAIL contains a crew cockpit and is treated as a fourth orbiter
with respect to all avionics and software changes.

Computer and Communications Security

The number of cyber attacks has grown considerably over the past few
years. This affects the shuttle because it is a vehicle largely controlled by
computers. The intended interference with either the software onboard
the vehicle or the software controlling various ground monitoring and
command activities poses a risk to the safe operation of the shuttle. In
September 1997 a hacker disrupted communications during a mission.
This was accomplished by attacking a computer on the ground at a NASA
location that was communicating with the shuttle. The communications
were only disrupted momentarily, and the safety of the shuttle was not

---

§§§Data available online of http://science.ksc.nasa.gov/Shuttle/technology/
sts-newsref/stsref-toc.html.
¶¶¶Data available online at http://www.space.com/missionlaunches/
sts108_imu_011213.html.

compromised in this situation because NASA was able to transfer almost immediately to a backup communications channel.

NASA made the following two statements on the incident:

1) "The transmission of routine medical information was slightly delayed due to a computer hacker. However, the transmission was successfully completed."
2) "At no time was communication between NASA and the astronauts compromised. The communication interruption occurred between internal ground-based computer systems."[****]

Although the safety of the astronauts was not compromised in this situation, it does serve to highlight that the security of the systems on the ground communicating with the shuttle, as well as the shuttle's system itself, requires high-level security measures to ensure uninterrupted communications.[††††]

Space Navigation Systems and GPS Applications

Because of the intrinsic worldwide coverage of the global positioning system (GPS), it is logical to implement GPS-based tracking and navigation architecture in order to support human spaceflight. However, experience with GPS in this arena is somewhat limited and lacks the sort of high-accuracy performance in space that is available in the terrestrial environment. Basically, there are only two GPS-based navigation systems with a history in NASA crew-based spaceflight; they are the Rockwell International Miniature Airborne GPS Receiver/Shuttle (MAGR/S) and the Honeywell Space Integrated GPS Inertial (SIGI) system (Fig. C.5).

The most advanced GPS system is the SIGI, which is considered to be a commercial-off-the-shelf (COTS) space-rated receiver. NASA has accepted this integrated inertial/GPS receiver as being operational for human spaceflight. The SIGI GPS Y-code subsystem is structured around a military Trimble Navigation Force 5 precise positioning service (PPS) receiver.

According to an unofficial NASA source we interviewed, but requested not to be identified, the only completely successful experience with SIGI has been limited to altitude regimes of 15.2 to 30.4 km (50,000 to 100,000 ft) (see Fig. C-5). In-orbit performance (at 300 to 550 km altitudes) has been less precise, and tracking data through reentry conditions are not available to our study team. The detailed engineering experience with the SIGI derives to large degree from the tests with the now-cancelled NASA

[****]Data available online at http://www.cnn.com/2000/TECH/space/07/03/nasa.hacker.02.
[††††]Data available online at http://science.ksc.nasa.gov/Shuttle/missions/sts-78/mission-sts-78.html.

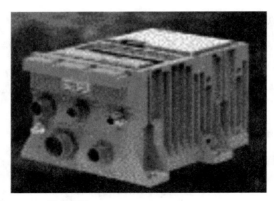

Figure C-5   Honeywell SIGI.

X38 crew return vehicle program. X-38 tests carried out prior to the cancellation of this program did not involve accelerations in excess of $2.5\,g$. (Tracking under higher acceleration conditions is certainly desirable.)

Both the MAGR/S and the SIGI GPS receivers rely upon the military cryptographic enabled Y-code for their operation. The availability of the Y-code receivers is tightly controlled according to the U.S. ITAR (International Traffic in Arms regulations). Under current law, neither MAGR nor SIGI is available to the Russians for their Soyuz capsules. There is also a concern that GPS in general might be vulnerable to electronic attacks such as jamming and/or spoofing, although having Y-code access makes the GPS operations less vulnerable than GPS civilian C/A code receivers.

The MAGR/S is intended to replace TACAN (a military tactical air navigation system) for the space shuttle and is currently undergoing certification by NASA. This five-channel receiver (a GPS architecture that is more than a decade old) was used to provide the space shuttle with real-time navigation acquired during STS-81 and STS-86, both space shuttle *Atlantis* flights to Mir, in January 1997 and September 1997, respectively. This is a Y-code receiver based on the military receivers developed by the GPS JPO (U.S. Air Force, Joint Project Office) and is manufactured by Rockwell Collins. NASA Johnson Space Center is using the receiver in its fully secure P(Y) code mode of operation. The receiver operates from a single rf input generated using an antenna combiner and does not support attitude determination (see Fig. C.6).

NASA, however, has experienced some difficulties with this receiver. To allow tracking in any orientation of the space shuttle, two antennas were installed (one top and one bottom, see Fig. C.7). Operation with these antennas has proved problematic because the selection of which communications satellites to use (five out of perhaps 14) has a built-in assumption of terrestrial applications and is not yet optimized for on-orbit operation. The lack of optimization means that the GPS receiver

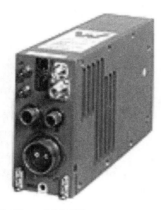

Figure C-6 Rockwell Collins, MAGR.

frequently experiences dropouts (failure to produce data) resulting in less than optimized navigation performance. This experience has led NASA to believe that another GPS user-equipment (UE) solution must be obtained before GPS tracking will be reliable for space operations.

Section 2. DTO Description

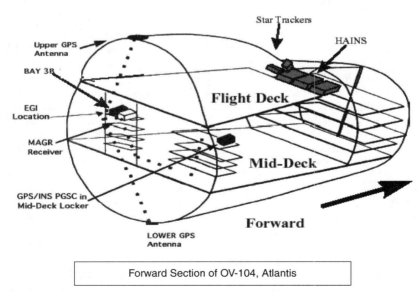

Figure C-7 Location of GPS and EGI systems on the space shuttle.

The embedded GPS receiver and inertial (EGI) navigation system, is a hybrid system that integrates GPS tracking and inertial measurements into a single line replaceable unit (LRU). The system is an all-attitude navigation system providing outputs of linear and angular acceleration, velocity, position attitude (roll, pitch and platform azimuth), magnetic and true heading, altitude, body angular rates, time tags, and time. When this EGI is installed in the host platforms in the appropriate configuration, the system provides the navigation functions of the equipment it replaces. The system uses the concept of open system architecture. Both Honeywell and Litton produce EGI systems.

The EGI is a modular system consisting of a subnautical mile (n mile)/hour-class inertial navigation system (INS) with three expansion slots, one of which contains an embedded GPS receiver. The EGI major subsystems are the inertial sensor assembly, GPS receiver, system processor, synchro circuit card assembly, and the dc power supply. It uses a digital laser gyro vehicle electrical power (28 V dc), turn-on and mode commands, initialization and altitude data, as well as GPS satellite inputs for GPS or GPS/INS operation, and is able to track five GPS satellites simultaneously. Being limited to only five satellites, when there might be as many as 14 GPS satellites simultaneously visible to the space shuttle, is a substantial limitation to accuracy and stability of operation that has been addressed in the SIGI design.

A space-qualified version of the EGI, the SIGI, has been developed for NASA by Honeywell for use on the ISS, and the CRV. This includes a 12-channel, L1 C/A code GPS receiver, and a Honeywell H-764G Inertial Navigation System.

Because the EGI includes a high accuracy INS, the integrated navigation solution will meet requirements during these drop-out periods (see Fig. C.7). However, this is a relatively expensive option for GPS metric tracking because of the cost of using the INS. A lower-cost option would be to use a lower-quality IMU and an all-in-view GPS receiver to maintain better satellite availability.

Large GPS data excursion indicates errors in the solution in the order of many kilometers. The periodic recovery of the solution to match the best-estimated trajectory (BET) suggests that the EGI software is detecting that a problem exists. However, another fault, possibly an erroneous acceleration, is causing the solution to diverge after being reset to the correct GPS position and velocity.

The Litton GPS/INS normally provides GPS, pure INS, and blended GPS/INS solutions for position and velocity. Litton GPS and blended position and velocity data were acquired during STS-86 ascent and early orbit, but no pure-INS data were available.

During ascent, Litton GPS position and velocity differences from the BET had a standard deviation or one-sigma value of 72 m and 1.14 m/s, and mean-plus-three-sigma values of 235 m and 3.75 m/s. The Litton blended position and velocity mean plus three sigma differences from the BET were 5800 m and 10.153 m/s. Semimajor axis mean-plus-three-sigma differences for a 30-s interval following MECO were Litton GPS, 2689 m and Litton blended, 13393.5 m. Litton rss attitude mean-plus-three-sigma difference from the shuttle GPC data for an interval from liftoff through 1 h was 0.19 deg with a 0.118 deg mean and a 0.034-deg standard deviation. Ascent powered flight was 8 min and 32 s, followed by external tank separation at 8 min and 51 s.

Litton GPS and blended position and velocity data acquired during STS-86 ascent were compared with a BET that was constructed by means of a batch filter that used cryptographic-keyed military GPS receiver position data to correct position and velocity propagated forward in time by means of measured velocity data from one of the three shuttle IMUs.

Potential Terrorists Threats

The first concern with regard to protecting the shuttle against terrorist attacks would logically focus on physical assaults on the spacecraft at the time of launch, landing, transport across the country on its especially adapted 747 transport vehicle or even within the shuttle maintenance facilities. Although there is a reasonable level of security maintained in shuttle-related facilities at all times and the takeoff and landing facilities at the Kennedy Space Center and Edwards Air Force Base are not easily accessible, the level of security could nevertheless be further increased. Even one individual with a rocket-propelled launcher could attack and potentially destroy a shuttle or leave it unable to fly.

It would appear desirable for further physical security and protection of the remaining shuttle fleet be studied and implemented as soon as possible. This would include direct physical attacks at any possible location as well as attempts to jam its controls or use radio surges to destroy the shuttle electronic or power systems by wider perimeter attacks.

There is perhaps an even greater danger that a shuttle could be attacked via digital assaults against its communications or navigational systems. This might involve the shuttle TTC&M system that provides vital ground-based commands, by interfering with voice or video communications with the shuttle crew, or electronically interfering with onboard computer systems during liftoff, landing, or other parts of its flight. The NASA inspector general did report on a so-called "cyber attack" on a shuttle mission, but this was not acknowledged until three years after the event occurred, and other unrecorded attacks might well have transpired. In September 1997, according to a BBC documentary made in the year 2000, a hacker overloaded NASA computer systems and threatened to disrupt communications with shuttle astronauts during a mission to link up with the Russian Mir space station.

As noted earlier, the official NASA statement about this cyber attack was that some routine medical information was slightly delayed because of a computer hacker, but that all data were eventually relayed. Specifically, a hacker began overloading NASA's computer facilities just as the shuttle docked at the Russian space station Mir and interfered with the data transmission of the computer system that monitors the heartbeat, pulse, and medical condition of astronauts aboard the spacecraft. Operation of the shuttle during docking operations is, of course, a particularly critical and sensitive to loss of ground communications.

Roberta Gross, NASA inspector general at NASA, was quoted on the BBC report stating that at one point "... a hacker was overloading our system ... to such an extent that it interfered with communications between the NASA center in the relay of some medical communications regarding the astronauts aboard the shuttle." This reportedly forced NASA communications to switch systems and talk to the astronauts via the Russian station Mir. A NASA statement on this event explained that the "communication interruption occurred between internal ground-based computer systems" and thus not with the communications uplink or downlink. It was further explained, without explicit amplification, that several fail-safe measures would have prevented any real danger. It was further acknowledged that in 1997 there were some 500,000 cyber attacks on NASA Web sites and networks. Today the reported number of such cyber attacks has grown into the millions. The NASA statement did acknowledge that in some circumstances more sophisticated attacks had the potential "... for doing some real damage to NASA's mission and astronaut safety."‡‡‡‡ Further electronic protection of shuttle telemetry and commands would appear to be desirable. This could be accomplished through coding, site diversity to verify commands, and enhanced security measures such as the use of GPS-based security systems to verify access to databases and to protect against spurious commands. These would all seem useful steps to take to augment protective systems for the shuttle program in both a physical and electronic sense.

Findings

A summary of the findings of the GWU review team is as follows:

1) All of the risk elements summarized in Appendix C should be examined by NASA with a view to determining how or if these concerns could be effectively addressed, or, alternatively, why no action is required at this time.

2) There should be a formal quarterly report independently prepared by the NESC (and in turn by the NASA independent technical authority if it is created in future months) indicating all waivers requested by contractors or NASA workers with regard to the shuttle and the actions taken with respect to each request.

3) The NESC should be further strengthened to perform its safety and risk-reduction functions. It should be given a clear proactive mandate to assess the safety and risk factors for the space shuttle, ISS, and other

---

‡‡‡‡Data available online at http://www.cnn.com/2000/TECH/space/07/03/nasa.hacker.02.

human-rated launch vehicles and not be simply a test and evaluation competency. The NESC and the NASA chief safety and mission assurance officer and staff should be given more autonomy and, potentially, be restructured to report independently such as with a formal briefing on a quarterly basis to the GAO, the OMB, and if established the space exploration steering committee. This would be in addition to providing weekly full reports to the NASA administrator, the associate administrators for space operations and exploration systems, as well as to the directors of all NASA centers. If the independent technical authority is created, then it should assume all of these responsibilities.

4) A formal congressional and OMB review should be made of the current and future safety of the shuttle program through 2010. This review should start with a truly independent assessment by a competent entity that is equipped to explore not only the basic management issues but technical program competencies as well. This review should be carried out in conjunction and cooperation with the NESC. This review should be a part of the overall review of NASA performance that comes with the departure of the NASA administrator and the independent report on NASA finance and operations as prepared by the NASA inspector general.

5) The independent assessment would provide a comprehensive list of all risk-reduction programs for the shuttle that have been deferred or decided against for either technical or cost-reduction purposes.

6) This independent assessment would also address and analyze the feasibility (in technical and cost terms) of using more robotic missions and expendable launch vehicles in lieu of manned space shuttle launches and to address the extent to which total manned shuttle launches could be reduced to a lesser number even if this meant certain elements of the ISS were not fully completed and more experiments were assigned to free flyers such as the Spartan.

7) BST, Inc., or another qualified contractor should systematically carry out surveys of NASA employees. The purpose of these surveys would be to determine if the agency's management culture has improved on safety-related measures. The specific objective would be to determine on an indexed annual scale whether higher priority is being given to safety issues and to soliciting employee input on such risk-related issues on a free and open basis.

8) Consideration should be given to further restructure of NASA and its centers as set forth in the final chapter of this report, taking into account the full nature of the review of all NASA programs, past, present, and future.

Space Shuttle Safety Survey—Interview Results

The results of the interviews showed a high degree of acceptance that the shuttle, even after the implementation of the CAIB recommendations, would still represent a launch vehicle of minimal safety integrity for a human-rated system. In short, no one disagreed that the shuttle even after refurbishment would represent a safety rating other than somewhere in the 1 in 60 probability of a category one failure. Thus everyone accepted the primary assessment of the CAIB regarding the overall safety of the shuttle. This is, of course, largely driven by the overall complexity of having some 30,000 plus constituent parts and the difficulty of consistent control over the manufacture, inspection, quality control, integration, and test of so many individual elements even if each of these were rated to many "nines" of reliability. In addition to the complexity factor, the CAIB and our own evaluation were also concerned with the issues of aging and degradation, quality control, and waivers in test and manufacturing operations and even management decisions involving schedule, budget, and overrides of safety officer concerns. These, and more, can all contribute to the overall shuttle safety situation.

Most of those interviewed also accepted the recommendations of the CAIB about steps that needed to be undertaken to return the shuttle to flight. On the order of 10% of the respondents, however, favored the immediate grounding of the space shuttle and rapidly moving to replace this system with a new and much more reliable launch vehicle that employs new technologies now available. These interviewees believed that the then projected 28 or so missions (as envisioned in mid-2004) to complete the space station was a fruitless effort to complete a multibillion project that had no remaining clear-cut U.S. objective, particularly in light of the proposed $400 million cutback in U.S. shuttle experiments. The great majority, however, felt that honoring U.S. international commitments to complete the ISS was a valid and "safe" space program goal even if it entailed 28 additional shuttle launches.

There was general agreement as to the key risks associated with the shuttle, which can be prioritized as follows.

Thermal Protection System

The 24,000 parts associated with the current ceramic-tile-based heat shield and other 2300 components of the thermal blanket system were considered risky and certainly elements that could be replaced with better technology on a new launch system—most likely a metallic TPS.

Lack of Launch-to-Land Escape System

The lack of a complete mission escape system was considered a major hazard that should be corrected with future launch systems. It was acknowledged that no viable redesign of the shuttle could achieve the objective of a complete launch-to-land escape capability.

Solid Rocket Boosters

The lack of a shutdown capability with a SRB once ignited prevents a viable escape option, and thus the clear majority felt solid-fuel systems should be eliminated from future human-rated launch systems. ("I don't like the SRBs because of their environmental pollution, but how about a blowout panel to instantly reduce pressure and shut the SRB down?")

Safety and Performance Margins

The design and use of human-rated vehicles should have greater safety margins and always maintain clear safety margins in determining payload size. This finding puts those surveyed in opposition to NASA's plans (as of mid-2004) to use essentially the full capability of the shuttle for 28 missions to complete the ISS and to launch five shuttles a year in contrast to the CAIB recommendation of no more than four launches a year. (Of course, NASA, as of early 2006, has now reduced the projected number of launches to around 18.)

Separate Crew and Cargo

The importance of this separation was emphasized a number of times. The cargo that needs no life-support system should be separated from the crew wherever possible. Robotically controlled cargo ships should be separated from human-rated vehicles or separate vehicle bays optimized for life-support systems.

Beyond these top issues, concern was expressed with regard to the performance, backup capabilities, and safety associated with many aspects of the space shuttle program. Anxieties were expressed with regard to IT and telecommunications systems, power systems, space suits, environmental controls and life-support systems, propulsion, etc., but these were clearly at a lower level of concern than the top five factors.

Comments made by those interviewed with regard to NASA's astronaut safety program varied over a wide spectrum of opinion. These views about "top things" to be done to improve safety are summarized and listed next. Sometimes comments were made several times, but these consolidated statements nevertheless attempt to capture the nuance of slightly different views.

Notes From Interviews[§§§§]

1) There needs to be clear safety objectives and probabilities of safe operation regarding the shuttle. This includes the application of a formal

---

[§§§§]"Notes from confidential interviews with space experts conducted in 2004 and 2005," Space Safety Study 2005, George Washington University, Washington, DC.

methodology of failure mode safety analysis (FMSA) and not "band-aids" that now seem to be the case.

2) There is a problem within NASA and Congress of thinking that economies can be achieved with shuttle at this point through taking some safety measures. Safety has to be designed by initial system margins. True safety will have to come from a next generation vehicle that designs safety in at the outset.

3) There needs to be a better system of monitoring the wear-out of materials or components, obsolescent sub-systems, and the implementation of all scheduled upgrades. Such efforts will include an automated self check system and an improved health countermeasures capability.

4) There needs to be new approaches and upgrades to the shuttle and especially to any follow-on human rated launch systems to enhance system safety. This approach would include: (a) better sensors, (b) better fuel tanks, (c) improved liquid fuel boosters, (d) better thermal protection, and (e) better external inspection capability. (This would include the ability to fly a video monitor around the space shuttle and inspect every part of shuttle exterior controlled by joystick.)

5) Always use robotic systems rather than EVAs wherever possible.

6) Instill an improved safety culture in NASA. Retrain all NASA and contractor staff with a different mindset. Safety is more than inspection and reaction to problems.

7) Create priorities in NASA. Revitalize centers and give them clear and specific missions. Allow money to be spent on actual space programs. (Too many staff without a clear mission).

8) Focus on key science, technology and especially launch vehicle development. Reduce number of NASA conferences. Money could be better spent. Safety could then be top priority.

9) Cut flight rate of shuttle to only four per year. More than four is dangerous.

10) Maintain adequate spares for quick change, update, and simple in-orbit repairs in designing future systems. (This approach clearly implies the need for modular design. This is why current TPS is so dangerous and expensive.)

11) Flight safety margins. Don't push performance. Also don't issue so many waivers but instead fix the problem wherever possible. The current "waiver system" is a risk to safety.

12) Separate crew and cargo. Use automated systems wherever possible. Develop automated heavy lift capability including the possibility of a robotically controlled shuttle.

13) Replace the solid booster rockets, and have a liquid propulsion system that could be shut down on the pad.

14) There should be consideration of a "blow out" panel that could allow the shut down of SRBs.

15) Always have another astronaut return option if there is a problem.

16) Adopt a realistic schedule as recommended by the CAIB.

17) Establish independent technical engineering authority that goes beyond limited capabilities of NESC.

18) Further develop contingency plans for problems detected while crew is in orbit.

19) Refocus on crew escape (e.g., HL-20 or X-38). Do not push performance, and thus keep high safety margins. Develop in-orbit free-flyer inspection capability. Have a contingency plan for all stages of mission. Identify options for all high-risk situations.

20) Always have expendable escape module to return to earth from ISS. This could be Soyuz for the time being and the ATV when available.

21) Design safety is first. (This means not only designing for high levels of safety but also setting sufficiently high standards and making budgetary commitments at outset.)

22) Don't design to ultimate performance. (Allow for under performance or partial system failure and still work.)

23) Don't use a greater systems tolerance/margin. (This means providing greater margins and tolerance to several system failures and not 'giving away' this margin by trade-off studies).

24) Need to have better initiatives with regard to health countermeasures. Astronauts in space face all sorts of health issues. Bone and muscle attrition, adverse affect on auto-immune system, cardio-vascular problems. Need on-board gravity and one g centrifuge for stem cell growth. Russians have a good deal of study in this area. NASA programs are minimal and do not take this subject seriously as a major issue.

25) NASA's policy and programs are too controlled by major aerospace contractors. Major progress is likely to come from innovative and entrepreneurial approaches such as Scaled Composites, SpaceDev, or others. If one compares progress of aeronautical industry in its first 40 years to current aerospace progress, there is not a similar rate of progress. Shuttle and ISS programs should be abandoned and shut down as soon as possible.

26) Shuttle was a budgetary compromise driven by White House in the Nixon years. It should have been a flying prototype and retired after no more than five years.

27) Shuttle has been the Model A of space transportation systems. Clearly, in designing for the future, we need to take into account what we have learned. The designs of the future need to be more modular for both safety and efficiency. Fully 30% of the reconditioning of a shuttle after a flight involves the thermal protection system (i.e., the TPS and the tiles). This should have been a modular system that could be replaceable on each shuttle. This would have increased safety and efficiency.

References

[1] "Space Shuttle Budget for FY2000," Letter from Daniel Goldin to Jacob Lew, Director, Office of Management and Budget, Washington, DC, 6 July 1999.

[2] Space Shuttle Independent Assessment Team, "Report to the Associate Administrator, Office of Space Flight, October-December 1999," NASA, 7 March 2000; also CAIB Document CTF017-0169.

3   Report of the Space Flight Advisory Committee, NASA Office of Space Flight, May 2001 Meeting Report, 1–2 May 2001, p. 7; also Space Shuttle Safety Budget CAIB Document CTF017-0034.

4   Space Shuttle Safety," Hearings Before the House Science Committee's Subcommittee on Space and Aeronautics, Washington, DC, 23 Sept. 1999.

5   Report of the Presidential Commission on the Space Shuttle *Challenger* Accident, NASA, Washington, DC, 6 June 1986.

6   *The Columbia Accident Investigation Report VI*, NASA, Washington, DC, 2003. pp. 1–17

7   Frosch, R., *"Examination of the Shuttle Program,"* NASA, 18 Aug. 1980.

8   "Meeting on the Space Shuttle," NASA Document NASA-SP-1023, 14 Nov. 1979.

9   Statement of Richard Blomberg, Former Chair, Aerospace Safety Advisory Panel before the House Subcommittee on Space and Aeronautics, Washington, DC, 18 April 2002.

10 "Space Shuttle Upgrades," General Accounting Office Testimony Before the Subcommittee on Science, Technology and Space, Committee on Commerce, Science and Transportation, U.S. Senate, Washington, DC, Sept. 2001.

11 Garman, J. R., "The Bug Heard Round the World," *ACM SIGSOFT Software Engineering Notes*, Vol. 6, No. 5, 1981, *also Formal Methods for the Specification and Design of Real-Time Safety Critical Systems*, URL: http://citeseer.nj.nec.com/ostroff92formal.html.

12 Ernie Reyes, Former Director of Quality Assurance, Kennedy Space Center, "Shuttle Heat Shields Have Flawed History," NASA Document, NASA-SPR-1861, 6 Feb. 2000, URL: http://www.nynewsday.com/chi-0302060357feb06, 0,1583634.story.

13 William F. Readdy Testimony, "Space Shuttle Safety," U.S. House of Representatives, Science Committee's Subcommittee on Space and Aeronautics, NASA Hearings on STS 93, Washington, DC, 23 Sept. 1999.

14 NASA Report to the Committee on Space Shuttle Upgrades, U.S. House of Representatives, Science Committee's Subcommittee on Space and Aeronautics Upgrading the Space Shuttle, Washington, DC, Sept. 2001, p. 48.

15 Schulze, N. R., and Prichard, R. P., "Occupant Safety in the Space Shuttle," NASA Report NASA-SP-813, Feb. 1978.

16 "Orbital Debris: A Technical Assessment," NAP, Technical Report, May 2004, URL: http://books.nap.edu/books/0309051258/html/index.html.

17 United Nations, Technical Report on Space Debris, Report adopted by the Scientific and Technical Subcommittee of the Committee on the Peaceful Uses of Outer Space, Corpuos 2003-237R, Vienna, Austria 2003.

18 "Space Program: Space Debris a Potential Threat to Space Station and Shuttle," Report to Congress, General Accounting Office (GAO), GAO/IMTEC-90-18, Washington, DC, April 1990.

19 Stich, J. S., "Conjunction Summary for STS-26 through STS-61," NASA JSC Memo DM42/93-010, Texas, Houston, 7 Feb. 1994.

20 NASA Johnson Space Center Flight Rules, Flight Rule 2-77, NASA, Houston, TX, 1993, p. 2-80a– 2-80b.

21 Golightly, G., "Biosensors May Revolutionize Space Life Support," *Space.com*, 26 Jan. 2000, pp. 1–3

22 David, L., "NASA's Aging Shuttle…," and "Shuttle Heat Shields Have Flawed History," *Space.com*, Feb. 17, 2003, pp. 1–5.

23 Iannotta, B., "On-Orbit Shuttle Repair Takes Shape," *Aerospace America*, Vol. 42, No. 8, Aug. 2004, pp. 30–34.

[24] Schwartz, J., "NASA Rescue Plan Is Reported to Have High Risk of Failure," *New York Times*, 9 July 2004, p. A-12.

[25] "Space Shuttle Transoceanic Abort Landing (TAL) Sites," NASA Report, NASA-SPR-1424, Washington, DC, 2000.

[26] Leary, W., "Oxygen Generator on Space Station Fails," *New York Times*, 10 Sept. 2004, p. A22.

[27] "An Assessment of Space Shuttle Flight Software Development Processes," ASEB Report, ASEB-21SF, Washington, D.C.

[28] "Shuttle Unable to Send Back TV Pictures," *Houston Chronicle*, Houston, Texas, 1 Aug. 2000, URL: http://www.chron.com/cgibin/auth/story.mpl/content/interactive/space/missions/sts91/stories/980603.html.

Appendix D
Detailed Technical Review of ISS Vulnerabilities

Chapter 5 provided an overview of technical concerns related to the International Space Station. Tables 5.1 and 5.2 presented a summary of the concerns, the degree of seriousness, the extent to which there have been related flight experiences, and suggestions as to how these problems might be addressed. This appendix provides greater detail from the GW study with regard to each of these issues.

Analyzing the ISS by Major Subsystems

The ISS has a very large number of subsystems crucial to its design and operation. Nevertheless those units that pose particular issues of safety, and constitute the largest areas of risk, are fewer than might be initially envisioned. The following sections highlight those subsystems in terms of their design as well as related operational and management issues concerning safety and risk minimization.

Gyro Systems and Orientation and Reboost

It is critical to the ISS mission both to keep the ISS properly oriented in space and to prevent the station from reaching too low of an orbit. Further, in the case of orbital debris it could, on occasion, be necessary to maneuver the station around such hazards. Proper orientation is particularly important at critical periods such as spacecraft docking or during EVAs. All of these safety issues are addressed in this section.

The ISS utilizes four control motion gyroscopes (CMGs) that control the attitude of the station. Consisting of spinning wheels that rotate at 6600 rpm, the CMGs can maintain or change the station's attitude by absorbing or generating torques that can be applied to the ISS. The four CMGs were assembled at the ISS as part of the Z1 Integrated Truss Structure in October 2000 and were activated the following year.* Figure D.1 shows a CMG before launch at the Kennedy Space Center.

In early June 2002 anomalies in the CMG-1 telemetry were noticed. Two days later, on 8 June 2002 one of two bearing assemblies in the CMG

---

*Data available online at http://www.shuttlepresskit.com/STS-92/payload76.htm.

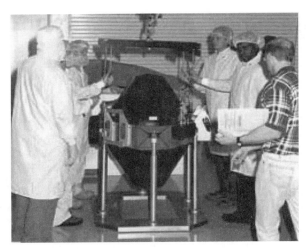

Figure D-1   Control motion gyroscope (courtesy of NASA).

apparently failed because of a believed lack of lubrication. This loss of lubricant could have occurred as the result of many scenarios. One of these might have been a micrometeorite "hit" on the gyro system, but it could also have been a design defect.

The faulty gyro system cannot be repaired in orbit. It requires that a replacement gyroscope must be launched on a shuttle mounted with a special carrier beam in the cargo bay. Unfortunately this replacement was not possible before the shuttle fleet was grounded in February 2003. At the time, Flight Director Paul Hill was quoted as saying,

> Losing a CMG is a big deal. It's a major component.... But from a risk perspective right now, we're in good shape. We're single-fault tolerant whether we're docked or not docked. So for the long haul on station, we can still lose one more CMG and still hold attitude on the station side and minimize the amount of propellant we use.[†]

On 8 November 2003, however, there was another incident with a CMG when flight controllers for the station detected current and vibration spikes in one of the three remaining CMGs. To prevent possible damage and allow engineers to evaluate the situation, the three remaining CMGs were only used for day-to-day attitude control for a month. In that time, Russian thrusters were used for major maneuvers. In early December 2003 all three CMGs were reported operational and functioning correctly.[‡] On 21 April 2004, NASA ISS controllers received an alarm

---

[†]Data available online at http://www.spaceflightnow.com.
[‡]Data available online at http://www.space.com/missionlaunches/ iss_thrusters_031206.html [cited 6 Dec. 2003].

reporting a failure in CMG-2. It was discovered that a failed circuit within the gyroscope's remote power control unit cut off power to CMG-2. Although not causing an immediate safety concern, it did result in the ISS being controlled by the minimum of two CMGs. Failure of one of the remaining two CMGs would have had the ISS relying on Russian thrusters for attitude control, of which there was only a 6–12-month supply of propellant.

This situation resulted in what *Washington Post* press accounts characterized as a "risky and unplanned EVA" executed in June 2004 by Expedition Nine crew members Gennady Padalka and Mike Fincke. (*Note*: as discussed elsewhere in the EVA section, the first attempt had to be abandoned when a leak was detected in Mike Fincke's space suit.) Further this EVA required that the station be fully turned over to ground control with no astronaut left within the ISS. This type of space-walk operation involved a change in "accepted ISS operational safety procedures." Had there been a problem with the air lock system or other such problems, this could have led to a loss of life and endangered the ISS itself [1,2]. The second EVA, however, was successful and allowed CMG-2 to be added back into the attitude control mix two days later after completing operational tests.§

Currently three of the four CMGs are operational on the ISS with the fourth due to be replaced once the shuttle resumes flight. The cause of the gyro system failure is still not clearly understood. In future design considerations, the addition of small intelligent sensors that can provide additional data about the gyro's operation as well as additional video monitors might well assist in detecting systems failures and perhaps even allow diagnostics to eliminate failures before they occur. It is also recommended that the design of the gyro system be reexamined for safety upgrades, possible easier in-orbit repair, and installation of sensors to predict wear-out and breakdown. Future space systems should employ a design that allows in-orbit repair and higher reliability.

ISS and Needed Orbital Corrections (i.e., Lack of Onboard Boosters)

The ISS orbits at more than 300 km above the Earth. Because of atmospheric drag and other influences, the ISS slows down and experiences orbital decay. As a result of this orbital decay, the station is periodically rebooted to its intended altitude of between 350 and 450 km with the use of the space shuttle, the Russian Progress vehicle, or the Zvezda service module. Without these periodic reboosts the ISS would slow down and could completely deorbit within months. The atmospheric drag of the ISS is dependent on the density of the atmosphere at that altitude and is primarily affected by the constantly changing solar flux and seasons.

---

§Data available online at http://www.nasa.gov/vision/space/
workinginspace/exp9_eva_advancer.html [2 July 2004].

Depending on the level of solar activity, the ISS can drop up to 300 m per day, and according to Robert Laine, the European Space Agency's program manager for the automated transfer vehicle, during periods of particularly intense solar activity the station can drop up to 1 km in a single day.[¶] The attitude of the ISS is also a factor as certain attitudes create more atmospheric drag.

To counter this orbital decay, the primary means of reboosting the ISS is with the Russian Progress/Soyuz vehicle, which is better equipped for this role than the shuttle or Zvezda service module. The shuttle was used for reboost early in the construction of the ISS, but is now largely ineffective because of the increased size of the station. The Progress and Zvezda service module propulsion systems were used to control the station's attitude in the early stages of construction.

Propellant can be used by the Progress spaceship or by the Zverda service module to boost the orbit of the ISS.[**] A Progress/Soyuz vehicle can stay inorbit with the ISS and complete reboosts for up to 180 days.

As the ISS nears completion, the frequency of reboosts is going to increase as the station itself increases in size. As long as there is a continual supply of Progress/Soyuz spacecraft and the shuttle can transport needed materials to carry out repairs, reboosting the ISS should not be a major challenge. Nevertheless, the recurring gyro problem, the long-term grounding of the shuttle, and the lack of a longer-term agreement with the Russian Space Agency post-2006 must all be considered elements of risk. Once the ATV spacecraft is available in 2005 to reboost the ISS (as well as to aid in avoiding orbital debris), this risk factor will be considerably reduced because the ATV has three times the thrust capability of the Progress/Soyuz vehicle and can provide this capability for six months at a time.

Environmental Control (Leaks and Monitoring for Noxious Gases)

The environmental control and life-support systems (ECLSS) provide the crew of the ISS with a habitable environment in which to live and work, but there is constant danger that many of these systems, which do not have full redundancy, could malfunction and thus create life-threatening conditions.

Control of the environment and provision of life support is organized into five subsystems[††]:

1) **The atmosphere control and supply** subsystem provides oxygen and nitrogen gases for a habitable environment for the astronauts.

[¶]Data available online at http://www.space.com.
[**]Data available online at http://www.shuttlepresskit.com/ISS_OVR/ assembly2_overview.htm [cited 6 July 2000].
[††]Data available online at http://www.boeing.com/defense-space/ space/spacestation/systems/eclss.html.

2) **The atmosphere revitalization subsystem** monitors oxygen and nitrogen levels while removing carbon dioxide and other contaminants.

3) **The temperature and humidity control** subsystem maintains the ISS atmosphere within a constant temperature range, circulates air, and removes humidity.

4) **The water recovery and management subsystem** recovers and recycles water from the sink, shower, urine, the shuttle's fuel cells, and condensation.

5) **The fire detection and suppression subsystem** consists of smoke detectors, alarms, extinguishers, shut-off systems, gas masks, and oxygen bottles.

The operation of these systems is imperative for the continued habitation of the ISS, and failure in any one of them could endanger the safety of the crew onboard the station. There have been incidents in the lifetime of the station where these systems have presented serious problems for the crew of the ISS. Astronauts from the STS-96 mission launched on 27 May 1999 suffered nausea, itchy eyes, and headaches while working in some parts of the space station. This problem of severe allergies was thought possibly caused by elevated carbon-dioxide (CO_2) levels. Thus part of the mission of STS-101 launched on 19 May 2000 was to undertake increased monitoring of the air quality inside the station, replace air filters, and increase circulation.[‡‡]

Problems also developed in two important environmental systems in November 2002. Two valves failed in the U.S. carbon-dioxide removal assembly (CDRA), which removes excess CO_2 from the station's atmosphere. The system remained partially functional, and the astronauts had an ample supply of lithium-hydroxide canisters to reduce the excess CO_2. The CDRA system was restored to full operation after the Space Shuttle *Endeavour*, launched on 23 November 2002 delivered replacement valves to the ISS.

At the same time, the Russian "Elektron" system that creates oxygen for the system failed. The crew of Expedition 5 relied on stored oxygen in the Progress while fixing the system by replacing components on the unit.[§§] In early September 2004, the oxygen generators again experienced problems. Unlike earlier problems involving excessive bubbling, the problem this time was thought to be associated with possible system blockage. Attempts to unblock the critical tubing have not been entirely successful, and the next launch of the shuttle will address the oxygen generator problem as a mission objective. Reliance on Progress module oxygen generators will supply adequate oxygen in the meantime, but the

---

[‡‡]Data available online at http://www.space.com/news/spacestation/ iss_sickair_805.html.

[§§]Data available online at http://www.aviationnow.com/content/publication/ awst/20021118/aw [cited 18 Nov. 2002].

failure of the oxygen systems in 2002 and again in 2004 remains a key element of concern [3]. Currently the greatest concern with regard to the ECLSS, beyond the oxygen generators, involves the environmental monitoring devices. These units measure contaminants in the air and water supplies and filters and environmental generators that are not working on the station. NASA medical specialists, according to press reports, expressed their concerns prior to the launch of Expedition 8 about the air and water quality and also other environmental concerns. However NASA managers concluded the station was sufficiently safe to proceed. Replacement parts to fix the monitoring devices are too large and can only be delivered with the use of a shuttle.¶¶ The fact that replacement parts can only be resupplied by the shuttle must thus be seen as a major safety concern that should be given high priority in safety reviews.

Fire onboard the ISS would be very dangerous for the crew, and thankfully the fire detection and suppression systems have not been used so far. NASA engineers have suspected that some smoke alarms were defective, but these and fire extinguishers are constantly replaced to ensure their correct operation.*** Tests with new "extremely fine mist" fire suppression systems tested on shuttle flights have shown that these work better in space to extinguish flames than earlier designs, and a retrofit of these systems is now planned, but this has not yet been accomplished.

The continued functioning of the ECLSS systems is vital to the ISS remaining inhabitable and operational. They provide an environment that allows the crew to live and work onboard. Failure of any of these systems would endanger the crew and could result in abandonment of the station.

Finally there is the problem reported in the press of the long-term very slow leak of the atmosphere on the ISS. This reported leak of atmosphere is sufficiently slow that there is no risk to the astronauts. Nevertheless, the fact that the source of these leaks has not been found after months of trying to detect their source is a potential source of concern. Additional smart instrumentation has been installed on the ISS to provide much greater sensitivity of detection of various types of environmental problems. This might provide the type of equipment needed to enhance the quality of the ISS atmosphere and to detect problems before they become large risk factors.

The environmental systems on the ISS would appear to be among the more "fragile" aspects of the ISS design for longer-term provision of a survivable environment. The addition of microsensors to determine subsystem-related performance issues such as leakage of oxygen and buildup of noxious gases would appear to be a useful upgrade to the ECLSS. Also the upgrade of the fire-fighting system with the previously tested extremely fine mist approach would also seem another way to increase ISS safety.

¶¶Data available online at http://www.cnn.com/2003/TECH/space/10/24/
station/safety/ [cited 24 Oct. 2004].
***Data available online at http://www.space.com/news/spaceshuttles/
space_station_life_000419.htm / [cited 20 March 2000].

Software Problems and Reliance on Ground-Based Control Systems

ISS software malfunctions are also a source of vulnerability during on-station operations. In November 2003, NASA Ames Research Center Human Factors and Systems Safety staff in conjunction with ISS flight controllers, Mission Operations Directorate (MOD) management, and the Operations Research Branch of MOD conducted a survey of ISS flight controllers. The results of the survey[†††] are intended to identify ISS organizational risks and produce solutions to mitigate them. The 191 ISS flight controllers who participated in the survey identified station program notes (SPNs) as a critical vulnerability to safe operations onboard the ISS. SPNs are written work-arounds for crew members to perform in order to bypass a known software malfunction. There are, according to press reports, a large number of different SPNs to handle these various software malfunctions, and flight controllers in survey report indicated having difficulty remembering them. One flight controller responded to the survey by writing: "I will be blunt—allowing the number of SPNs to get to where they are is NO different from allowing repeated foam strikes on the tiles to be considered OK since we have survived it before."[†††]

The results of the survey identify software-related issues in addition to the high number of SPNs and the difficulties in remembering them as follows: 1) "the relatively low rating given to the adequacy of the development and testing of the software," and 2) "the difficulty in ensuring that a software problem will ever get fixed."[†††] This survey, which is intended to discuss organizational risks, identifies an organizational communications problem as well, which is related to the software on the ISS. This is that the boards that control and manage the ISS software are located in a different directorate. The survey results document the response of one PHALCON (a power, heating, articulation, lighting control officer) as follows:

> "There are too many independent boards, all working in their little areas, and no one is coordinating all of the problems at the big picture level to make sure that a bunch of smaller problems don't add up to a big one." As the CAIB report has shown, organizational issues are critical in ensuring the proper identification and mitigation of identified technical risks. This relates to ensuring that the organization can properly identify and communicate the risk and allocate resources to correct and manage the vulnerability.

The improvement in software as well as system management and training for flight controllers should be given high priority to the extent that key upgrades have not yet been completed.

[†††]Data available online at http://www.spaceref.com/news/viewsr.html?pid=12128 [cited Feb. 2004].

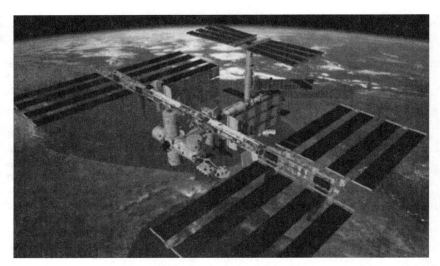

Figure D-2   Impression of completed ISS with solar arrays (courtesy of NASA).

Power Systems

Electrical power is arguably the most important resource for the ISS because the power system enables everything from the life-support systems and flight-control computers to the experiments conducted onboard. The ISS uses a combination of solar arrays utilizing photovoltaic cells and banks of rechargeable nickel-hydrogen batteries to provide a continuous power source to the station. Figure D.2 provides an artist's impression of what the completed ISS will look like with deployed solar arrays.

The ISS orbits the earth every 92 min, which means there are periods of up to 36 m in where there is no direct sunlight to the station. During periods where there is sunlight, the ISS uses the photovoltaic cells on the solar arrays to extract this energy and supply power for the running of the station. Electrical energy is also supplied to 38 rechargeable nickel-hydrogen batteries that are discharged during times without sunlight in order to keep a continuous supply of power. The switching back and forth between the solar-generated power and the stored battery power has to be seamless and reliable to keep continuous current flow to all of the important systems on the station, especially the computers that control vital operations and the life-support systems.‡‡‡

The design for the fully completed the ISS includes eight flexible solar wings that when deployed will each consist of a mast and two solar-array

---

‡‡‡Data available online at http://www.nasa.gov/www/PAO/PAIS/ fs06grc.htm.

blankets of photovoltaic cells. These arrays measure 107 × 38 ft (or approximately 32.5 × 11.5 m) and when fully deployed are designed to provide a continuous supply of 110 kW of power for all onboard operations and have a lifetime of 15 years.

The arrays can be oriented so that they face the sun to achieve optimum power production. They are also feathered with the object of minimizing the potential for damage as a result of construction and assembly of the ISS and particularly to avoid collision damage by an arriving or departing spacecraft. The first two of these solar arrays were launched onboard Space Shuttle *Endeavor* in November 2000 and were assembled as part of the P6 integrated truss structure in December 2000. The following three pairs of solar arrays are planned for launch early in the assembly schedule, once the shuttle resumes flight.

The 38 nickel-hydrogen batteries are stored in an enclosure called an orbital replacement unit that is designed for simple removal and replacement of the battery cells. These batteries are recharged during the sunlit phase of each orbit and have a life expectation of five to six years in orbit. Replacement of these battery cells well before their projected end of life is clearly a major safety concern now that the reliability of the shuttle service missions has been questioned and the shuttle grounded for 25 months. In short another shuttle failure before the battery cells are replaced would result in this becoming an increasing safety concern.

Figure D.3 shows banks of these rechargeable batteries used to discharge power to the ISS during nonsunlit periods.

The use of solar arrays and the battery storage system clearly involves several identifiable hazards. Storing electricity in batteries builds up excess heat that can damage important equipment; this requires liquid

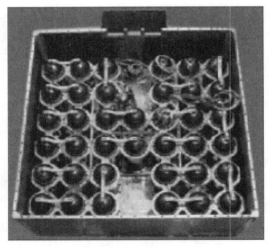

Figure D-3   Banks of nickel-hydrogen batteries on ISS.

ammonia radiators to be used to dissipate heat away from the station. The solar arrays also produce a strong electric field. Unless action is taken, this can leave the hull of the ISS electrically charged. Plasma contactors and circulation isolation devices can be employed to neutralize the charge on the hull and allow space-walking astronauts to complete EVAs without risk of electrical shock. This neutralization of the charge is considered to be key to astronaut safety when undertaking an EVA.§§§

It is suggested that improved means of separating astronauts from charged metallic surfaces through insulative materials or discharge needs to be explored and implemented for both the ISS and future in-orbit structures that are to be manned. There are no documented problems with the power system identified by the research team up to this point in the ISS's operation. The solar arrays are of a feathered design and are very fragile. Several fault developments in the solar arrays, the transmission lines, or the battery banks could result in the station receiving reduced power. The solar arrays have been designed so that a puncture caused by micrometeorite debris will not propagate through the array and cause a short. This assumes that the micrometeorite would be of relatively small dimensions. The earlier discussion on micrometeorite vulnerability presented in the Environmental Control Section indicates that the larger the micrometeorite the larger the element of significant risk.

Almost any micrometeorite impact will reduce the array's ability to produce power, although it would require a more sizable hit to do appreciable damage.¶¶¶ Contamination of the arrays from the space environment or thruster fuel could also reduce the effectiveness of the photovoltaic cells in producing electricity from the sunlight. Over time this could significantly reduce the power available to important systems on board the station.

Finally there is the problem of radiation damage to the solar cells that comes from the outer-space environment. The low Earth orbit of the ISS is well designed to be below the lowest of the Van Allen belts, and thus the risk of the radiation damage is lower than for satellites in higher orbit. Additional glass shielding of the solar cells is thus not indicated for this orbital location. Adding solar-cell capabilities rather than protective coating would be the best protection against radiation damage.

The design of the power system (first developed in the 1980s) is in some ways out of date in terms of solar-cell performance, insulation, battery performance, and the method of reduction of electrical charges on the ISS surface. These are more of a performance issue than a safety issue. There is nevertheless concern that battery heat will become an increasing issue over time, and thus battery upgrades might be appropriate. Further electrical charge reduction might be addressed by improved insulation measures as modification and upgrades are possible. It is suggested that

---

§§§Data available online at http://www.nasa.gov/WWW/PAO/PAIS/fs06grc.htm.
¶¶¶Data available online at http://www.cnn.com/2000/TECH/space/ [cited 2 Dec. 2000].

such upgrades and improved power systems need to be included in any space-station system of the future.

External Inspection and Monitoring Capability

NASA implemented extended capability to undertake more extensive exterior inspections of the ISS in November 2003 and continues to make other safety upgrades to its ISS safety procedures as the result of a post-*Columbia* safety review. Specifically, in the fall of 2003 NASA developed a new plan for safely keeping a skeleton crew of two astronauts onboard the space station without the help of the remaining three shuttles that are grounded until 2005. This plan entails the use of smaller Russian space-craft to take new crews and supplies to the station.

The update of the plan, in the form of an 84-page report released in March 2004, highlighted the need for more and better inspections of space-station wiring, equipment, and outside surfaces. This report also noted the need for improved shielding of the ISS against orbiting debris and more complete monitoring of problems.**** In response to the CAIB report, extensive new monitoring capabilities exist on the retrofitted space shuttle and will also exist on the ISS.

The visual monitoring of the ISS as recommended by the CAIB is considered to be adequate, but there is a need for improved systematic review of ISS wiring, key equipment, and other subsystems (plus external debris damage) to be conducted on a regular and routine inspection process. This is an operational/QC issue as opposed to a hardware upgrade.

Docking with Shuttle and Other Spacecraft

The International Space Station is designed for docking with a variety of launch systems. The purpose of such docking is many-fold. This is not only to take on new cargo and experimental equipment and adding new structural elements of the ISS, but also exchanging crews, disposing of waste, and even maintaining the ISS in orbit. As just noted, in the most extreme cases of intensive solar activity the ISS can descend up to 1 km in orbital height in a day and thus reboost capabilities from external vehicles is of critical importance. The flexibility to dock with a half-dozen different vehicles is thus vital to the ISS's operation.

A docking accident involving the Mir has clearly demonstrated the importance of such docking to the safety to both space shuttle and ISS. A higher level of automation and improved software in the docking process and redundancy in the controls and control overrides to such docking

****Data available online at http://msnbc.msn.com/id/3404496/[cited 3 March 2004].

procedures, as well as improved laser guidance and alignment tools as noted earlier, should be seriously considered.

Debris and Micrometeorites

There has already been discussion of problems associated with orbital debris and the associated need for improved space navigation systems for tracking and avoidance of such debris. This is obviously even more crucial for the ISS. This previous discussion included issues such as the use of space navigation systems by these vehicles that are so critical as a source of supply to the ISS. In the case of the Soyuz, this also serves as an escape vehicle. Therefore the discussion of the hazards represented by orbital debris and micrometeorites and the role of tracking this debris and the need to use global positioning system (GPS) navigational systems to support collision avoidance by the ISS are critical.

Because of the intrinsic worldwide coverage of the GPS, it is obviously appealing to implement a GPS-based tracking and navigation architecture in order to support all human-based spacecraft including the ISS. It is not widely understood that the GPS, when applied to a low-Earth-orbit system such as the ISS, lacks the sort of high-accuracy performance available in the terrestrial environment. These reasons include atmospheric and ionospheric distortions and various software issues. Further, GPS systems can be jammed by relatively low-level transmissions and mobile power sources that make them difficult to locate [4].

The extent of the "GPS challenge" to support of the ISS (or for that matter the space shuttle, Soyuz, or ATV) was very recently reported by NASA Johnson Space Center staff in abstracts presented to the Institute of Navigation. The NASA engineers reported problems as follows:

> These problems caused NASA to pursue re-writing the attitude determination code using a code standard. Plots are shown comparing the attitude output from SIGI [i.e., the Honeywell developed Space Integrated GPS Inertial (SIGI) system] prior to and after the code rewrite. The problems in the navigation code were more subtle. The GPS receiver was tracking satellites through the Earth's atmosphere, which caused significant navigation errors. The health messages from the GPS receiver were out of sync with the actual navigation message, causing ISS to use solutions that it should have screened. The ionosphere was also causing significant errors that were not anticipated. Plots are shown comparing the navigation output from SIGI prior and after the code rewrite. The problems caused by the ionosphere have not yet been solved.
>
> In conclusion, the code residing in the GPS receiver for ISS is equally as complicated as the code residing in the ISS flight computers. The code within the GPS receiver should have been developed with the same rigor as the code residing in the flight computers that was developed to the specification of a man rated space vehicle. Since the GPS receiver code was not written to such a specification, it had to be rewritten [5].

GPS will likely be critical to future in-orbit maneuver strategies to avoid forecast risk to any human crew vehicles on the ISS. GPS capability, however, is not a panacea in this respect, and tracking is yet another dimension of the problem. Detection of debris remains a very significant hazard for the ISS. Space surveillance by USSPACECOM radar for debris is limited to approximately $10\,cm^2$ of radar cross section (equivalent to a 3.2 by 3.2 cm) and only for metal objects.[††††]

The ISS or other human-rated spacecraft can avoid collisions by maneuvering around the larger debris, but only if there is sufficient alert time and if the thrust capability is available onboard the ISS. The USSPACECOM regularly examines the trajectories of orbital debris to identify possible close encounters. If a catalogued object is projected to come within a few kilometers of the ISS, then a maneuver away from this object is undertaken. Smaller particles, however, are not tracked by radar. Fortunately, small particles pose less of a catastrophic threat, but they do cause surface abrasions and microscopic holes and possibly might be the source of slow leaks in the ISS atmosphere. The greatest challenge is medium-size particles (objects with a diameter between 1 mm to 10 cm) because they are not easily tracked and are yet large enough to cause catastrophic damage, especially for the largest of these debris objects. Because the relative velocity of these debris particles is typically on the order of approximately 16 km/s, they can do extensive damage. This is to say that avoidance of space debris is one of the most important safety issues and that risk factors here, just as in the case of the space shuttle, are, over a period of time, quite high.

One of the largest problems is that the catalog of hazardous objects that potentially pose a threat to the ISS is not complete. Counterorbital, nonmetallic objects of substantially larger equivalent cross section than $10\,cm^2$ and a mass much larger than a paint chip are a real concern. The detection and orbit determination involving such objects will be difficult. One solution to this problem would be for NASA to invest resources to develop effective detection methods in order to form a more complete catalog of the actual space debris hazards. This, however, seems unlikely in the current budgetary constraint cycle that applies to the U.S. government, which is projected to run significant deficits for coming years. The study team suggested that NESC (and the ITA once established) should assume responsibility for seeking improvement of debris-tracking and debris-avoidance capability for the ISS and future manned craft.

Health and Medical Systems

The quality of health and medical systems onboard the ISS has represented another area of concern among NASA safety officers who have

---

[††††]Data available online at http://www.wstf.nasa.gov/Hazard/Hyper/debris.htm [cited Oct. 2004].

spoken to our team anonymously. These concerns, as attributed to NASA safety engineers in a *Washington Post* story, have been called "risk creep." It has been alleged that high-level NASA officials have asked if certain "risky" procedures could be accomplished given the special circumstances of a having just a two-man crew onboard the ISS. Those concerned have suggested that the current absence of a full crew has allowed more and more of the previously agreed safety rules to be rewritten or reinterpreted. The safety officers who have commented on these concerns have indicated that these decisions have at times been driven or pressured by Russian schedule concerns that are triggered by milestone payments (such as European milestone payments related to the ATV) [6,7]. Concerns about the ISS onboard safety as far as health and medical conditions currently include the following: the performance of the oxygen generators that have had to be repaired (because of faulty valves); past levels of carbon dioxide and toxic gases buildup in some parts of the ISS; overall air- and water-quality monitoring systems; other parts of the life-support system as already discussed; concerns about the performance of the spacesuit's oxygen supply units; the makeshift "lifeboat" arrangements if the use of the Soyuz vehicle were to be required; what has been characterized as failing medical equipment for monitoring the health of astronauts; the need for improved medical treatment capability onboard the ISS; ongoing concerns about radiation dosage and the fact that the ISS design offers limited shielding against "high-rad"-level solar storms (During "normal" radiation conditions, astronauts receive radiation levels in two weeks that are typical of annual dosages on Earth. During major solar storms, the levels are greatly increased.); and the current limited ability to offer advanced medical services to astronauts in the case of a serious medical problem even though NASA has major research programs ongoing to upgrade this capability.

In light of the fact that NASA is strongly focused on the return of the space shuttle to flight and the budgetary pressures on efforts to develop new systems for the moon, Mars, and beyond program, there appear to be limited resources in the near term to upgrade ISS medical and health facilities or to upgrade the environmental equipment in a significant way. Systems such as those that could provide artificial gravity against bone loss and other low-*g* maladies are currently not planned nor are any expanded radiation protection or expanded telemedical services planned.

Congressional hearings during the summer of 2004 have sought to explore what might be done with regard to reports of failing medical equipment and air- and water-quality monitoring devices onboard the ISS. But according to press reports, these reviews have not led to any specific safety improvements [8].

Interviews with NASA employees off the record have shown continuing concerns regarding the override of safety officer concerns related to both space shuttle and ISS missions.

According to the study team, there appeared to be merit in the creation of an independent technical authority as recommended by the CAIB so that both the quality control and the safety officers (including for both the shuttle and the ISS programs) could then be transferred to a separate chain of command with the safety and QC personnel units reporting directly to the ITA and thereby the administrator. This would not only give safety findings and recommendations higher visibility but would also make the administrator the directly responsible person for key safety and QC decisions including the granting of waivers. This would mean that mission control officers could not simply sign off on mission decisions over safety officer objections by signing of the requisite forms.

Result of Survey and Interviews Relating to the ISS

The interviews and survey questionnaires returned to the study team indicated that there were indeed a number of areas of concern with regard to ISS safety. Among the top concerns were those discussed in the following subsections.

Maintenance of Necessary Environmental Conditions

There were, in this respect, a number of concerns that included the inability to find and correct the long-term slow leakage of atmosphere, concerns about the oxygen generator, the carbon-dioxide removal, and noxious gas monitors and the lack of backup for these systems, as well as the performance of valves in the ISS air lock.

Gyro System and Stabilization of the ISS

The gyro system and stabilization of the ISS included concerns about the performance and reliability of the gyro system, questions as to whether one or more gyros had been impacted by micrometeoroids or debris, and the need for EVAs to repair gyro subsystems.

Reliance on Skeletal Maintenance Crews to Operate the ISS

This reliance concerns included the view that there should be at least three crew at the ISS at all times so that in the event that an EVA was necessary, such as to repair the gyro system, etc., two crew could back each other up for the EVA and one crew could remain onboard rather than putting the ISS on ground-based automated control. In the event of problems with the air lock, an astronaut could be inside the ISS to deal with emergency maneuvers. These concerns also extended to critiques suggesting that having committed to constructing a $100-billion ISS, not having sufficient crew to then use the facility for scientific experimentation, for space-related health, and for life-support tests and data gathering, seemed a poor use of resources. (**Researcher's note**: *The new agreement to* *keep four crew onboard the ISS after the return to flight of the shuttle would appear to respond effectively to these concerns.)*

Health, Medical Services, and Space-Suit Systems

Several respondents stated a concern that the onboard delivery of health services on the part of NASA was not as robust as Russian programs that were more intensive and more serious in their practical ability to provide near-term care to astronauts in medical distress. Also there were concerns about space-suit malfunctions as seen on recent EVAs and the feeling that EVAs should be minimized wherever possible by developing robotic technology for surveillance, reconnaissance, and even repair of modular systems.

Pressures on Budgets and Schedules

Respondents rated this as a high concern with regard to both the shuttle program and the ISS. Detailed comments noted that pressure from Congress and the Office of Management and Budget was constantly driving NASA to reduce operational costs to meet schedules and increase productivity.

Beyond these top concerns there were a number of observations with respect to better protection from radiation, micrometeoroids, debris, escape systems that can handle a full crew, stabilization and orbital boost capabilities, and the need to change NASA culture with a renewed focus on safety. There were mixed opinions about how soon or how viable in-orbit repair of the shuttle at the ISS might be and how soon it could be accomplished, but there was strong agreement that video reconnaissance via robotic systems was very feasible. There was perhaps the greatest division about the reasonable operational lifetime for the ISS. Some believed the ISS should be virtually immediately abandoned as a "white elephant" with no clearly defined purpose despite its enormous cost, while others believed that this enormous investment should be used for as long as possible to recoup the value of the investment, and thus many respondents projected operational lifetimes to the 2020–2025 time period. Certainly the sizable investment made by Japan and Europe into the JEM, CAM, and Columbus Laboratory modules is premised on the idea that decades of useful experimentation can be obtained from these space infrastructure investments and therefore could be available for use through the 2020–2025 timeframe.

The great majority of those interviewed believed that NASA and the U.S. government should give more encouragement to private entrepreneurial development of new technology, and some even favored private space platform initiatives such as those represented by current planning by Bigelow Aerospace with launch of deployable spacehabs via Space X rockets. These respondents noted that the public would support a much higher level of risk for private space programs (both in terms of mission success and private astronaut safety) as indicated by the recently highly publicized X-Prize initiatives. It was noted that the FAA has been more supportive of such new approaches, in contrast to NASA.

The following were explicit observations provided concerning the ISS and safety-related concerns:

1) Develop new and better radiation and micrometeorite protection. (This would largely apply to any future human space mission because the ISS design leaves only modest opportunities for improvements.)

2) Restructure NASA, and place key people on critical tasks. Train new people, and retire people who have become bureaucratic and slaves to budget and schedule pressures.

3) Change NASA culture to put priority on safety in deeds rather than just words.

4) Enhance and fund a serious safety and health study program for longer-term stays in space. Create a truly serious health countermeasures program. Astronauts in space face all sorts of health issues: bone and muscle attrition, adverse affect on autoimmune system, and cardiovascular problems. There is a need for onboard gravity and 1-g centrifuge for stem cell growth.

5) Develop a reliable and complete escape capability. This could be Soyuz for the time being, but this is inadequate for full ISS crew. Therefore NASA should immediately return to development of a crew return vehicle.

6) For safe operations and full experimentation program ISS should return to a full crew of at least five members.

7) Continuation of the ISS for the longer term only makes sense if new objectives are developed such as test and deployment of large-scale solar-power satellite technology, space tourism free-flyer modules, or test bed for high thrust nuclear propulsion system such as under development at Goddard Space Flight Center.

8) Pursue more critical evaluation of worth and merit of ISS experiments. Do not do stupid experiments.

9) There is no clearly defined U.S. mission for ISS. Thus the ISS should be turned over to another competent entity or deorbited as soon as feasible.

10) Because the ISS is not even complete, there is very little in terms of a track record of safety issues/concerns. At a minimum, any of the CAIB findings applicable to the ISS should be implemented, such as the formation of an independent technical engineering authority.

11) NASA cannot accomplish U.S. space goals as demonstrated by performance over the last 40 years. New programs should look to private initiatives and restructured U.S. governmental programs.

References

[1] Gugliotta, G., "Faulty Air Switch in Astronaut Suit Ended Spacewalk for American," *Washington Post*, 26 June 2004, p. A2.

[2] Gugliotta, G., "Spacewalk Aborted After Suit Malfunction," *Washington Post*, 25 June 2004, p. A9.

[3] Leavy, W., "Oxygen Generator on Space Station Fails," New York Times, 10 Sept. 2004, p. A22.

[4] "Global Positioning System/Inertial Navigation System, Development Test Objective (GPS/INS DTO)," NASA Report, NASA SP-868, Sept. 1998.

[5] Gomez, S. F., and Lammers, M. L., "Lessons Learned from Two Years of On-Orbit Global Position System Space Station," Experience on International, Abstract for the Inst. of Navigation Meeting, No. 37, Sept. 2004.

[6] Coledan, S., "Space Station Crew Aborts a Spacewalk," *Washington Post*, 25 June 2004, p. A20.

[7] Sawyer, K., "Crew to Exit Space Station in Exercise," *Washington Post*, 23 Feb. 2004, p. A1, & A9.

[8] Reinert, P., "Ask NASA About Space Station Safety," *Houston Chronicle*, Washington Bureau, 17 Aug. 2004, URL: www.chron.com/cs/CDA/printstory. mpl/space/ 2176718.

Index

Supporting Materials

For a complete listing of AIAA publications, please visit http://www.aiaa.org.